Fundamentals of Pediatric Anesthesia

Fundamentals of Pediatric Anesthesia

Third Editon

Arun Kumar Paul
BSc MBBS DA MS (Anesth)
Ex-Professor
Department of Anesthesiology
Medical College and Hospital
Kolkata, West Bengal, India

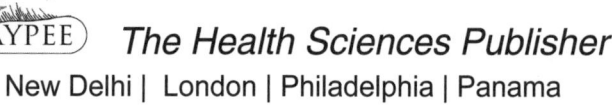

JAYPEE   *The Health Sciences Publisher*
New Delhi | London | Philadelphia | Panama

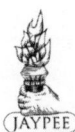 **Jaypee Brothers Medical Publishers (P) Ltd**

Headquarters

Jaypee Brothers Medical Publishers (P) Ltd
4838/24, Ansari Road, Daryaganj
New Delhi 110 002, India
Phone: +91-11-43574357
Fax: +91-11-43574314
Email: jaypee@jaypeebrothers.com

Overseas Offices

J.P. Medical Ltd
83 Victoria Street, London
SW1H 0HW (UK)
Phone: +44-2031708910
Fax: +44 (0)20 3008 6180
Email: info@jpmedpub.com

Jaypee-Highlights Medical Publishers Inc
City of Knowledge, Bld. 237, Clayton
Panama City, Panama
Phone: +1 507-301-0496
Fax: +1 507-301-0499
Email: cservice@jphmedical.com

Jaypee Medical Inc
The Bourse
111 South Independence Mall East
Suite 835, Philadelphia, PA 19106, USA
Phone: +1 267-519-9789
Email: jpmed.us@gmail.com

Jaypee Brothers Medical Publishers (P) Ltd
17/1-B Babar Road, Block-B, Shaymali
Mohammadpur, Dhaka-1207
Bangladesh
Mobile: +08801912003485
Email: jaypeedhaka@gmail.com

Jaypee Brothers Medical Publishers (P) Ltd
Bhotahity, Kathmandu, Nepal
Phone: +977-9741283608
Email: kathmandu@jaypeebrothers.com

Website: www.jaypeebrothers.com
Website: www.jaypeedigital.com

© 2016, Jaypee Brothers Medical Publishers

The views and opinions expressed in this book are solely those of the original contributor(s)/author(s) and do not necessarily represent those of editor(s) of the book.

All rights reserved. No part of this publication may be reproduced, stored or transmitted in any form or by any means, electronic, mechanical, photocopying, recording or otherwise, without the prior permission in writing of the publishers.

All brand names and product names used in this book are trade names, service marks, trademarks or registered trademarks of their respective owners. The publisher is not associated with any product or vendor mentioned in this book.

Medical knowledge and practice change constantly. This book is designed to provide accurate, authoritative information about the subject matter in question. However, readers are advised to check the most current information available on procedures included and check information from the manufacturer of each product to be administered, to verify the recommended dose, formula, method and duration of administration, adverse effects and contraindications. It is the responsibility of the practitioner to take all appropriate safety precautions. Neither the publisher nor the author(s)/editor(s) assume any liability for any injury and/or damage to persons or property arising from or related to use of material in this book.

This book is sold on the understanding that the publisher is not engaged in providing professional medical services. If such advice or services are required, the services of a competent medical professional should be sought.

Every effort has been made where necessary to contact holders of copyright to obtain permission to reproduce copyright material. If any has been inadvertently overlooked, the publisher will be pleased to make the necessary arrangements at the first opportunity.

Inquiries for bulk sales may be solicited at: jaypee@jaypeebrothers.com

Fundamentals of Pediatric Anesthesia

Third Edition: **2016**

ISBN 978-93-5250-041-3

Printed at Rajkamal Electric Press, Plot No. 2, Phase-IV, Kundli, Haryana.

Preface

The book was published several years back, and so a need was felt to revise the book and include the advances that have been made since then in the field of anesthesiology. A new chapter entitled 'Anesthesia for Pediatric Trauma' is also included.

This book *Fundamentals of Pediatric Anesthesia* intends to provide a concise source of information regarding anesthetic management of pediatric patients for the students of anesthesiology. It also aims to develop greater interest in this superspecialty among all concerned with anesthetic care, including the established practitioners. The book is written in a style that makes it easy to read and assimilate the practical points. The book provides essential and comprehensive theoretical and practical coverage of most aspects of pediatric anesthesia.

Materials have been drawn freely from the books indicated in bibliography. I intend to express my indebtedness and appreciation to their authors and publishers. The drug doses and other data have been largely taken from standard textbooks. In spite of our best efforts, it is possible that some errors may have crept in. The readers are strongly urged to consult the product manuals and drug literature of the manufacturers before using them.

I express my sincere thanks to all those who helped me directly or remotely in preparation of this book. My special thanks are also due to my wife, Kanyakumari, and daughter, Sushmita, for their endless patience and constant inspiration in this endeavor.

I am grateful to Shri Jitendar P Vij (Group Chairman), Mr Ankit Vij (Managing Director) and Mr Tarun Duneja (Director-Publishing) of M/s Jaypee Brothers Medical Publishers (P) Ltd, New Delhi, India, for publishing this book.

I sincerely hope the book will satisfy the needs of the students of anesthesiology for better understanding and management of pediatric anesthesia, and also appeal to all anesthetists, in general, seeking a practical guide in their everyday pediatric anesthetic service.

Arun Kumar Paul

Contents

Chapter 1: Respiratory Physiology   1
- Anatomical considerations 1
- Respiratory mechanism 3
- Respiratory distress in neonates and infants 6

Chapter 2: Cardiovascular System in Infants and Children   11
- Fetal circulation 11
- Changes in circulation after birth 12
- Preanesthetic evaluation of cardiovascular system 16
- Disorders of the heartbeat 18
- Arrhythmias caused by conduction block 20

Chapter 3: Thermoregulation in Infants and Children   21
- Temperature regulation during pediatric anesthesia and surgery 25
- Pyrexia in children 27
- Management 29
- Inadvertent hypothermia during anesthesia 30
- Prevention of inadvertent hypothermia in operation theater 31
- Treatment of accidental hypothermia 32

Chapter 4: Renal Function and Fluid Balance   33
- Renal function 33
- Fluid and electrolyte balance 34
- Fluid management during pediatric surgery 36
- Objectives of intravenous fluid therapy 37

Chapter 5: Psychological Problems Associated with Anesthesia and Surgery   42
- Somatic factors producing perioperative psychological disorders 42
- Surgical and anesthetic factors 43
- Common psychological reactions in perioperative period 43
- Management of psychiatric problems 46

Chapter 6: Pediatric Anesthesia Equipment   47
- Anesthetic machine 47
- Breathing circuits 48
- Pediatric anesthetic set 53
- Bain circuit 54
- Choice of anesthetic circuit in pediatric anesthesia 55

- Components of the breathing attachments 56
- Airways 68
- Endobronchial anesthesia in children 72

Chapter 7: Monitoring 79
- Direct clinical monitoring by the anesthetist 79
- Noninvasive monitoring 80
- Invasive monitoring 88
- Miscellaneous methods 91

Chapter 8: Anesthetic Pharmacology 95
- Inhalational agents 97
- Intravenous induction agents 100
- Neuroleptanalgesia/neuroleptanesthesia 102
- Opioids and related drugs 103
- Anticholinergic drugs 105
- Antiemetic drugs 106
- Muscle relaxants 107
- Antagonism of muscle relaxants 113
- Local anesthetic drugs 114

Chapter 9: Preanesthetic Assessment 116
- History 116
- Physical examination 117
- Respiratory system 119
- Other systems 119
- Routine investigations 119
- Special investigations 120

Chapter 10: Preanesthetic Preparation and Premedication 121
- Preanesthetic preparation 121
- Premedication 122

Chapter 11: Anesthetic Management 127
- Induction of anesthesia 127
- Endotracheal intubation 130
- Maintenance of anesthesia 132
- Recovery 134
- Special considerations in the case of neonates and small infants 136
- Difficult intubation 138

Chapter 12: Postanesthetic Care and Complications 141
- Transport to recovery room 141
- Postanesthetic recovery score 141
- Postoperative analgesia 143
- Postoperative sedation 143
- Common postanesthetic complications 145

Chapter 13: Anesthesia for ENT Surgery   153
- Anesthesia for tonsillectomy 153
- Anesthesia in ear surgery 157
- Anesthesia for nasal and sinus surgery 160
- Endoscopy 162
- Laser microsurgery 165
- Anesthesia for tracheostomy 166

Chapter 14: Anesthesia for Ophthalmic Surgery   169
- Specific problems 169
- Anesthetic management 171

Chapter 15: Anesthesia for Dental Surgery   175
- Anesthetic management 175
- Filling and reconstruction of teeth 177
- Common complications following dental procedures 178

Chapter 16: Anesthesia for Plastic Surgery   179
- Anesthesia for repair of cleft lip and palate 180
- Burns 182
- Neck contracture 184
- Anesthesia for craniofacial dysostosis 184
- Excision of cystic hygroma 185
- Craniectomy 186
- Major oral and maxillofacial surgery 186
- Anesthesia for condylectomy 187

Chapter 17: Anesthesia for Day Case Surgery   188
- Selection of patients 188
- Preanesthetic assessment 189
- Preanesthetic preparation 189
- Anesthetic management 190
- Recovery 192
- Discharge 192

Chapter 18: Anesthesia for General Surgery   194
- Anesthesia in congenital diaphragmatic hernia 194
- Anesthesia in tracheoesophageal fistula 197
- Anesthesia in congenital pyloric stenosis 199
- Anesthesia in surgery of abdominal wall defects 201
- Anesthesia in biliary atresia 206
- Anesthesia in bowel obstruction 207
- Anesthesia in 'acute abdomen' 210
- Anesthesia for splenectomy 211
- Anesthesia in pheochromocytoma 212
- Anesthesia for minor surgery in children 213

Chapter 19: Anesthesia for Urological Surgery   216
- Voiding cystourethrograms 216
- Hypospadius 216
- Pyeloplasty/ureteral reimplantation 217
- Wilms tumor 217
- Anesthesia in children with chronic renal diseases 218

Chapter 20: Anesthesia for Neurosurgery   223
- Cerebral blood flow (CBF) 224
- Intracranial pressure (ICP) 224
- Cerebrospinal fluid (CSF) 225
- Anesthetic management 226
- Anesthesia for neuroradiology 228
- Hydrocephalus 230
- Myelomeningocele/encephalocele 231
- Craniosynostosis 232
- Cerebral tumor 233
- Head injuries 233

Chapter 21: Anesthesia for Cardiothoracic Surgery   236
- Special problems related to lung surgery 236
- Anesthetic management 237
- Congenital lobar emphysema 238
- Mediastinal tumors 239
- Anesthesia for cardiac catheterization 240
- Anesthesia for cardiac surgery in children 241
- Patent ductus arteriosus 243
- Coarctation of aorta 244
- Anesthesia for noncardiac surgery in children with congenital heart disease 246

Chapter 22: Anesthesia for Pediatric Trauma   248
- Basic resuscitation 249
- Intravenous access 250
- Fluid resuscitation 250
- Blood transfusion 251
- Secondary survey 252
- Head injuries 253
- Neck injuries 254
- Chest injuries 254
- Abdominal injuries 255
- Genitourinary tract injuries 256
- Orthopedic injuries 257

Chapter 23: Regional Anesthesia for Children   259
- Local or subcutaneous infiltration anesthesia 260
- Ilioinguinal and iliohypogastric nerve blocks 260
- Penile block 261
- Intercostal nerve block 262
- Brachial plexus block 263
- Intravenous regional anesthesia (the Bier block) 264
- Femoral nerve block 264
- Spinal anesthesia 265
- Caudal block 266
- Lumbar epidural block 268

Chapter 24: Miscellaneous   271
- Croup 271
- Laryngospasm 273
- Anaphylaxis 274
- Down's syndrome 274
- Retinopathy of prematurity 274
- Bronchopulmonary dysplasia 275
- Malignant hyperthermia 275
- Cardiopulmonary resuscitation 276

Bibliography   *281*
Index   *283*

CHAPTER 1

Respiratory Physiology

The fetus may be taken as a biological parasite of the mother that lives in the aqueous environment of the amniotic fluid, but as soon as it is delivered from the mother's womb and its umbilical cord is tied, almost immediately it behaves as a separate individual and lives in atmospheric, airy environment. The most vital and dramatic change of environment occurs just after its birth. It no longer gets gaseous exchange from the mother's circulation and its lungs expand almost immediately.

The first 28 days of life after birth are regarded as the neonatal period. A newborn is an infant in the first 24 hours of life. Neonatal period includes the newborn period. The newborn is about one-third the length, has one-ninth the body surface and one-twentieth the weight of the adult. But the newborn should not be taken as a mere diminutive form of the adult. The neonates differ in many respects from the adult both morphologically and physiologically, and they have problems of their own in addition to their small size and shape.

ANATOMICAL CONSIDERATIONS

In neonates the thorax is of cylindrical shape with a circular cross-section. Ribs are relatively small and arranged horizontally. The oblique position of the ribs starts at the end of first year and ends at the end of fourth year of life. The thoracic cavity is relatively small in comparison with the abdominal cavity of the newborn. The small thoracic cavity is mostly occupied with a large-sized heart and its big vessels. There is relatively little space for the two lungs for adequate expansion. The cardiothoracic ratio is 0.55 as compared to that in the adult, which is 0.5. Due to this anatomical configuration, the anteroposterior and transverse diameters cannot be increased during inspiration. Only there is a piston-like up and down movement of the diaphragm during respiration in neonates.

The intercostal muscles are less active and the diaphragm is the main muscle of respiration in infants. At birth, it is placed higher at the level of

T_8/T_9, and its left dome is a little lower than the right, partly due to the presence of a large-sized liver of the neonates. The diaphragmatic movement is thus limited by a large liver, spleen and other viscera. Thus, the respiration of neonates is usually shallow, rapid and mostly diaphragmatic. There may be intercostal sucking during crying.

The newborn has an interesting peculiarity in that the baby is unable to breathe through mouth and is thus accustomed to nasal breathing. Nares is relatively large and may be of same size as cricoid ring. They are edentulous. The tongue of the infant is of a large size. The buccal pad of fat provided for sucking makes the cheeks large and mobile. The bulky tongue comes in close contact with hard palate and may cause a valve-like obstruction of the airway. It is life-threatening specially when there is nasal obstruction, as in cases of enlarged adenoids, postchoanal atresia and so on. It sometimes causes distressed breathing when the nose is pressed during breastfeeding.

Neck and occiput of a newborn have features that may affect the airway. A large occiput makes the head to be flexed anteriorly and this may cause a difficult airway management. During endotracheal intubation, optimum positioning of the head, neck, and shoulders can be obtained by placing a small rolled towel transversely at the level of shoulders.

The larynx of the neonates is placed more cephalad, lying opposite to the 3rd and 4th cervical vertebrae. Epiglottis is more stiff and V-shaped. The hyoid and thyroid cartilages are close to each other. There may be stenosis at the level of cricoid.

Anatomic differences of the neonatal head and airway compared with those of the adult include narrow nares, large tongue, high glottis, slanting vocal cords, narrow cricoid ring, and large occiput.

Glottis is one-half cartilagenous and one-half ligamentous. Cords are more concave and they are of the small length in both sexes. Cricoid plate is inclined posteriorly so as to make the larynx funnel-shaped. Arytenoid cartilage is inclined inferiorly as compared to that of the adult where it is horizontal.

In the newborn, trachea lies slightly to the right of midline. It is easily shifted on either side. The bifurcation of trachea lies between T_3 and T_4 in the first year of life; between T_4 and T_5 during 2 to 6 years; and between T_5 and T_6 during 6 to 12 years of age. Sagittal diameter at birth is 5 mm and in adult it is 16.5 mm. So the trachea is relatively wider in neonates. Hence, the dead space of the neonates is greater. In the neonates, the tracheal cartilages are soft and immature. The tracheal glands are not so well-developed. That is why anticholinergic drugs may be avoided in newborn except in cases where vagal reflexes are to be inhibited.

Trachea divides into bronchi, right and left, at about equal angles. Therefore, the longer endotracheal tube may enter in either bronchus easily, and cause one-lung anesthesia. In the early neonatal period, the bronchioles are very delicate, and alveolar ducts and alveoli are not so mature. At birth, the alveoli are thick-walled and their number is only about 10% of the adult total. Alveoli multiply with the growth of lung until the age of 6 to 8 years. The relatively narrow airway results in high airway resistance. There are enough connective tissue surrounding them. Relatively, there are little elastic tissue in newborn lung. So there is more chance of atelectasis and pulmonary infection with minimum etiological factor. The total respiratory surface of the newborn lung is relatively smaller. The postanesthetic pulmonary complications can be minimized, if the operation can be delayed for several weeks after birth when the alveolar ducts are better dilated.

RESPIRATORY MECHANISM

In intrauterine life, the respiratory center is inhibited as there is no need of respiration through the lungs. But in animal experiments it has been shown that there is some degree of respiration in fetal life due to its muscular movements on tactile stimulation. Earlier, in the stage of segregation, there is a rhythmical type of respiration. But later, there is a stage of quiescence in which respiration is almost inhibited by the growing central nervous system. In this stage, the fetus is more sensitive to the effects of lack of oxygen.

In intrauterine life, gas exchange takes place through the placenta. Maternal blood enters from the uterine arteries into the intervillous sinusoids. Fetal blood is supplied through the umbilical arteries to capillary loops which protrude into the intervillous space. Gas exchange takes place there across the blood-blood barrier which is roughly 3.5 microns thick. But the mechanism is not much efficient for gas exchange in comparison to that in the adult lung.

The delivery of the baby into the outside world is the most crucial part of his life and he is suddenly exposed to a variety of external stimuli. Moreover, the process of birth interferes with placental gas exchange resulting in hypoxemia and hypercapnia which stimulate the respiratory center through chemoreceptors. As a consequence of all these factors, the baby takes his first breath.

The fetal lung is not collapsed but is inflated with liquid upto about 40% of the total lung capacity. This fluid is secreted by the alveolar cells. Some of this fluid is squeezed out during the birth process and the rest may have some role in the subsequent inflation of the lung. The intrapleural pressure may fall to 40 cm water pressure during the first breath. This is partly caused by the high viscosity of the lung liquid compared to that of air. Expansion of the lung and ventilation become uniform within several days of birth. But the adequate gas exchanging surface is established within a few moments due to the presence of pulmonary surfactant and removal of lung liquid by lymphatics and capillaries.

When the center is depressed by anesthetic or analgesic drugs given to the mother prior to delivery, the sensory stimulus may not be sufficient to initiate first breathing. Chemical stimuli, after a short period, may cause some gasps in the baby and if the oxygen is given at that time it may initiate a regular rhythm of respiration. Carbon dioxide excess, anoxia, increased H-ion concentration or a combination of these factors may stimulate the respiration or release the inhibition of respiratory center.

Oxygen lack depresses the respiratory center by its direct action and indirectly through the carotid and aortic bodies which stimulate the center. These chemoreceptors have an immense role in starting the first breath in severely anoxic babies. The hypoxic baby, whose center is already depressed, is unresponsive to carbon dioxide, but in well-oxygenated baby, carbon dioxide increases both the rate and depth of respiration. The chemoreceptor activity of neonates is similar to that of adult.

Some babies show automatic respiration immediately after birth or even when the head is delivered keeping the baby still in the birth canal. Some babies may not respire for 1 or 2 minutes after birth. The most interesting point is that the baby can tolerate hypoxia more than the adult. The baby who is apneic for 10 minutes after birth, may survive after treatment whereas the adult will not tolerate the anoxia for more than 5 minutes without cerebral damage.

The first breath of the newborn may be as high as and a pressure of 35 cm of water is usually enough to inflate the lungs.

The respiratory patterns in neonates may be of various types. These are as follows:
1. Regular type: Inspiratory phase and expiratory phase are of equal lengths with no pause.
2. Periodic type: It may or may not be associated with apneic pause between the periods. This type of breathing is almost similar when the adult respires in oxygen deficient atmosphere, in alkalemic states, or when the respiratory center is depressed by anesthetics or analgesics. It is very characteristic of premature babies. This type of breathing may be due to temporary hypoxia of brain of the newborn. Immaturity of respiratory center may also be a factor. This may not be associated with dyspnea or cyanosis and may be corrected by administering oxygen to the breathing air.
3. Cogwheel type of breathing: Here the expiration is rather jerky and prolonged and usually followed by a pause.
4. Completely irregular pattern: It may be seen in some neonates specially in prematures.

During sleep there may be slowing and deepening of respiration. Some sort of periodicity is often found in normal mature babies. The neonate may not have a single pattern of respiration. It may be of mixed type of breathing. If there is no obvious sign of hypoxemia, this particular type of breathing may not be harmful to the baby and need not cause worry. But small doses of analgesics may impair the ventilatory response to carbon dioxide. Progressive hypoxemia will ultimately lead to respiratory arrest.

The normal term baby is born both hypoxic and hypercarbic. During first 24 hours of life, pH of arterial blood goes up from 7.26 to normal adult level of 7.34 to 7.4; arterial CO_2 tension is reduced from 55 to 35 mmHg and oxygen tension comes upto 71 mmHg. Venous admixture of arterial blood is higher in a 24 hours old baby due to right-left shunt and may be 20 to 25% of cardiac output. There may be the contribution of bronchial veins or patent foramen ovale or ductus arteriosus, but the common factor is the perfusion of completely unventilated alveoli. A normal arterial oxygen tension in the newborn is approximately 70 mmHg.

Respiratory Rate

In newborn, it is about 40/minute. The infant cannot respire deeply because of relatively small size of thoracic cavity and its configuration and low muscle tone. Respiration is mostly diaphragmatic. During emergency, the rate is increased in order to overcome hypoxia and hypercarbia. It may be upto 100/minute in normal resting condition. The respiratory rate at 2 years ranges from 20 to 30/minute, at 6 years it is 15 to 20/minute and at 12 years it is 12 to 15/minute. The metabolic result of the large surface area of the neonate increases rate rather than the depth of the breathing. The metabolic cost of respiration is higher and may be about 15% of total oxygen consumption.

Tidal Volume

This is the amount of air inspired or expired during each breath. It is about 20 ml in neonates. It may be increased during crying upto 180 ml, which is near to its vital capacity. Tidal volume is usually 7 ml/kg. Dead space is equal to tidal volume multiplied by 0.3 ml.

Dead Space Volume

It is the volume of the air extending from nostrils and mouth down to but not including alveoli. It is 2.2 ml/kg body weight. It is greater in comparison with that of the adult as the trachea is more wide in neonates and baby is usually nose breather.

Minute Volume

Due to increased rate of respiration of minute volume of the neonate is much higher than that of the adult when compared on weight basis.

Vital Capacity

It is maximum volume of air that can be expelled from the lungs forcefully following maximum inspiration. It is about 33 ml/kg of body weight (crying).

Lung compliance in neonates is low being 5 ml/cm H_2O when in adult it is 200 ml/cm H_2O. Functional residual capacity is about 24 ml/kg of body weight. The ratio of tidal volume to functional residual capacity is about 0.20 whereas in adult it is 0.21. The ratio of alveolar ventilation to functional residual capacity is about 0.14 (same as in adult). In infants there is small functional residual capacity but oxygen consumption rate is high, so little respiratory inadequacy even for a short period may cause hypoxia in the baby. The poor elasticity of the infant lung causes the closing volume to be greater than functional residual capacity until the age of 6 to 8 years. The respiratory muscles of the neonate are composed of a lower percentage of slow twitch, high oxidative muscle fibers which are capable of sustained activity. Thus, they are prone to early respiratory muscle fatigue.

In the newborn infant, total lung weight is about 50 g. Alveolar surface area is about 4 square meter. The oxygen consumption rate is higher, about 6 ml/kg/minute. The negative intrapulmonary pressure is 40 to 50 cm H_2O. Negative pressure may suck large amount of air into stomach and may cause respiratory distress in neonates. A pressure of 35 cm H_2O is usually needed to inflate the lungs in neonates. High intratracheal pressure specially in positive pressure ventilation, may cause rupture of alveoli. Controlled ventilation may upset the circulatory mechanism of the neonate more easily. In premature infants there may be rupture of alveoli spontaneously causing interstitial emphysema by own respiratory efforts specially during crying. It may not occur in normal lung, but not uncommon in premature babies. Premature infants and those with bronchopulmonary dysplasia also have problems with increased lung water.

RESPIRATORY DISTRESS IN NEONATES AND INFANTS

There are various conditions in neonates and infants which may call for emergency treatment to relieve the respiratory distress. Some of them are as follows:
- Nonpotency of the posterior nares or *postchoanal atresia* may cause respiratory obstruction in neonates. The condition is more worse by

the bulky tongue of the baby which is pressed against the hard palate causing complete obstruction of the airway. Establishment of an oral airway either by oropharyngeal airway or through endotracheal tube is mandatory.
- Cyst or tumor in the base of the tongue may cause obstruction in the airway. Maintenance of clear airway is necessary until the condition is treated surgically.

The Pierre Robin Syndrome

It is due to gross underdevelopment of the mandible, and the placement of bulky tounge backwards to the posterior pharyngeal wall. Other associated features are retrognathos, glossoptosis, small epiglottis, high arched palate usually with cleft and small mouth orifice. There may be respiratory obstruction. The face down position with head extension may give relief. Endotracheal intubation should be done in severe cases.

Enlarged adenoids and hypertrophied tonsils causing respiratory obstruction should be treated surgically for permanent relief.

Foreign bodies, mucus, secretions, blood and so on in the airway may be sufficient enough to cause respiratory distress. This should be removed or sucked out in no time.

The angioneurotic edema causing respiratory distress may need emergency tracheostomy. Endotracheal intubation in these patients carries a great risk.

Laryngomalacia with incomplete development of epiglottis causes inspiratory obstruction. Enlarged inflamed epiglottis may also cause respiratory distress. Tracheostomy should be done immediately. Attempts of intubation in these cases may be fatal.

Edema of larynx may be caused by the injury to larynx due to clumsy endotracheal intubation. The distress usually occurs within a few hours of injury. Patient should be kept upright in bed. Cool humidified mist inhalation is helpful. Adrenaline through a nebulizer, corticosteroids and antibiotics are needed. Tracheostomy is done in extreme cases. Further endotracheal intubation is not recommended.

Aspiration and regurgitation may cause laryngospasm and pneumonitis. Clearance of the airway and positive pressure ventilation under mask may help. Relaxant drugs may be necessary to break the spasm. Bronchodilators are needed in presence of bronchospasm. Aspiration pneumonitis should be treated with adequate bronchoscopic suction, intermittent positive pressure ventilation, bronchodilators, antibiotics, hydrocortisone and tracheobronchial toilet.

Congenital anomalies like vascular rings may result in respiratory obstruction. Endotracheal intubation and assisted respiration are required until the condition is relieved surgically.

Treacher Collins Syndrome

It is a rare condition in which various characteristics such as receding chin, obtuse angled mandible, high-arched palate with or without cleft, abnormal maxillae, coloboma of eyelid or iris, deafness, choanal atresia, micrognathia, etc. are seen. Maintenance of airway and endotracheal intubation are difficult in these cases.

Mechanical impairment caused by various factors like multiple fracture ribs, exomphalos repair, repair of diaphragmatic hernia, abdominal distension, thoracotomy or sternotomy, intrathoracic tumors or cysts, etc. may cause respiratory distress. These patients may need IPPV until the conditions are treated effectively.

The evaluation of pulmonary physiology is essential in the preanesthetic period in neonates, infants and children. Simple history, thorough physical examination and radiographic examination are usually sufficient in most cases. Blood gas analysis is important in some cases. Pulmonary function tests are not always practicable in small pediatric cases. Hence the anesthesiologist should have some knowledge of pulmonary complications and their effects on respiration.

Increased intracranial pressure or cerebral trauma causes slow and shallow respiration with subsequent hypoxia. These babies should be given the premedication very cautiously. Cerebral damage due to hypoxia, or trauma, or infection causes neuromuscular impairment and impairs ventilation. Spinal cord injury, acute cerebral compression and cerebral hemorrhage may cause respiratory failure. Epilepsy and neuromuscular disorders, either infective or degenerative, may also impair ventilation.

In excessive vomiting or prolonged gastric suction as in case of pyloric stenosis there is a chance of metabolic alkalosis. It causes a compensatory slow and shallow respiration. Sedatives may further deteriorate the condition. Hyperventilation during anesthesia in these cases may result in alkalotic tetany.

Profound hypothermia depresses the respiration and there is metabolic acidosis. It may be associated with hypoglycemia. So the baby should be kept in humid warm atmosphere in the operation theater and recovery room. The room temperature, the airflow rate and the relative humidity of the baby ward and operation theater should be kept in comfortable range for the babies.

The babies suffering from poliomyelitis, myasthenia gravis, etc. may suffer from respiratory inadequacy. The sedative and the relaxant drugs should be given carefully, or better be omitted. IPPV and tracheobronchial toilet may be needed even before anesthesia. Postoperative close observation of the respiration should be maintained.

Birth injury, specially in Erb-Duchenne syndrome where the phrenic nerve component may be damaged, may cause diaphragmatic paralysis and thereby respiratory distress in neonates. These patients should be intubated and IPPV may be necessary.

The deformities of thorax and of spine may limit the thoracic movement during respiration and more so by depressant and anesthetic drugs. Scleroderma and sclerema cause hardening of the subcutaneous tissue and may involve the respiratory muscles.

The neonates very often suck large amounts of air during their own respiratory efforts and this may result in abdominal distension, sufficient to cause respiratory distress. Aspiration through Ryles tube is beneficial in relieving the symptoms.

Pleural effusion or pneumothorax limits the lung expansion and may even cause collapse of the lungs. The air or the fluid should be aspirated before anesthesia and even the water seal drainage may be needed. Pneumonia, bronchiolitis and lung contusion may also cause cardiopulmonary failure.

Associated heart diseases and failure of the heart may cause cardiomegaly occupying most of the thoracic cavity. Pericardial effusion may cause respiratory difficulty and cardiac tamponade in severe cases. Cardiac patients with pulmonary hypertension are prone to the development of respiratory insufficiency.

Tracheoesophageal Fistula

There is always contamination of lung parenchyma with gastric fluid or with feeding material. Pneumonitis is a common feature. Prematurity and associated other congenital abnormalities add more risk to the baby. The abdomen is highly distended due to sucking of air during rapid respiratory efforts. There may be paradoxical movements of thorax and abdomen. Initial gastrostomy may relieve the distension and prevent further aspiration and/or regurgitation.

Diaphragmatic Hernia

The baby may be cyanosed. There is respiratory distress as the abdominal contents enter through the congenital gap on one side of the thoracic cavity and make the lungs to collapse shifting mediastinum to contralateral side. In these cases the baby should be intubated in head up slanting position. Acidosis should be corrected. Ventilation should be done carefully; otherwise, more pressure may rupture the alveoli and may even cause internal bleeding in lung parenchyma which is collapsed for a long time.

Hyaline Membrane Disease

It is idiopathic respiratory distress syndrome of the newborn. Predisposing factors are prematurity, baby born through cesarean section, maternal diabetes and amniotic fluid in the respiratory passage. There is hypoxia associated with right to left shunt. Clinical features include low Apgar scores at birth, chest retraction during inspiration, expiratory grant, poor muscle tone, hypoxemia, hypercarbia, hyperkalemia, hypothermia, acidosis and hypotension. Arterial blood gas analysis reveals hypoxemia and acidemia. Acidosis is both respiratory and metabolic in origin. Chest radiography shows classic ground glass appearance with scattered air bronchograms throughout both the lungs. The exact cause is not known. But it may be due to deficiency of the surfactant material, poor stability of lung expansion and hypoperfusion of lungs. Surfactant is a lipoprotein and maintains stability of terminal air spaces and acts as an antiatelectasis factor. Treatment should include IPPV, IV glucose infusion, hydrocortisone in massive doses and sodium bicarbonate for correction of metabolic acidosis. Baby should be nursed in an incubator with humid atmosphere at 35°C to minimize oxygen consumption. These infants need longer inspiratory times and higher levels of inspiratory pressure and positive end-expiratory pressure (PEEP) for better oxygenation and ventilation. Exogenous surfactant material is useful in premature infants either at birth or with the onset of respiratory distress. Surfactant replacement therapy improves oxygenation and pulmonary compliance immediately. It reduces the complications such as barotrauma, bronchopulmonary dysplasia and pulmonary interstitial emphysema.

Some useful data on pulmonary and cardiovascular variables in neonates and adults on average or range		
Characteristic	Neonate	Adult
Body weight (kg)	3	70
Respiratory rate/min	35	15
Tidal volume, ml/kg	6	6
Vital capacity, ml/kg	35	70
Alveolar ventilation, ml/kg/min	130	60
Functional residual capacity, ml/kg	25	40
Tracheal internal diameter, mm	4	16
Tracheal length, mm	57	120
Oxygen consumption, ml/kg/min	7	3.5
Systolic blood pressure, mmHg	65	120
Heart rate, beats/min	130	80
Blood volume, ml/kg	85	65
Hemoglobin, g%	17	14
PaO_2, mmHg	65–85	85–95
$PaCO_2$, mmHg	30–36	36–44
pH	7.34–7.40	
CO_2 production, ml/kg/min	6	3

CHAPTER 2

Cardiovascular System in Infants and Children

The human baby who is in mother's womb, gets all its nourishment from the mother through placenta. Placenta is the main organ of fetal nutrition and excretion. But as soon as it comes out of the mother's womb, its umbilical cord is tied and cut and is thus completely separated from the mother. Now the baby has no other means than to depend on his own body organs to maintain the vital signs of life. The most important and vital transitional changes occur in respiratory and cardiovascular mechanisms.

FETAL CIRCULATION

Without entering into the complex development of heart and blood vessels from the embryonic rudiments, let us consider the circulation of blood in intrauterine life which is very much peculiar and differs considerably from the normal postnatal circulation.

The oxygenated blood of the mother passes from the placenta through the umbilical vein. In the undersurface of liver, it is divided into two parts. One part passes through the liver and then to inferior vena cava. The other part directly passes through the ductus venosus into inferior vena cava and it also receives blood of portal vein and from the lower part of the fetal body. The blood of inferior vena cava reaches the right auricle which also receives the blood of the head and neck through the superior vena cava. The two sources of blood usually do not mix except in small quantity. The less oxygenated blood from the superior vena cava passes through auriculoventricular opening into right ventricle. The blood of inferior vena cava passes through the foramen ovale in left auricle and then in left ventricle and thence to aorta from where the whole body, specially the head and neck receive blood. The blood of superior vena cava passes in small quantity through pulmonary veins. The greater part, of course, passes through the ductus arteriosus from pulmonary artery to aorta and thence to other parts of the body. Lastly, through the umbilical arteries it returns to placenta. From the placenta it is returned to umbilical vein from where the circulation started.

Fetal circulation thus consists of three physiological shunts—Placenta, foramen ovale and ductus arteriosus. Pulmonary bed has a high vascular resistance as the alveoli are mostly closed and filled with fluid and the blood vessels are compressed. The ductus arteriosus is a low pressure system as it is dilated, secondary to a low PaO_2.

Both the ventricles pump blood through systemic circulation to all parts of the fetal body and ultimately to placenta for oxygenation through umbilical artery. But after birth right ventricle is meant for pulmonary circulation and the left ventricle is for systemic circulation.

Persistent pulmonary hypertension may sometimes occur, mostly due to hypoxia and acidosis along with various other factors. It usually occurs in cases of meconium aspiration, neonatal respiratory failure and diaphragmatic hernia. It may lead to right to left shunt through the foramen ovale and the ductus arteriosus.

CHANGES IN CIRCULATION AFTER BIRTH

Immediately after birth lungs expand. Ventilation decreases the pulmonary vascular resistance and thus lowers the pulmonary arterial pressure. Just after clamping of the umbilical cord, aortic pressure is increased due to the closure of umbilical arteries. Closure of sinus venosus may be due to rise of blood flow through the portal vein after clamping of umbilical vein.

Closure of Foramen Ovale

It is closed by the hemodynamic changes after birth. After the stoppage of circulation through the cord, the blood volume and hence the blood pressure in the inferior vena cava are reduced and the momentum of the blood is less to the vena caval side of the valve of the foramen ovale. Thus, there is a reduction in pressure difference between the two sides of the valve. The increase in pulmonary venous return also alters this pressure difference. These factors may be responsible for the closure of foramen ovale. On the whole, rise of left atrial pressure above that of the right atrial pressure results in this closure. In the presence of patent foramen ovale, there is a right to left shunt.

Closure of the Ductus Arteriosus

The ductus arteriosus is a large channel connecting the pulmonary artery and the descending thoracic aorta at an acute angle. The mechanism of closure of this large vessel within a day or two after birth is very interesting. The closure occurs in two stages. In the first stage, there is a rapid constriction of the ductal tissue after birth which is functional closure of the ductus arteriosus. Later, in the second stage, there is anatomical obliteration of the ductus within a few weeks. But the intermittent closure is not uncommon. The closure may be due to rise of arterial oxygen tension which immediately stimulates the closure just after birth. The incidence of patent ductus arteriosus is common in the babies ually associated with fetal distress or the babies delivered at high altitudes.

In patent ductus arteriosus, the direction of blood flow depends on cardiac output, systemic and pulmonary vascular resistance, and the degree of constriction and the length of the ductus. The cause of patency is chiefly hypoxemia, but the children with cyanotic heart disease may not be necessarily associated with the patent ductus arteriosus as their arterial oxygen tension may still be raised well above the fetal level. In the patent ductus there may be the shunt in either direction depending upon the pressure of pulmonary artery and aorta. In normal term babies after birth there may be the bidirectional flow through the ductus, specially during crying for about 6 hours after birth. Then the flow is mainly from left to right upto 15 hours of age. With hypoxia there is pulmonary vasoconstriction and associated increase in pulmonary artery pressure above systemic pressure, this will again cause right to left shunt. In severe hypoxia, the release of catecholamines may also constrict the ductus.

The usual type of murmur may not be heard on auscultation during first month because the pressures of pulmonary artery and aorta are very close enough not to produce any murmur. The murmur in neonate may not indicate any associated heart lesion; on the other hand, presence of heart disease may not produce any murmur. Murmur is more common in asphyxiated and premature babies.

Heart Size

It is usually large, more so in asphyxiated babies. The relatively small-sized thoracic cavity is more occupied by the heart as if there was little space for the lungs to expand. Cardiothoracic ratio is greater in children. When there is no associated heart disease or respiratory distress, the heart size returns to normal within 1 to 3 days. Shape of the heart is conical and it is obliquely placed in the thorax. In the newborn, right atrium is larger than the left. Right and left ventricles are of equal thickness and weight, but the left one grows more rapidly. It is said that fetal and neonatal myocardium contains lower percentage of contractile mass than mature myocardium. Neonatal myocites may support cell growth, but do not take part in mechanical work. However, these noncontractile elements are subsequently replaced by mature myofibrils in first several months of age.

Heart Rate

The heart rate of fetus is about 140 to 160/minute, but at birth it may be upto 180/minute. Within 8 days it comes down to 124 to 130/minute. In first and second year, it is 100 to 110/minute. In 4 to 10 years of age, it is 80 to l00/minute. and at 12 years, it is about 80/minute. Vagal stimulation, distension of stomach with air, which is common in neonates, may cause bradycardia. Activity, crying, change of posture, etc. may cause tachycardia. Heart sounds are readily audible on placing the small diaphragm of a stethoscope. Low audibility may be due to cardiac dilatation or low cardiac output. Radial pulse may not be readily palpable due to the tiny size of the vessel. Babies may tolerate heart rates of upto 200/minute without evidence of cardiac failure.

Heart Volume

On the day of birth the average heart volume is 48 ml approximately. During the next 4 days, the volume diminishes and, thereafter, there is a gradual increase. The decrease is more marked in prematures.

Cardiac Output

Just after birth the baby may have a high cardiac output of approximately 200 ml/kg/minute which is 2 to 3 times the adult value. The small ventricles result in poor ventricular resistance, thus large cardiac output is maintained by increasing heart rate.

Ordinarily, cardiac output range is wide, being 180 to 850 ml/minute and the average is 540 ml/minute. Cardiac index is 2.5 liters/minute. Stroke volume is roughly 4 ml. The minute volume is equal to stroke volume multiplied by heart rate, average being 5 liters. Stroke volume output per ventricle per beat, normal value is 70 ml. Cardiac index is cardiac output per minute/square meter of body surface and the normal value 3.2 liters. The output in two ventricles is almost same.

Blood Volume

In neonates, blood volume is an average about 85 ml/kg of body weight. The range may vary from 68 to 115 ml/kg. A large amount of blood is present in the visceral venous system in the newborn. Blood is not equally distributed, being particularly less in periphery due to ill development of anastomotic channels. Blood volume in the infant and young child (2 to 6 years) decreases to about 80 ml/kg and comes to the adult level of 75 ml/kg at the age of 6 to 8 years. In children blood losses greater than 10% must always be replaced with blood.

Circulation Time

The range is wide and may be within 4.4 to 15 seconds. Circulation time may not have any relation with blood pressure, pulse, respiration, sex, weight, activity or crying.

Blood Pressure

Arterial blood pressure

The average systolic blood pressure at birth is low, 40 to 60 mmHg, and thereafter there is an increase (60 to 80 mmHg) within the first week. In the first year, it comes to 80 to 85 mmHg and gradually increases to 90 to 105 mmHg within 6 to 12 years of age. The adult level of blood pressure, 120/70 mmHg reaches at approximately 16 years of age. On the whole, blood pressure of a newborn is 70/45 mmHg, at 2 years 80/60 mmHg, at 6 years 90/60 mmHg and at 12 years 110/65 mmHg. Blood pressure may be reduced due to shock, respiratory distress syndrome, accidental hypoglycemia, or cold injury of newborn or in neonatal hypoglycemia. Low blood pressure is observed in cases of fetal distress or in babies born through cesarean section. High blood pressure may be observed during crying, after cerebral trauma and in babies delivered after high forceps. Pre-eclamptic toxemia usually do not cause high blood pressure in newborn as the toxic material most probably is destroyed after birth.

Venous pressure

The pressure in the vein is usually subjected to two opposite forces. One is the positive pressure of arterial side and the other negative intrathoracic pressure. The first one is prominent in peripheral veins but centrally the second one is predominant. The central venous pressure is usually 3 to 6 mmHg below atmospheric pressure. It can be detected roughly by lowering down the infusion set to see the blood is coming through the needle. The distance from the level of the heart is the venous pressure.

Peripheral Vessels

The veins are usually inaccessible in neonates. For intravenous fluid therapy often cut down is necessary. The peripheral vessels may not show any dilatation in the first 3 days after birth. The cause may be asphyxia or hypothermia. On tilting into feet down position, there may not be any change of blood pressure in the first 4 days, but thereafter there is increased heart rate and rise of blood pressure suggesting that the baroreceptors are active.

Hemoglobin

In newborn, 75 to 80% of hemoglobin is fetal hemoglobin. Adult hemoglobin hemopoiesis is well-established at about 6 months. Fetal hemoglobin has a greater affinity for oxygen as it contains less 2, 3-diphosphoglycerate and the dissociation curve is shifted to the left. This greater affinity for oxygen is overcome to some extent in the tissues of newborn because of low tissue oxygen tension and a metabolic acidosis which usually persists in the newborn. Respiratory alkalosis due to hyperventilation may reduce the oxygen availability. At birth the hemoglobin concentration is usually 15 g/dl and it becomes 11 g/dl by 6 weeks. Hemoglobin concentration declines progressively causing physiological anemia of infancy which is more marked in prematures.

PREANESTHETIC EVALUATION OF CARDIOVASCULAR SYSTEM

History and Physical Examination

History of mother is often important. Mothers suffering from hypertension, diabetes, asthma, etc. may reflect the disease to their children. History of retarded growth, cyanosis, syncope and convulsions may be the eliciting factor. History of acute rheumatic fever, viral infections like smallpox, mumps and measles may require postponement of operation for at least 3 months due to associated myocarditis. Diphtheria toxin may also cause myocarditis.

Some endocrine disorders may affect the heart. *Hyperthyroidism* is rare in infants but may occur before 12 years of age. There may be tachycardia, high cardiac output and hypertension. Heart may not show any abnormality in the initial stage. *Hypothyroidism* causes cretinism. There may be bradycardia, low blood pressure, cardiomegaly and associated anemia and retarded growth. *Hyperparathyroidism* may be primary or secondary to renal disease. Associated hypercalcemia may increase cardiac irritability. There may be bradycardia with shortening of QT interval. *Hypoparathyroidism* will produce the opposite effect and may show myocardial depression. Pituitary disorders are rare in children. *Cushing syndrome* may cause hypertension. Gigantism may be associated with dilated heart and hypotension. *Simmonds disease* is usually associated with hypothyroidism and hypotension. *Addison's disease* may be congenital and usually related with hypotension and hyperkalemia. *Pheochromocytoma* is common in children. It is the tumor of adrenal medulla or of any chromaffin tissue of the body. It is characterized by hypertension and symptoms associated with it. There is increased irritability of myocardium due to large secretion of catecholamines in circulation. The child with juvenile diabetes may present metabolic acidosis and hypokalemia, and in severe cases it may be associated with hypertension due to arteriosclerotic changes.

Some disorders of vitamin metabolism may affect the cardiovascular system. Vitamin B deficiency causes beriberi and there is hypertrophy of adrenal cortex. It is characterized by edema, tachycardia, hepatomegaly and cardiac failure. Vitamin C deficiency may cause anemia and cardiomegaly. Vitamin D deficiency causes rickets in children. There may be deformity of chest, enough to cause cardiac compression. The excess of vitamin D causes hypercalcemia with increased cardiac irritability.

In anemia there is tachycardia, chronic hypoxemia and low myocardial activity. Correction of anemia is essential before elective surgery. Renal disease may cause uremia and hypertension. In pericardial effusion there may be cardiac tamponade. The fluid is better removed through paracentesis before the onset of anesthesia.

Clinical Examination

Clinical examination of cardiovascular system should be done with extreme care. Pulse and blood pressure should be recorded. Auscultation of heart sounds and murmurs, if present, should be carefully done.

Arterial pressure should be measured with a sphygmomanometer. The cuff size should be 2.5 to 4 cm for better and reliable results.

Radiological Examination

Plain X-rays of chest will determine the size of heart, cardiothoracic ratio, pulmonary vascular patterns and cardiac chamber analysis.

Angiocardiography and aortography

Serial X-rays are taken after specification of the chambers of the heart and great vessels by injection of a radiopaque medium. Selective angiography is done by IV injection of dye through a catheter in peripheral vein in the desired position. This is an important technique in cyanotic congenital heart diseases where cardiac catheterization alone cannot show the defect clearly. Aortography can demonstrate the status of aortic valve, coronary arteries, patent ductus arteriosus and coarctation of aorta. Hypersensitivity of the contrast medium may occur and there may be shock, hypotension, dyspnea, cyanosis, bronchospasm, confusion and convulsion.

Electrocardiography

It is a useful monitoring technique by which the cardiac activity can be studied in detail. Myocardial status and cardiac arrhythmias can be better by ECG study than the clinical methods as it indicates the site of origin.

Cardiac Catheterization

Catheterization may be necessary to detect the abnormal channels of heart or for pressure and gas analysis at different chambers of the heart and great vessels. Right heart catheterization is done through a systemic vein into the right heart chambers and pulmonary arteries. Left heart catheterization may be done by retrograde insertion through a peripheral artery. The technique may induce cardiac arrhythmia of which ventricular fibrillation may cause death. Extreme caution and continuous ECG monitoring are essential.

Routine Blood Examination

This includes examination of TC, DC, Hb%, bleeding time, clotting time, blood group and blood biochemistry.

Urine Examination

Examination of specific gravity, glucose, albumin and microscopic studies.

DISORDERS OF THE HEARTBEAT

The cardiac action is controlled by cardioinhibitory center which is a part of dorsal nucleus of vagus and cardioacceleratory center, which in turn is intimately connected with dorsal sympathetic outflow. Both of them are situated in the floor of 4th ventricle. Sympathetic nervous system supplies the heart in general, and parasympathetic nervous system supplies the SA and AV nodes and is limited to supraventricular regions of the heart. The heart rate is controlled by the balance of the two systems but the vagal effect is more dominant. The heart muscle has peculiar physiological properties like automaticity, rhythmicity, conductivity, excitability and refractoriness. In general, the impulse originates in SA node, then passes to AV node and then through the bundle of His, the bundle branches and the Purkinje network of the ventricular muscle. Normally, the SA node is the pacemaker with its property to undergo spontaneous depolarization in highest rate, although some tracts of atrial tissue and the His-Purkinje system are the potential weak pacemaker sites. The normal resting cardiac rhythm is said to be the normal sinus rhythm.

Sinus Tachycardia

It is the rapid regular rhythm of the heart. In infants, the resting rate is normally high. It may be found in hypermetabolic states, like thyrotoxicosis, fever, exercise, emotional disturbances and after atropine injections. Muscle relaxants like gallamine and pancuronium may also cause tachycardia.

Sinus Bradycardia

It is slow regular rhythm of the heart. Here the PR interval is longer, P waves are rather low. It may be due to vagal stimulation, increased intracranial tension, gastric dilatation, jaundice and so on. It is not always suggestive of cardiac disease and may be found normally in athletes.

Sinus Arrhythmia

Here the SA node is on cyclic change of rate. The rate changes with respiration, rapid during the end of inspiration and slow at the end of expiration. It is common in cardiac surgery but requires no treatment.

Ectopic Beat

The impulse originates outside SA node, may be in other parts of auricle or ventricle and the beat is necessarily premature, because it may come from AV node and ventricle.

Extrasystoles: These are the extra beats in between the two normal beats.

Auricular Paroxysmal Tachycardia

This is a common form of tachycardia but another form of tachycardia may occur in paroxysms. Here the repeated attacks of rapid beating occur. The impulse arises in auricle at a single ectopic focus and possibly there is a circus movement in the heart thereby causing rapid regular beats. The paroxysmal tachycardia may also originate in the AV node (nodal paroxysmal tachycardia) or ventricle (ventricular paroxysmal tachycardia).

It is rare in infancy. But if it occurs and persists for a longer period, congestive failure may result. Quinidine, carotid sinus pressure and vagal stimulation may help. Paroxysmal ventricular tachycardia occurs in organic cardiac disease and sometimes precedes ventricular fibrillation. For treatment, quinidine is the drug of choice. Paroxysmal ventricular tachycardia and ventricular flutter are not differentiated in electrocardiogram.

Atrial Flutter

It is dangerous and caused by organic heart disease. Here the ectopic focus is always from SA node and there is a single circus movement in the auricle around the vena caval openings producing a circular path of auricular depolarization. Digitalis and quinidine are used to treat it.

Auricular Fibrillation

It is characterized by a rapid irregular rate with pulse deficit between apex and radial pulse. It is probably due to many active circus movements at one time or variations in refractoriness in different sites of auricular musculature or a combination of these factors. Carotid sinus pressure cannot stop this though there is a decrease in ventricular rate. Digitalis is the drug of choice.

Ventricular Fibrillation

It is grave amongst all cardiac irregularities. Clinically, it will lead to cardiac arrest.

ARRHYTHMIAS CAUSED BY CONDUCTION BLOCK

SA Block

Here SA node fails to generate impulse occasionally, so the heart misses one beat. Digitalis intoxication may cause it.

AV Block

It is due to either delay or failure of impulses to pass from atrium to ventricle.
- 1st degree: It is the prolongation of atrioventricular conduction. PR interval is prolonged.
- 2nd degree: The impulse occasionally fails to reach the ventricles. Here the rhythm is regular. Every 2nd, 3rd or 4th impulse is conducted.
- 3rd degree: It is corresponding to complete AV block. All the atrial impulse fail to reach the ventricle, so the auricle and the ventricle beat at their own rhythms. Pulse rate will be about 30/minute as the ventricular beat is 30/minute. The block may be produced by poisons, drugs, and fever.

CHAPTER 3

Thermoregulation in Infants and Children

In intrauterine life, fetus is warmed and insulated in the uterus, but as it comes out naked and wet, it is at once exposed to the temperature of the labor room. The modern labor room is usually air-conditioned and the room temperature usually varies from 20° to 30° C. The baby, following this sudden exposure to cold, rapidly loses heat. Hence proper care should be taken to maintain the body temperature; otherwise, prolonged hypothermia may lead to mortality and morbidity.

Thermoregulation in infants is imperfect. Human baby is rather poikilotherm due to immaturity of the heat regulating center, lack of subcutaneous tissue, relatively larger surface area and relatively low ability to lose heat by sweating or conserve heat by shivering. Environmental temperature largely influences the body temperature of infants.

Just after birth the baby increases his metabolic rate and hence heat production and tries to minimize heat loss during cold stress by vasoconstriction. Similarly, when the baby is subjected to hot atmosphere, heat loss is augmented by panting type of respiration, vasodilatation and sweating. Sweating in infants is, however, minimal.

The environmental temperature does not depend solely on the room temperature. It will also depend on movement of air, relative humidity and cooling power of ambient air. All these factors should be kept at comfortable level in the labor room or in wards. At one stage of environmental conditions, the baby will neither lose heat nor gain heat; this may be taken as neutral thermal environment. In this range of neutral thermal environmental conditions, there is minimum oxygen consumption. The upper limit of this range can be determined by measuring oxygen consumption. It depends on various factors and the condition of the baby, whether he is awake or asleep. The lower limit is regarded as the critical temperature.

Heat production can be measured by simply measuring the oxygen consumption rate. The oxygen consumption of normal adult at rest is about

3.5 to 4 ml/kg of body weight per minute. The oxygen consumption in newborn baby is about 6.5/kg body weight per minute.

Heat production in neonates can also be measured by direct calorimetry. It may vary with body size, activity and some other factors like state of digestion, etc. When the activity is reduced to minimum and factors like digestion can be eliminated the heat production will be equal to basal metabolic rate. But the factor of digestion cannot be removed in case of infants, because the babies are always digesting and feeds are given at more frequent intervals. If the fluids are withheld for some hours, there will be dehydration and the baby cannot be expected to behave as normal. So in infants the heat production can be better taken as the minimum metabolic rate. On an average, heat production in infants is 42 calories/kg/day (1.75 calories/kg/hour) in the first month of life. Later on upto 3rd year of age, it may be upto 2 calories/kg/hour. In the adult, it is about 1 calorie/kg/hour. In prematures, the heat production is high in comparison with the term baby.

In relation to surface area of the baby, the newborn produces heat to the extent of about 25 calories/sq meter/hour. At the age of 2 years it may increase upto 50 calories/sq meter/hour. In an adult, it is about 35 calories/sq meter/hour. The premature baby produces more heat than the full term baby.

Total calorie requirement in the newborn is about 92 calories/kg/day of which basal metabolic requirement is 48 calories/kg/day. The calorie requirement is highly increased during crying or other activities.

The source of energy in fetal life is mainly carbohydrate, but after birth, body fat plays an important role in metabolism. Later, carbohydrate and fat may be the sources of energy. In this respect, the premature infants depend more on fat than the full term babies, but when milk is given, they are more dependent on carbohydrate and less on fat.

Normal newborn shows a greater rise in oxygen consumption rate on the first day. There may be no rise in the next 2 or 3 days. During this period, there may be hypoglycemia. On the 4th day, there is again rise. The prematures may not show any rise in the first week of life. The baby usually spends more hours of the day in sleep. Oxygen consumption is low in deep sleep, but high during light sleep.

Regarding the glycogen reserves in the body of neonates, liver, muscle and heart are the chief reserves. Since the baby does not usually get mother's milk for first 2 days of birth, the baby is more dependent on the stored muscle and liver glycogen. If it is already depleted, the baby suffers to be in a bad metabolic state and cannot withstand hypoxia and hypothermia. During early neonatal period, the body weight decreases. This loss of body weight can be minimized by free supply of water and glucose. The baby can survive without any food for certain length of time, if kept in a warm comfortable condition. But if kept under cool environment, the baby will die earlier due to hypoglycemia. Metabolic response to cold environment is decreased in hypoxia. It is also reduced in intracranial hemorrhage, by various drugs and in severe hypothermia.

The body temperature of the newborn at the time of birth is the same as that of the mother. Just after birth there is an immediate fall of temperature which may be of the order of 1° to 3° C even when the baby is wrapped and kept in a warm room. But soon after 8 hours, the temperature tends to rise approximately to 37°C.

The temperature regulating mechanism in infants is not perfect, yet the infant tries to keep the core temperature near to its normal limits by a balance of heat gain and heat loss.

Heat gain depends on several factors of which metabolic rate of the baby is the most important. Metabolic rate depends on basal metabolism, muscular activity, and assimilation of carbohydrate and fats. Sympathetic activity increases the BMR upto 50% above normal. Increased thyrotoxin may raise BMR upto 100%. The increased body temperature increases BMR by 13% for each degree of rise of centigrade temperature. Heat may be gained from high ambient temperature by physical processes like radiation, conduction and convection.

Heat loss may occur in several ways. There is some requirement of heat to warm inspired air and ingested food. The body can lose heat by conduction, convection, radiation and evaporation. *Radiant heat loss* or gain occurs in transmitting heat in the form of infrared rays. It depends on radiant temperature of surroundings and effective radiating area exposed. Convection is the heating of air, which rises and is replaced by cooler air which in its turn is warmed. *Convective heat loss* will depend on mean surface temperature of the body, air temperature, air flow and effective convective area. The rate of heat loss is modified by changes in posture. Heat loss from the body increases with the square root of wind speed. *Conductive heat loss* occurs by transfer of heat directly to a substance in contact with the body. *Evaporative heat loss* occurs from the surface and depends on the degree of sweating, vasodilatation and skin temperature. The rate of evaporation depends on the pressure gradiant between the vapor pressure of skin and the surrounding air. Vasodilatation and skin blood flow increase evaporative heat loss. Sweating is regulated by anterior hypothalamus and by autonomic nervous system.

The heat-sensitive receptors are said to be present both in the skin and in the hypothalamus. The central thermal center in hypothalamus regulates reflex activity of the autonomic nervous system which controls sweat secretion and shivering. Normal temperature is maintained by a delicate balance in the release of adrenaline, noradrenaline and 5-hydroxytryptamine in the hypothalamus. Adrenaline and noradrenaline lower and 5-hydroxytryptamine raises the temperature. Change in temperature disturbs the balance. There is another view that the temperature regulation is not dependent on the release of amines normally but their release can upset the balance. Extracellular fluid plays an important role in maintaining body temperature. In dehydration, there may be rise of core temperature which is more common in infants.

In response to heat stress, the baby shows vasodilatation which favors increased rate of heat loss by convection and radiation. A little sweating and hence evaporation may occur. In cold stress, the normal baby tries to conserve body heat by cutaneous vasoconstriction and maintain body temperature by increasing heat production in the body. The baby usually relies on nonshivering thermogenesis.

The brown adipose tissue is the main site of heat production in neonates. The embryonic fat is yellow in color and finely lobulated with rich blood and nerve supply. It is found in the neck, back of the axillae, mediastinum and around thoracic and abdominal viscera. The brown color is due to high concentration of iron in mitochondria. The histological appearance varies with the fat content. In granular cytoplasm, there are rounded nucleoli and small vacuoles of fat. The small vacuoles may fuse to form a big one as seen in babies of diabetic or obese mothers. When the cell is depleted of fat, the vacuoles decrease in size and lastly disappear. The main function of brown adipose tissue is the heat production by nonshivering mechanism. Nonshivering thermogenesis begins with the liberation of catecholamines as skin and mucosal temperatures decrease. Noradrenaline induces the metabolism of fatty acids in brown adipose tissue causing heat production. Heat production is also controlled by sympathetic system. Noradrenaline is the mediator of metabolic response to cold stress and it helps in splitting the triglyceride molecules into glycerol and fatty acid. Fatty acid is locally metabolized and this triggers the cycle of heat production and increases oxygen consumption. Its role in an adult is uncertain though it may be detected in adult body. The neonates who are underweight because of their prematurity or due to intrauterine malnutrition, may lack the brown adipose tissue. They cannot maintain the body temperature in heat losing environment.

A clear knowledge of thermoregulation in neonates and the physiological effects of environmental temperature on them is essential for all concerned with the care of the baby, whether in a labor room, in an operation theater or in a baby ward. Proper maintenance of the thermal environment and adequate care of the babies will surely reduce the incidence of neonatal mortality and morbidity and save many of them from cold injuries.

Prolonged cold stress elevates metabolic rate and depletes energy stores and causes metabolic acidosis. Exhaustion of fat and glycogen stores may occur and there may be hypoglycemia. Special care should be taken for premature and small-for-date babies.

TEMPERATURE REGULATION DURING PEDIATRIC ANESTHESIA AND SURGERY

During general anesthesia, the thermoregulation is usually depressed and more so in the case of children. Heat regulating center in hypothalamus is depressed and muscle tone and body metabolism are diminished. On the whole, the children become poikilothermic and are unable to maintain the body temperature. The naked pediatric patients are particularly confronted with the problem of thermal control principally because environmental factors which influence heat loss or gain are variable in operation theaters, recovery rooms, oxygen tents, incubators and hospital wards. There may be hyper-or hypothermia according to the high or low ambient temperature in operation theater. All these may be due to small body mass, relatively larger surface area, inadequate body insulation (principally subcutaneous fat) and immaturity of heat regulating center of the children.

The range of ambient conditions within which the core temperature can be kept fairly constant by vasomotor reactions alone is narrow in adults and this is more so in children. During anesthesia, the children are immobilized and unable to change the effective surface area by altering posture and this may restrict the regulatory range.

The fall of body temperature may be due to the direct effect of anesthetic agents on the heat regulating center at hypothalamus. It is not clearly understood whether the anesthetic agents render the hypothalamus insensitive to amines or hypothalamus retains its sensitivity under anesthesia.

The premedicant drugs like atropine and hyoscine cause rise of body temperature. Atropine directly acts on temperature regulating center and increases basal metabolic rate. Atropine also inhibits sweating by 40 to 50% and produces 'atropine fever'. Atropine also helps in heat loss by increasing minute ventilation and causing vasodilatation. The heat loss may be enhanced in presence of low ambient temperature. Hyoscine is more likely than atropine to cause pyrexia. When morphine or pethidine is added to atropine or hyoscine, there is less rise of body temperature but complete prevention of pyrexia may not be possible.

Usually, all the anesthetic drugs cause depression of heat regulating center, relaxation of skeletal muscles, reduction of basal metabolic rate and produce vasodilatation which aids heat loss, specially when the subject is exposed in low ambient temperature. Halothane causes profound vasodilatation which favors heat loss. Ether may reduce body temperature owing to depression of central thermal center and decreased metabolism. Muscle relaxants cause profound muscular relaxation and hence less heat production. Succinylcholine in the initial stages causes fasciculations of muscle fibers and may lead to rise in body temperature.

Heat loss is said to be more in the open drop method (300 calories/minute) than that in the semiopen administration of ether (250 calories/minute) and in carbon dioxide absorption technique circle method (180 calories/minute), but the carbon dioxide absorption with to-and-fro method results in negligible heat loss and may even conserve heat. The cold temperature of ether-air mixture during open drop administration may disturb its smooth induction pattern. However, the ether vapor when delivered through corrugated rubber tube from Boyle apparatus or through Oxford inflating bellows is warmed upto the room temperature at the patient's end. Thus, the patient inhales the gas mixture at room temperature.

When soda lime is used in the anesthetic circuit, heat is liberated because of the reaction between carbon dioxide and soda lime. If to-and-fro system is used, the inspired gas becomes heated and saturated with water vapor, so that it scatters heat to lungs. When the circle system is used, the temperature of inspired gases is the same as the room temperature although they remain saturated with water vapor and no cooling effect is obtained by evaporation.

Hypercarbia, in the initial stages, increases the body temperature. In shock, there is overall depression of metabolism and hence reduction of body temperature. In the case of dehydration, there may be rise of body temperature specially in children.

During surgery, when the body cavity is opened, larger surface of the viscera is exposed to the low environmental temperature of air-conditioned operation theater and thus loss of body temperature may occur. Irrigation with cold solutions of the peritoneal cavity or bladder after prostatectomy in adults may reduce body temperature. Infusion of cold fluids or refrigerated blood may cause inadvertent hypothermia. Surgical draping may also influence the body temperature. Skin preparation with alcoholic antiseptics, if it involves large areas of the body surface, may produce significant heat loss. Surgical drapes, particularly heavy clothing, rubber materials, etc. entrap some air around the body surface and produce a separate ambient atmosphere (microclimate) which is necessarily different from the room atmosphere. This microclimate will essentially preserve body heat. In addition, heat loss by evaporation and convection will be minimized. Application of plaster of Paris jackets may increase the body temperature initially due to chemical reaction of the plaster but when it dries, it losses water. As a result the cast as well as the patient may lose temperature. The proximity of surgeon with his assistants and operating room lights should also be accounted for in estimating further heat load.

PYREXIA IN CHILDREN

Fever accompanies various diseases and is a valuable indicator of disease activity. The cause of the fever should be determined and treated accordingly. Fever itself adversely affects the body systems causing increased tissue catabolism, dehydration, precipitation or exacerbation of heart failure, delirium and convulsions. Hyperpyrexia occurs in certain conditions with a core or internal body temperature usually exceeding 40.6°C (105°F). Heat stroke and malignant hyperpyrexia are really life-threatening conditions.

In pyrexia there is a marked failure of thermoregulatory mechanism to maintain proper balance between heat gain and heat loss. The factors responsible for pyrexia may be as follows:
1. Decreased heat loss: Lack of sweat glands, inhibition of sweat glands as for example by atropine or hyoscine, insufficient peripheral circulation, high ambient temperature with increased humidity.
2. Increased heat gain from high environmental temperature.
3. Increased heat production due to:
   a. Endocrine disorders like thyrotoxicosis and pheochromocytoma.
   b. Increased muscular activity as in shivering in response to cold stress struggling during induction of anesthesia and rigor.
   c. Abnormality of the central heat regulating mechanism in hypothalamus.
   d. Increased body temperature itself results in increased metabolism and heat production and may further elevate body temperature and metabolism.
4. Besides these, there are other causes of hyperpyrexia like heat stroke, enteric fever, septic meningitis, tubercular meningitis, encephalitis and cerebral malaria.
5. Pyrogens either exogenous (bacteria) or endogenous (from body tissue usually granulocytes) may raise body temperature.
6. Altered energy metabolism like uncoupling of oxidative phosphorylatio can produce enormous rise in body temperature.
   The salient features of pyrexia can be summarized as follows:
   a. Basal metabolic rate: It is greatly increased with the rise of body temperature. Oxygen consumption increases 7%/°F rise of body temperature. So there is always demand hypoxia. If extra oxygen is not supplier vital organs will suffer. Liver and brain tolerate hypoxia very badly and necrosis may occur.

b. Cardiovascular system: Heart rate increases 5 to 10 beats/°F of temperature. There is decrease in blood volume and fall in peripheral vascular resistance resulting in low blood pressure. The diastolic cardiac work is increased, resistance that there is further need of oxygen for myocardium. Coronary dilatation usually protects the myocardium from ischemia. Circulation time is decreased because of increase in cardiac output. There may be dehydration due to excessive sweating and hemoconcentration may result. All these may cause peripheral circulatory failure. Bleeding diathesis may be encountered. Cardiac irregularities or failure may also occur.
c. Respiratory system: Respiratory rate increases 5%/°F rise of temperature in order to meet the increased demand of oxygen. There may be respiratory alkalosis and kidney tries to compensate by excreting alkaline urine. Increased water loss through hurried respiration may further lower the circulatory blood volume. Aspiration and bronchopneumonia may occur.
d. Central nervous system: Usually, there is stimulation and increased demand of oxygen. Muscular twitching and convulsion may occur, specially in children. Electroencephalogram pattern may be abnormal.
e. Liver: Hyperpyrexia may cause increased hepatic glucose metabolism, glycogen depletion, increased lactic acid outflow, deceased bile flow and increased oxygen consumption. Hepatic blood flow may be increased and bromsulphthalein clearance may be reduced. Jaundice and even hepatic failure may occur.
f. Kidneys: Kidneys try to compensate water loss and urine becomes concentrated, high colored and of small quantity.
g. Water and electrolytes: There may be dehydration due to sweating and hurried respiration. Hemoconcentration and peripheral circulatory failure usually result. There may be large loss of sodium and chloride due to sweating, which may cause tissue exhaustion.
h. Blood catecholamines: Blood catecholamines increase due to overactivity of sympathetic system during hyperpyrexia. Histamine levels may also increase. The catecholamines may be of adrenal origin. Noradrenaline may induce the increase in histamine level which may cause cardiovascular collapse.
i. Anesthetic requirements: These are increased.
j. Tissue damage: There may not be any specific lesion on gross or microscopic examination of the organs. The changes that occur in various tissues are due mainly to associated hypoxia. Liver is sensitive to hyperthermia and there is marked destruction of liver cells reflected by the elevation of enzymes. Increased body

temperature will increase the metabolism of all the cells of the body which ultimately results in greater oxygen consumption. This causes relative hypoxia and an increase in waste products. Due to severe vasoconstriction or cardiovascular collapse there is poor tissue perfusion which leads to acidosis. The direct damage of the tissues may be due to protein denaturation, enzyme degradation, alteration in physical structure of the cell membrane and change in viscosity of the cell protoplasm. All these factors together with decreased responsiveness to catecholamines will ultimately lead to cardiovascular collapse and death.

MANAGEMENT

The primary aim should be to lower the body temperature and bring it towards normal, and support vital organ systems. Thereafter, the proper diagnosis should be made to treat pyrexia accordingly.
1. Cooling may involve continuous ice water sponge baths and ice sponging. Ice bags over the head, axillae and groins will help. Chlorpromazine, IM or IV in small doses may be needed to stop shivering. Active cooling should be discontinued when the internal body temperature reaches 102°F; otherwise, hypothermia may result.
2. Oxygenation is essential. Endotracheal intubation is indicated in patients with inadequate ventilation or with convulsion and in comatose patients.
3. Intravenous fluid therapy should be adequate; otherwise, fluid and electrolyte imbalance and even cardiovascular collapse will occur. Monitoring of pulse, blood pressure and central venous pressure is always helpful.
4. Sodium bicarbonate IV may be needed for correction of metabolic acidosis.
5. In presence of convulsion, diazepam should be given to stop it. Phenytoin may be needed in severe cases.
6. Oliguria, if present, should be managed with the infusion of mannitol.
7. Other measures against bleeding diathesis, infection and so on should be taken accordingly, if present.
8. Elective surgery should better be delayed when the patient is febrile. Every attempt should be made to make the patient afebrile at the time of elective anesthesia and surgery.
9. Prevention of pyrexia should be tried by avoidance of belladonna drugs like atropine and hyoscine, using the nonrebreathing anesthetic circuits, using light drapes and properly controlling the temperature and humidity of the operating room. Monitoring of core temperature at frequent intervals is recommended.

INADVERTENT HYPOTHERMIA DURING ANESTHESIA

Induced hypothermia is an adjunct to anesthesia and surgery. The procedure lowers the overall metabolism and reduce the dangers of hypoxia and cellular damage resulting from the circulatory occlusion of the brain, heart, liver, and legs for a limited period of time. Accidental hypothermia may also occur when the core or internal body temperature is less than 35°C (95°F). This may be due to exposure to severe cold, specially of infants and aged during winter in cold countries. Intoxication, debilitating diseases, exhaustion, head injuries, insanity, malnutrition, etc. may be the precipitating or predisposing factors. Accidental hypothermia is a well known complication of hypoglycemia, myxedema, hypopituitarism and hypoadrenalism. Neonatal cold injury may also be due to accidental exposure to cold. Mortality in hypothermia is high and mostly related to the presence of associated diseases.

Accidental hypothermia may occur in neonates and infants when they are operated in air-conditioned theaters at low ambient temperature. It may also occur in the aged and thin persons who have little fat to act as insulation or as a heat depot. The factors leading to hypothermia during anesthesia are vasodilatation, depression of heat regulating center in hypothalamus, absence of muscular activity, lack of insulation, lengthy operation, exposure of body cavities, viscera, and large muscle mass, infusion of cold solution, transfusion of refrigerated blood, irrigation of body cavity with cold solution, inadequate draping and so on. The use of muscle relaxants and controlled ventilation aid heat loss in anesthetized children. The undernourished ill children, premature and small-for-date babies are prone to develop hypothermia. Another factor responsible for considerable heat loss is the diathermy pad. The electrode covered with a towel soaked with saline is usually placed under the lower half of the body and this leads to considerable heat loss.

Clinical signs of hypothermia are not so obvious as those of hyperthermia. Body surface is cool and skin is pale. There may be cyanosis due to peripheral vasoconstriction. Shivering may occur in older age group but is rare in neonates. It ceases at core temperatures below 90°F. Blood pressure is low due to reduced cardiac output from bradycardia and there is unusual flaccidity of muscles. Heart rate and respiration are depressed. Pupils are dilated. The clinical signs resemble those of cardiac arrest or severe hypotension.

Profound hypothermia is usually associated with cardiac arrhythmia, metabolic acidosis and increased bleeding tendency due to coagulation defects. There is depression of central nervous system. In neonates prolonged hypothermia may cause sclerema and increase the incidence of neonatal mortality or morbidity. During hypothermia, anesthetic requirements are reduced and thus a relative overdose is common even with usual doses. Certain drugs used in anesthesia are not destroyed in hypothermic state when overall metabolism is reduced. These drugs may become effective in the postoperative period in normothermic state resulting in a dangerous situation for the patient.

During hypothermia, oxygen consumption decreases 6%/°C. But shivering increases oxygen consumption. Oxygen dissociation is retarded as temperature falls and the curve shifts to the left. Basal metabolic rate is reduced. Glucose consumption is reduced to a greater extent and hyperglycemia may result. Hepatic and renal functions are severely depressed. Cerebral blood flow and cerebral oxygen consumption decrease. In mild hypothermia, nervous system may be hyperactive and convulsions are not uncommon. Coronary blood flow is reduced, but coronary arteriovenous oxygen difference remains essentially unchanged. Blood volume decreases and there is pronounced shift of fluid out of the vascular tree to tissue spaces. A true anhydremia occurs, There is increased concentration of proteins in blood and there is hemoconcentration. Viscosity of blood also increases.

Complications of accidental hypothermia may include cardiac arrest, respiratory arrest, arrhythmias, aspiration, bronchopneumonia, pulmonary edema, acidosis, pancreatitis, acute renal failure, intravascular thrombosis leading to cerebrovascular accident, myocardial infarction, cardiovascular collapse, gastrointestinal bleeding and so on.

PREVENTION OF INADVERTENT HYPOTHERMIA IN OPERATION THEATER

1. The operation theater should have optimum air temperature and relative humidity, so that heat loss may be minimized. During neonatal surgery, air-conditioning may have to be stopped totally.
2. The infusion fluids should be warmed to approximate body temperature. Refrigerated blood should never be used before warming. 500 ml of blood at 4°C can reduce the body temperature upto 1°C given rapidly.
3. The use of closed circuit can reduce water loss from respiration. An open circuit with humidifier can also prevent water loss.
4. The draping should be adequate to minimize heat loss. Surface area of head is comparatively greater in children and it must be wrapped in cotton wool.
5. Constant monitoring of body temperature during anesthesia should be a routine. Any fall of body temperature should be detected and treated

immediately. Careful monitoring of vital signs, central venous pressure (CVP) and arterial blood gas is also required.
6. The patient may be placed in a water mattress through which water circulates. The temperature of water should be according to the need to the patient. Cold water circulates in hyperthermic patients. Care should be taken not to injure the skin of the patient as hypothermic patient may suffer burns at relatively low body temperatures.

TREATMENT OF ACCIDENTAL HYPOTHERMIA

It should include intensive supportive care, rewarming and treatment of associated and complicating disorders.
1. Oxygenation is essential to prevent hypoxia. Humidified oxygen is preferred. Endotracheal intubation is necessary, if the patient is unconscious.
2. Intravenous fluids should be given preferably with CVP monitoring. Temperature of fluid should approximate the body temperature.
3. Sodium bicarbonate IV may be needed to combat metabolic acidosis.
4. Hydrocortisone may also be helpful.
5. Vasoconstrictors like noradrenaline or mephentermine or dopamine may be given in hypotensive cases to raise blood pressure, to prevent renal cortical necrosis and irreversible damage to brain.
6. Antibiotics may be needed to combat infections. It is better to be guided by culture and sensitivity tests.
7. Rapid active rewarming is prohibited in children as it may cause cardiac irregularities and even death due to circulatory collapse.
8. Slow rewarming with blankets and hot water bottles is preferred. Use of warm humidified oxygen and IV fluids is helpful.
9. Hypothermia with cardiac arrest needs rapid core rewarming. Cardiopulmonary resuscitation (CPR) should be continued. These patients tolerate prolonged CPR due to the protective effect of hypothermia on the central nervous system. No patient should be declared dead while hypothermic. It can only be done when the patient fails to survive with rewarming at 32°C and appropriate resuscitative measures.
10. Underlying and associated complications should be carefully diagnosed and treated accordingly.

CHAPTER 4

Renal Function and Fluid Balance

RENAL FUNCTION

The kidneys are immature at birth and both glomerular filtration and tubular reabsorption are somewhat reduced until the age of 6 to 8 months. Initially, the number of cells increases and then the size. Until about 4 months of age, there is low cortical blood flow and relatively high intrarenal vascular resistance. Eventually, 80 to 90% of renal blood flow occurs in the cortex and 10 to 20% in the medulla. The autoregulatory abilities of the infant kidney are not known. This possible lack of autoregulatory mechanism may be a contributing factor to acute renal failure in premature infants. In fetal life, the kidney is essential as it excretes copious amounts of dilute urine which maintains the amniotic fluid volume during pregnancy. During gestation, the fetal kidneys receive 3 to 7% of the cardiac output while mature kidneys receive roughly 20% of the cardiac output. This level is usually achieved by about 2 years of age.

In the fetus, glomerular filtration is usually less than 1 ml/minute, but in the full term baby glomerular filtration rate is 2 to 4 ml/minute, within the first few days it is 8 to 20 ml/minute and is said to be mature by 1 year of age. This rapid increase in glomerular function is mostly due to increase in systemic blood pressure and decrease in renal vascular resistance. The pores of glomerulus of an infant kidney are about half the size of those in adults. However, for normal functions, the immature kidneys are usually adequate for the infants, but under abnormal stress the baby may be adversely affected. Thus, the neonates are more susceptible to nephrotoxic drugs like aminoglycosides. The doses of filtered drugs like digoxin, tubocurarine, etc. should be adjusted accordingly in neonates and infants.

Tubular function in newborn is depressed in comparison to that in adults. Small-for-date babies have decreased tubular reabsorptive capacity for glucose and may have glycosuria with osmotic diuresis and dehydration. Albuminuria is also common in premature infants. On the whole, in infants the capacity to excrete water and retain sodium or to concentrate urine is somewhat restricted. The maximum urine osmolarity is about half compared to that of adult. The permeability of the tubular membrane and the colloidal osmotic pressure are usually low in the early weeks of life.

In view of all these factors, there is inability to handle excessive water loads, and over infusion or over transfusion may lead to edema and cardiac failure. Abrupt increase of sodium, as in cases with administration of sodium bicarbonate, is also handled poorly. Urinary obstruction, hypothermia, excess catecholamines, high arterial oxygen tension, etc. increase the disability to handle abnormal loads. Infant has a low threshold for bicarbonates and does not rapidly excrete acids or ammonia; thus, a mild acidosis and raised blood urea nitrogen are normal. Infants have persistent metabolic acidosis though the urine is alkaline, the pH being 5 to 7. Urine excretion in newborn is about 15 to 60 ml/day, at 6 months 250 to 450 ml/day, at 1 year 500 to 600 ml/day, at 5 year 650 to 1000 ml/day, and at 12 years 700 to 1500 ml/day. In this connection, it should be borne in mind that the full bladder rises higher out of the pelvis in infants and children than in adults.

Renal insufficiency is not uncommon in children. Acute renal failure in children as in adults is divided into prerenal, renal and postrenal causes. Prerenal causes are mostly due to low circulating blood volume, low cardiac output, hypotension, hypoxia and serious infection. The most common causes of intrinsic renal failure are acute glomerulonephritis following bacterial, viral, mycoplasmal, fungal, protozoal, helminthic or spirochetal infections, and nephrotoxic drugs and chemicals. Glomerulonephropathy may also occur in Henoch-Schonlein purpura where there is vasculitis attacking joints, kidneys and the gastrointestinal system. In children, acute tubular necrosis may occur due to renal ischemia and from nephrotoxic drugs. Postrenal failure usually occurs as a result of bilateral obstruction of the kidneys, obstruction at the bladder level, urethral obstruction or in unilateral obstruction in presence of evere hypofunctioning of one or both kidneys. Chronic renal failure may occur above the age of 5 years and is mostly due to obstructive uropathies, or congenital malformations of the urinary tract.

FLUID AND ELECTROLYTE BALANCE

At birth, total body water in a full term baby is about 80% of his body weight. It decreases to about 70% of body weight by the age of 3 months and then to adult levels of 60 to 65% at the age of 1 year. The extracellular fluid in the case of neonate is about 40% of total body fluid. It decreases to 30% of total body fluid by 3 to 6 months and then gradually decreases to adult levels of about 20%. Fluid status in the neonates, infants, and children is mainly governed by the kidney. The infant kidney readily excretes dilute urine but there is limitation of its power to concentrate and/or to conserve water. Infants have also limited ability to cope with excess water and sodium.

The rapid rate of fluid turnover in infants and children is mostly due to their high metabolic rate and high oxygen consumption. On the weight basis, an infant may lose water at about twice the rate of an adult and thus rapidly becomes dehydrated. It is said that in an adult if there is no intake by mouth for a day, there is weight loss of about 4%, but in an infant it may be about 10% of his body weight. Fluid imbalance in neonates, infants and children may cause more immediate and adverse reactions than in adults and this has important implications for perioperative fluid therapy.

Blood volume in relation to weight in neonates and infants is always greater than that in adults, but it remains a similar proportion of total body fluid. Blood volume in newborn is 90 to 100 ml/kg body weight and within 1 to 2 years it decreases to about 80 ml/kg and then gradually attains the adults level of 75 ml/kg at the age of 2 to 3 years. It is said that a moderate loss of blood volume of about 10% indicates blood replacement in pediatric patients and when 15% of blood volume is lost the infant is potentially in danger.

Blood components change mostly in the first week; fetal hemoglobin is rapidly lost with relatively slow replacement by the adult type. Protein level is usually low in infants, which may lead to reduced plasma osmolarity. Thus, the extracellular fluid easily collects in interstitial space and there is increased possibility of edema in case of excessive extracellular fluid accumulation.

Water Balance

Water balance is maintained through a delicate balance between water loss and gain in the body. Water loss usually occurs by evaporation through lungs and skin, in the form of urine and from alimentary tract. Water loss in infants is most variable depending on metabolic rate, insensible loss through lungs and skin, ambient temperature and so on. At a temperature of 34°C with relative humidity of 45%, infant loses water at the rate of about 20 ml/kg body weight per 24 hours by evaporation. It is gradually reduced with advancing age. The amount of water lost through alimentary tract is usually about 10 ml/kg/24 hours. In growing children, there is some retention of water for growth. It is very small, amounting to about 5 ml/kg/24 hours. There is also loss of water through urine. The infants are mostly on fluid diet. Infants excrete very dilute urine as the infant kidney is less able to concentrate urine. Absolute minimum water output to allow excretion of urea and electrolytes is usually 35 ml/kg/24 hours in case of infants upto 4 weeks of age, about 25 ml/kg/24 hours in infants and about 10 ml/kg/24 hours in older children.

Water intake is usually by mouth and alimentary tract, through infusion and by oxidative metabolism of the body. Input should always be well in excess to cover for insensible loss, urinary loss and alimentary tract loss and also retention for growth. Allowances should also be made for water produced in metabolism. In infants, it is about less than 1 ml/kg/24 hours. Minimum water requirement for healthy children is about 60 ml/kg/24 hours in cases of infants upto 1 month of age, 50 ml/kg/24 hours in infants of 1 to 3 months of age. In older children, it steadily falls to 25 ml/kg/24 hours. The input of water should be maintained as follows: upto 10 kg, 100 to 130 ml/kg/hours; 10 kg to 20 kg, 75 to 100 ml/kg/24 hours, and over 20 kg 25 to 50 ml/kg/24 hours.

Electrolyte Balance

Electrolytes are essential for life and for adequate growth. The excretion of electrolytes through urine and insensible water loss, should always be replaced. In children as in adults, the kidney does not recover all the potassium content of the glomerular filtrate, thus urinary loss is usually substantial. In malnutrition, tissue catabolism further increases potassium loss.

Minimum requirements of electrolytes are as follows: Sodium 2 mmol/kg/24 hours, potassium 1 mmol/kg/24 hours and calcium 1 mmol/kg/24 hours.

FLUID MANAGEMENT DURING PEDIATRIC SURGERY

Fluid management during pediatric surgery is most vital and many times it dictates the outcome of surgical procedure and reduces the incidence of mortality and morbidity of surgical patients. Infants and children tolerate blood loss very badly, particularly during anesthesia and surgery. Acute and/or inadequately treated blood loss causes cardiovascular insufficiency very easily in children. The distribution of blood in the child body differs from that in adults and there is much less amount in peripheral venous pools in upper and lower extremities.

During surgery, the child may have a deficiency of extracellular fluid due to various reasons such as prolonged preoperative fasting, evaporative fluid loss from skin, gut, pleura, peritoneum, dry anesthetic gases and so on. Major surgery is associated with an apparent reduction in functional extracellular fluid volume because of sequestration. Any operation which may result in blood loss exceeding 5% of estimated blood volume should have intravenous fluid therapy. Blood loss above 10% of blood volume should indicate blood transfusion.

Stress of surgery and anesthesia has its implications on fluid balance. Surgery and anesthesia may cause acute reduction in renal function and urinary output. In the postoperative period, there is usually retention of sodium and water as a consequence of metabolic response to injury. Oliguria is mostly due to reduction and redistribution in renal blood flow caused by increased sympathetic activity and catecholamine release, and partly due to an increase in plasma antidiuretic activity due to ADH, adrenocortical hormones and hormones liberated in the kidney.

Anesthesia may influence the fluid and electrolyte balance. Vasodilatation caused by most volatile anesthetics maintains the renal blood flow and provides renal excretion of excess water and electrolytes, provided no severe hypotension occurs. Some volatile anesthetic agents may reduce renal blood flow by causing renal vasoconstriction. Hypocarbia from any cause may also reduce renal blood flow by causing vasoconstriction. Narcotic analgesics in large doses may depress catecholamine, plasma cortisol and growth hormone response to surgery. It may also reduce ADH release.

Excessive fluid therapy should always be avoided; otherwise, pulmonary congestion and even edema may occur. However, the kidneys of children are able to excrete excess amount and thus embarrassment of the child may not be a problem. On the other hand, active diuresis may protect against renal shut down resulting from shock or trauma.

OBJECTIVES OF INTRAVENOUS FLUID THERAPY

a. To provide adequate fluid volume in presence of dehydration.
b. To replace the predicted loss of fluid (blood).
c. To provide an excess fluid volume to act as protection buffer against blood loss.
d. To prevent hypotension caused by vasodilatation of various drugs used in anesthesia like halothane.
e. To provide nutrition.

Fluid Therapy

During fluid management, the volume of the fluid should be calculated and the type of the fluid should be selected carefully considering preoperative dehydration either by usual fasting or abnormal losses as in pyloric stenosis, burns, etc. maintenance requirements, surgical trauma and body temperature.

Preoperative dehydration

It may be due to prolonged period of fasting or secondary to increased losses due to vomiting, diarrhea, pyrexia, etc. The amount of deficit can be assessed by physical examination, body weight loss and hematocrit. The percentage of the normal body weight in kg can be converted to ml.

Clinical assessment of dehydration

- Mild dehydration: 5% loss of body weight. Child is pale, dry mouth and tongue, skin and subcutaneous tissue are less elastic, fontanelle is less tense, pulse—normal, blood pressure—Normal, urine output becoming less, specific gravity 1010 (normal 1006 in infants).
- Moderate dehydration: 10% loss of body weight. General condition becoming worse, pyrexia, mucous membrane and tongue are dry, sunken fontanelle, tachycardia and hypotension. Urine volume is scanty, specific gravity is 1010 to 1015.
- Severe dehydration: Over 15% loss of body weight, child in shock, hypovolemic, skin is gray, mottled, lax and inelastic. Slow capillary refilling, eyes are sunken, fontanelle are depressed, veins collapsed, marked tachycardia and hypotension, pulse is feeble, anuria or severe oliguria and respiratory distress.

Some investigations should help in the diagnosis and these are hemoglobin concentration, hematocrit, urea and creatinine estimation, electrolytes, urine and blood osmolality. Blood pressure, central venous pressure and urine output should be monitored during replacement of losses. Physiological saline, dextrose saline or even blood may be needed depending upon the type of fluid loss.

Maintenance fluids

These are the fluid losses occurring normally through the kidney, bowel, skin and lungs. The simplest way to calculate the maintenance fluid of average child is approximately 4 ml/kg/hour for the first 10 kg body weight, adding 2 ml/kg/hour for the next 10 kg and then 1 ml/kg/hour for body weight above 20 kg. Dextrose 4%/saline 0.18% is used normally, except in neonatal period where one-third to one-fifth dextrose saline can be used. In addition, potassium 2 mmol/100 ml may be given provided urinary output is adequate.

Replacement of losses (other than blood loss)

This is due to abnormal losses not covered by maintenance fluids and during operation it accounts for the evaporative losses from the operating site, *third spacing* and respiratory water loss due to dry anesthetic gases and lack of humidification in the ventilator circuit. Fluid may also be lost by evaporation if overhead radiant heaters are used. For minor surgery, it is 1 to 3 ml/kg/hour, for moderate surgery it is 3 to 5 ml/kg/hour and for major surgery it is 5 to 7 ml/kg/hour. Respiratory water loss due to dry gases may be 2 ml/hour. A rise of body temperature by 1°C can increase fluid loss by 12%.

Blood loss replacement

When more than 10% of the estimated blood volume is lost, blood should be replaced. If crystalloid solution is used to replace the blood loss, the replacement volume is 3 to 4 times the blood loss. When blood is given, it should be replaced milliliter for milliliter. In case of blood loss, hypotension indicates a loss of more than 20% blood volume. Following return to normal blood pressure, urine output should be at least 1 ml/kg/hour.

The following may be considered as another useful guide: In the first hour of operation 15 ml/kg. Subsequently, basic 2 ml/kg/hour + for mild surgery 2 ml/kg/hour or for moderate surgery 4 ml/kg/hour or for major surgery 6 ml/kg/hour + blood replacement.

An alternative regime may also be taken into account as follows: Initially Hartmann solution should be given at the rate of 20 ml/kg/hour in the first hour or so of the operation. This solution closely approximates the composition of interstitial fluid. Hartmann solution is Ringer lactate solution and its one liter contains sodium 130 mEq, potassium 4 mEq, calcium 4 mEq, chlorides 100 mEq and lactate 28 mEq. Infusion is then to be continued according to the need of the child. Prolonged preoperative starvation may cause hypoglycemia and it is recommended to administer 5% dextrose solution. It may be continued for 24 hours to make up the rest of normal requirement of water of the child. Potassium may also be added to fulfil maintenance need for which serum potassium concentration should be measured often. In presence of significant trauma, blood loss, and prolonged surgery additional Hartmann solution, 20 ml/kg/hour, may prove useful.

Half-strength Hartmann solution in 5% dextrose solution can also be given intraoperatively. Blood losses of 10 to 20% of blood volume can reasonably be replaced by plasma substitutes like dextran, hemaccel, etc. without restoring to blood transfusion. Some anesthesiologists prefer to maintain the hematocrit at 30%. Routine blood loss measurement is essential as it dictates the need of blood transfusion and many times it avoids unnecessary blood transfusions. Blood loss can be easily monitored by weighing the swabs, measuring the suction volumes and by visual evidence.

Blood loss below 5% of estimated blood volume can be ignored and usual infusion can be maintained. Losses from 5 to 10% of blood volume should be adequately replaced by an additional equivalent volume of Hartmann solution. Blood loss of 10 to 15% of blood volume may need but 70,000 molecular weight dextran or hemaccel can be replaced satisfactorily. Blood loss above 15% should always be replaced by blood. But for all practical purposes, in case of above 10% blood loss, blood transfusion is indicated.

During intravenous therapy, following measures should be adopted:

i. All infusions should be well-recorded particularly the type of fluid and its volume. Intake and output chart must be maintained. Blood group should be noted and well-checked before transfusion.
ii. Full aseptic measures should be adopted.
iii. Careful monitoring of vital signs such as pulse, respiration, blood pressure and body temperature is essential.
iv. Blood loss should be assessed carefully.
v. Dehydration, if present, should be clinically assessed.
vi. Central venous pressure monitoring, urine volume, plasma electrolytes, hemoglobin estimation, hematocrit, blood gas analysis and so on may be helpful in selected cases. Blood glucose estimation may have to be done in some cases. Dextrose solution in excess of 10 ml/kg/minute may lead to hyperglycemia and osmotic diuresis. Hyperglycemia is usually associated with hypertonic dehydration.
vii. Progress of therapy should be carefully judged by clinical findings and laboratory investigations.
viii. Whenever children are given intravenous fluids, it is essential to have a burette system available. In setting up a drip, meticulous care is needed to avoid the entry of any air bubbles into the bloodstream.
ix. Catheterization of any vein particularly the cut-down technique should be done with full aseptic measures. Intravenous infusions may lead to phlebitis, if kept for prolonged period.
x. The drip rate should be well-controlled even to very small volumes. Drip controllers of either mechanical or electrical type may help in the administration of small volumes.
xi. Drugs used in infants are usually given well diluted. Overdilution should be avoided, since excessive fluid intake or overload may result. The drug and dilution should be well recorded.

Some basal fluid volumes in neonates and adults on average or range		
	Neonate	Adult
Urine volume, ml/kg/hour	1–4	1–4
Urine osmolality, mOsmol/liter	100–600	50–1600
Extracellular volume, % body weight	35	20
Intracellular fluid volume, % body weight	40	40
Plasma, % body weight	5	5
Total fluid volume, % body weight	80	65
Blood volume, ml/kg	80–90	65–70

CHAPTER 5

Psychological Problems Associated with Anesthesia and Surgery

The psychology of surgical patients plays a prominent role on the outcome of surgical procedures. In addition to the organic stress of illness and operation, psychologic stress may produce a wide spectrum of reactions covering almost whole of the common psychopathologic disorders ranging from mild neurasthenia to severe depressive states, often with life-threatening sequelae. Since the earliest days of modern anesthesia, the patients have been manifesting mad, delirious, sad, psychotic and even odd behavior in the early weeks following operations. Most of the surgeons and anesthetists tend to ignore the psychological problems as long as they can and simply hope that the sequelae will disappear.

The psychological response to surgery and anesthesia seems to be always present, whether identified clinically or not. It is as true as the metabolic response to injury following operation. But mental functions are difficult to judge and quantitate and there is limited ability to assess and estimate the prevalence of psychological complications. Surgical patients, particularly the young children, are most likely to experience gross psychological stress.

SOMATIC FACTORS PRODUCING PERIOPERATIVE PSYCHOLOGICAL DISORDERS

1. Fluid imbalance.
2. Acid-base imbalance.
3. Electrolyte imbalance such as hypokalemia, hyponatremia, hypochoremia, calcium imbalance and hyperosmolar states.
4. Inadequate cerebral perfusion with oxygenated blood and hypoxemia.
5. Extensive physical trauma.
6. Hypoglycemia.
7. Liver failure.
8. Uremia and renal failure.

9. Cerebral anoxia: Following acute or prolonged chronic hypoxia several manifestations may be seen such as acute psychosis, increased psychomotor activity, decerebrate states, parkinsonism, blindness or visual agnosia. It may also occur following circulatory arrest.
10. Drug withdrawal.
11. Endocrine disturbances.
12. Hyperpyrexia.

SURGICAL AND ANESTHETIC FACTORS

1. Prolonged anesthesia and surgery: It may be mostly related to complexity of surgery and to the likelihood of fluid shifts.
2. Hyoscine and atropine can cause anticholinergic syndrome. Symptoms range from sedation and stupor to anxiety, restlessness, hyperactivity, disorientation and hallucinations.
3. Ether anesthesia: State of excitement and delirium is notorious. Behavioral changes may also occur in postoperative period following prolonged anesthesia with halothane or isoflurane.
4. Intraoperative awareness particularly in older children may cause psychologic changes postoperatively. Various features like apathy, indifference, mute, excitement, hallucinations, dreams and fantasies may occur for several days following operation.
5. Ketamine: Psychological disturbances due to ketamine may occur in older children. These may include hallucinations, dreams, inability to coordinate thought with word expression, floating sensation and physical movements.
6. Cyclopropane may cause emergence delirium during recovery from anesthesia.
7. Barbiturates may cause bad dreams and emotional upset in the postoperative period. Phenothiazines alone, particularly in presence of pain, may make the patient more restless and painful.
8. Patients undergoing emergency surgery are more likely to be excited postoperatively. Certain surgical procedures like cardiac surgery and plastic surgery and major orthopedic surgery may be associated with significant emotional stress.
9. Changes in mental status and orientation may be induced by sedatives and narcotics and often precipitate confusion and delirium.

COMMON PSYCHOLOGICAL REACTIONS IN PERIOPERATIVE PERIOD

Fear and Anxiety

Fear is an unpleasant sensation and bad emotion, but anxiety itself is not pathologic. It is a normal and healthy reaction to danger and is the expected response when facing a major operation. It is not the presence of anxiety, but its extent and the manner in which the patient copes up with anxiety that are important. Undue anxiety produces maximum stress and affects the patient's physiological status significantly. Fear activates sympathetic, parasympathetic and endocrine systems, thereby increasing the secretion of thyroxine, adrenaline and noradrenaline. So there may be increase in metabolic rate, pulse rate and blood pressure. Dysrhythmia is not uncommon. The endogenous catecholamines may sensitize the myocardium to some anesthetics like halothane and trichlorethylene. Anxiety makes the patient resistant to anesthesia and requires more anesthetics to tackle. Panic states may be manifested by shaking, dilated pupils, cold wet palms, tachycardia, hyperventilation and a state of doomed condition. In the postoperative period, these patients are mostly noncooperative and with low pain threshold. The extreme cases may experience a stormy recovery course.

Psychotrauma in children is very common. A child entering the hospital is always fearful and apprehensive particularly due to separation from home and parents. The new hospital surroundings, pain, needles and unpleasant medicines aggravate the situation. The discomfort of other children in the wards also reflects on the mind of the child. All these produce a detrimental effect on the child's subsequent behavior and emotional status. Undue apprehension causes resistance to anesthesia, increases the anesthetic risk and affects the surgical outcome seriously.

Even children below 4 years are emotionally disturbed for several months after operation and may manifest personality changes, nightmares, bed wetting and so on. The causative factors of preoperative fear are usually many and most of the children cannot pinpoint a single cause of fear. The younger children bother little about what is going to happen to them. The older children, of course, are additionally anxious about the discomfort during and after operation and have active fear of needles. The children who have experience of previous anesthesia, may dislike the smell of gases particularly ether and may describe it as frightening one.

The main factors contributing to psychotrauma in children are as follows (Rees and Gray, 1980):
1. Related to age: Separation, anxiety, fear of mutilation and fear of death.
2. Related to child specific: Vulnerable personality, personal backgrounds, and private misconceptions.
3. Related to parents: Misconceptions, personalities; no child is entirely self-sufficient. No appraisal can ever be complete without some reference to parental role. Thus, parents should always be included in any program related to child care.
4. Related to hospitals: Anesthesia technique, premedication, induction, injection and poor preoperative briefing.

The alleviation of preoperative fear should always be dealt with adequate briefing involving the patient and his parents. The ensuing operation and anesthesia should be explained sympathetically in simple languages and his liking about injection, inhalation or oral medicines should be cared duly. An informed patient is usually a tranquil patient. Persuasion and reassurance are most important in worried children. Hidden fears should be brought to the surface in the patient and parents. It should be freely discussed and dispelled than suppressed. "Bottling" increases the tension. Pharmacological approach with administration of a proper sedative drug is always complementary and in combination with psychic approach produces a better result than either method used singly.

Mental Depression

The mood of the patient is one of grief and misery, and he is in a state of helplessness and sadness. The patient has little interest in pleasure and is always down hearted. The depression is mostly associated with disturbances in sleeping, eating and bowel habits leading to insomnia, anorexia, constipation and ill health. Depressed patients mostly show delayed convalescence, more perioperative complications and increased death rate. Depression is not common even in older children, but if present, it should be properly evaluated and treated adequately before subjecting to elective surgery. Psychiatric consultation is often helpful.

Distrust and Anger

Usually the patient places his life and health in the hands of the surgeon and anesthetist and submits himself to painful, dangerous and even life-threatening procedures. But some patients may manifest acute crisis resulting in extreme anger and frustration at the prospect of dependency and ill health. These patients are mostly noncooperative and refuse to follow the medical advice. The best prevention of such psychiatric reaction is a close doctor-patient rapport with an empathic, kindly, caring but confident and direct manner on the part of the doctor. Cultivation of confidence and trust for prevention of psychotrauma is said to be as important as the sterile operating room technique for prevention of infection.

Excitement and Delirium

These are common in early postoperative period. There may be restlessness, irritability, confusion, disorientation, crying, moaning, irrational talking, shouting or screaming. It may be due to premedicant drugs like barbiturates, hyoscine or anesthetic drugs like cyclopropane, halothane, ketamine, etc. or cerebral hypoxia, pain, hypoglycemia and so on. Systemic metabolic disorders, endocrine disturbances, electrolyte abnormalities, liver failure, kidney failure, brain dysfunction, head trauma, etc. may also cause delirium.

MANAGEMENT OF PSYCHIATRIC PROBLEMS

1. Prevention: Prevention of psychiatric illness is most important in the case of children as in adults and it should be based on a solid patient-anesthetist and patient-surgeon relationship. Preanesthetic visit is of immense value to evaluate the patient's psychological status. Patients prone to psychotrauma should be identified, their emotional needs should be responded adequately thereby establishing a good rapport, trust and confidence.
2. Early identification: Early identification of psychiatric illness is essential. The presence of abnormal emotion, fear, anxiety, depression, and distorted reality will need full investigations on psychological aspect and therapeutic measures in the preanesthetic period. In severe cases, expert psychiatric consultation may be needed. Sometimes, the elective procedure may have to be deferred till the condition improves.
3. Assurance: Surgeons and anesthetists should listen to their child patients effectively, respond with adequate empathy and express specific understanding of the patient's discomfort. Patient's belief or expectations are often far from reality and such disparity should be minimized as far as practicable. Hidden fears should be brought to the surface and dispelled as far as practicable rather than suppressed.
4. Psychic support: Coping styles of individuals and their modes of adaptation may vary widely. The anesthetist should judge all the factors and assure firm and kind management and psychic support accordingly.
5. Environmental prophylaxis: The patient should be in a healthy, homely and safe atmosphere and in a supportive and stimulating environment. Television, radio, books, pictures, diversional occupational therapy, visitors, relatives, particularly parents of children—All can help the patient pastime which otherwise might be filled with morbid fantasy, anxiety, fear and discomfort. Relaxation training may be helpful in older children.
6. Good management: Good management can certainly minimize the prevalence, duration, intensity, consequences and complications of perioperative psychiatric problems.

CHAPTER 6

Pediatric Anesthesia Equipment

While anesthetizing pediatric patients, certain physiological and anatomical differences between adults and children should be borne in mind. In neonates and small infants, the respiratory rate is high and the tidal volume is low. The dead space, both physiological and mechanical is usually high in proportion to tidal volume. Thus, the ventilation may easily become inadequate. These children need accurate flow rate of gases and avoidance of undue resistance to flow of gases. The alveolar ventilation in infants is also high, may be double that in adults on a body weight basis. The type of respiration in neonates is usually sinusoidal with no expiratory pause. The air passages of infants are usually narrow, so the lumen of the endotracheal tube automatically becomes small. Care should be taken against obstruction, kinking and compression. The narrowest part of the larynx in infants is at the cricoid ring and is circular in cross-section. The plain endotracheal tube is always preferred in the case of infants.

Considering all these factors, a scaled-down version of appropriate breathing circuit should be used in pediatric anesthesia. But the circuit should be simple, with minimum dead space and the resistance to laminar gas flow should be minimum. Turbulance of gas flow should be avoided as far as practicable. Rebreathing should be either nil or negligible. Adequate care should be taken to warm the inspired gases, ambient atmosphere and infusion solutions, particularly in cold air-conditioned operation theater for prevention of hypothermia. Dry gases may also cause heat loss. Prolonged anesthesia might require warming or humidification of the gases.

ANESTHETIC MACHINE

Pediatric patients can be satisfactorily anesthetized with any standard anesthetic machine. The Boyle anesthetic machine is the commonly used machine in India. It is a standard continuous flow type apparatus which provides the sources of oxygen, nitrous oxide and vapors of volatile anesthetic liquids. Intermittent flow type of anesthesia machine or draw-over machines are not suitable for children and these need too much inspiratory effort by the patient. There should be a pressure relief valve at the end of back bar which will open at a relatively low pressure of about 60 cm water pressure. Usually, the regulated pressure is about 60 lb/square inch. Vaporizers used for children should give an accurate percentage of vapor even at a low flow rate. Flow meter should have a full scale of low flow calibrations.

Pediatric anesthesia machines may be equipped with a flow meter and cylinder yoke for air. Providing the capability to dilute oxygen with air and thus nitrous oxide can be avoided in cases where it is contraindicated. An on-line oxygen analyzer is needed to quantitate the inspired oxygen concentration. In sophisticated machines, a pulse oximeter and a carbon dioxide analyzer should be provided for assessing ventilation in the cases of neonates, infants and children as these play a vital role in routine anesthetic management of pediatric patients.

BREATHING CIRCUITS

Magill Semiclosed System (Mapleson A System) (Fig. 6.1)

The standard Magill semiclosed system or Mapleson A system which is used in adult patients is quite satisfactory for spontaneously breathing children who weigh over 25 kg. Here the fresh gas flow should be at least equal to the patient's minute volume or somewhat higher. The standard adult size (2 liter) reservoir bag should be replaced by a smaller bag. But its capacity should be at least equal to the patient's tidal volume. The volume of the connecting hoses should also be modified. The standard expiratory valve may not be much efficient in the case of smaller children. It may be replaced by a Ruben nonrebreathing valve to change the system into a nonrebreathing attachment. This Magill attachment is not recommended for prolonged intermittent positive pressure ventilation. In such cases, a mechanical ventilator is better employed. This system should not be used in the case of smaller children weighing less than 25 kg when Mapleson E system is the circuit of choice.

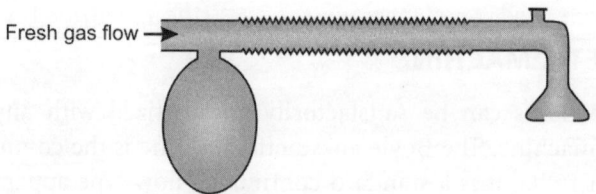

Fig. 6.1: Mapleson A system

Mapleson D System (Fig. 6.2)

The system consists of face mask or endotracheal tube, fresh gas inlet nearer the face mask, a corrugated rubber tubing one end of which is connected with the expiratory valve and then a reservoir bag connecting the valve. The system is mainly used in anesthesia with assisted or controlled ventilation, but can also be used in spontaneous ventilation. The Bain coaxial system is the most commonly used modification of the Mapleson D system where the inflow tube is housed conveniently inside the corrugated tube. During IPPV there is little chance of rebreathing in this Mapleson D system. Even in spontaneous breathing, rebreathing can be minimized by increasing the fresh gas flow to 2 to 3 times the minute volume of the patient.

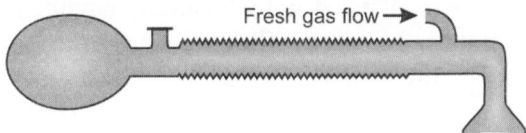

Fig. 6.2: Mapleson D system

The system may also be used even in the case of infants weighing 10 kg or less. The degree of rebreathing will depend on the volume of the expiratory limb, the fresh gas flow and the amount of tidal volume. However, greater fresh gas flow prevents rebreathing during spontaneous respiration. The system has a lower circuit volume; its compression and compliance losses are less and it provides rapid induction of anesthesia due to rapid transmission of inspired anesthetic concentration to the patient. The disadvantages of the system include the waste of anesthetic gases, unnecessary pollution of environment, loss of patient's heat and humidity to anesthetic gases and greater risk of anesthetic overdose.

Mapleson E System (Fig. 6.3)

The system is identical with the Ayre's T-piece anesthetic system. Here the fresh gas inlet is nearer the face mask or endotracheal tube. It is then connected with a corrugated tubing at the end of which no reservoir bag is attached. No expiratory value is incorporated in this system. The system is most popularly used in pediatric anesthesia. As the system has no expiratory

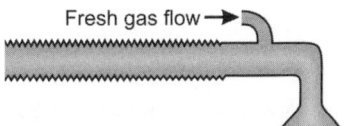

Fig. 6.3: Mapleson E system

valve, resistance to expiration is usually very low. To prevent rebreathing, the fresh gas flow should be 2.5 to 3 times the patient's respiratory minute volume.

Ayre's T-piece System (Figs 6.4 to 6.6)

It was introduced by Dr Philip Ayre in 1937. It is a small T-shaped metallic system comprising a straight tube with a side arm. The horizontal limbs are longer and of bigger diameter. One end of this limb is connected with the endotracheal tube and the other end with a short rubber tubing which acts as a reservoir. The vertical limb is connected with fresh gas supply from the anesthetic machine.

It is the most commonly used anesthetic breathing circuit for pediatric patients. This is flow-controlled nonrebreathing circuit. But rebreathing can occur, if it is not used correctly. The circuit has a single inspiratory and expiratory gas limb. The system relies on the pressure of the continuous incoming fresh gas flow to expel the expired gas to the open ended limb in the T-piece system.

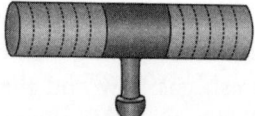

Fig. 6.4: Ayre's T-piece

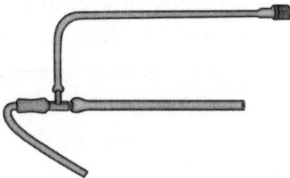

Fig. 6.5: Ayre's T-piece with its connections

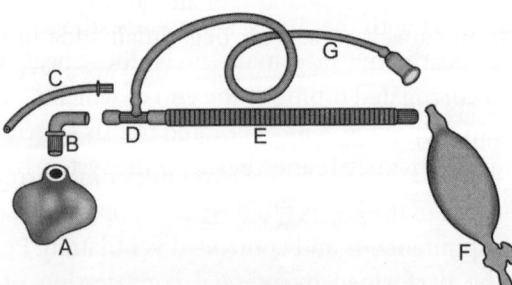

Fig. 6.6: Ree's modification of Arye's T-piece [A = Rendell-Baker-Soucek face mask, B = metal adaptor, C = endotracheal tube, D = T-piece, E = corrugated rubber tube, F = rat-tailed reservoir bag with stop-cock, G = fresh gas intel tube]

This system is mainly used for endotracheal anesthesia in neonates, infants and children and it offers the least resistance to respiration. The diameter of the T-piece should not be less than 10 mm. The system is light and can be satisfactorily used in all cases upto 25 kg body weight. To prevent rebreathing with spontaneous ventilation and to prevent air dilution of inspired gas, the flow rate of fresh gas should be in excess of 2.5 to 3 times the minute volume of the patient or at least 4 liters/minute. The volume of the reservoir tube should be at least one-third of the tidal volume of the patient. The internal diameter of the tube should be preferably 1 cm in the case of neonates and infants, and 1.25 cm the case of adults. One inch length of the 1 cm diameter tube contains nearly 2 ml of gas and in case of 1.25 cm tube about 3 ml. These measurements should be strictly followed, otherwise increased dead space will result. Too large a diameter may cause mixing of the fresh gas with alveolar gas and lead to inefficiency of the system.

In this system, rebreathing is nil or minimal as only fresh gas is inspired from the anesthetic machine and from the reservoir tubing as a little supplement during the time of peak inspiratory flow. Resistance to respiration is also low as the respiratory pathway is of wide bore. The disadvantages of the system include gas wastage and a small increase in resistance to outflow caused by turbulence at the T-piece.

The lungs may be ventilated by intermittent occlusion of the end of the expiratory tube with the thumb. However, the pressure generated in the circuit with this technique cannot be assessed. Excessive pressure may sometimes develop. A pressure limiting device may be incorporated in the system to obviate such a problem. Chest inflation by occluding the end of expiratory limb may be faulty and even cause pneumothorax. As it is very close to the patient, its use during head and neck surgery may cause problems.

Recently there have been various modifications of Ayre's T-piece; one modification uses a Y-piece and attaches an expiratory valve and an open ended 500 ml capacity reservoir bag. Small soda lime canisters (in miniaturized form with 85 g and 175 g capacities) are also used for efficient carbon dioxide absorption.

The most popular and widely used modification is that of Jackson Rees. It adds a double ended bag to the end of expiratory limb through corrugated tubing. The open end of the bag is fitted with an adjustable tap. The bag can be used for both spontaneous and controlled ventilation. Positive pressure ventilation can be performed by manual compression of the bag with simultaneous adjustment of the open end. The circuit seems to be the most efficient for pediatric anesthesia when the child is below 5 years of age or below 25 kg body weight. If the patient needs no endotracheal intubation, the T-piece can be used in conjunction with an angle mount and a face mask.

The circuit has several advantages over the Ayre's T-piece. Bag movements indicate the breathing of the child. It provides some continuous positive pressure or positive end-expiratory pressure instead of allowing the child to breathe out at atmospheric pressure. It can also provide a better assisted or controlled ventilation.

In the T-piece, the fresh gas inlet limb is usually at right angle to the body. But if it is at an angle facing towards the patient, there will be continuous positive pressure, causing some resistance during expiratory phase. On the other hand, if the angulation is directed towards the reservoir limb, a negative pressure may be caused by venturi effect.

If there is no expiratory limb in T-piece system, there will be no rebreathing. Air dilution is possible during spontaneous respiration, but can be pervented by increasing the fresh gas flow to 3 to 5 times the respiratory minute volume of the patient. However, in controlled ventilation, no air dilution is possible.

When the volume of the expiratory limb is greater than the tidal volume of the patient, there may be rebreathing in spontaneous ventilation, but it can be prevented by increasing the fresh gas flow to 2.5 to 3 times the minute volume. In controlled ventilation, by simply occluding the end of expiratory limb, there will be no rebreathing. Air dilution is usually absent here.

When the volume of expiratory limb is less than the tidal volume, limited rebreathing may occur in spontaneous ventilation. Rebreathing can be pervented by increasing the fresh gas flow to 2.5 to 3 times the minute volume. During controlled ventilation there is no rebreathing and no air dilution. However, air dilution is possible in spontaneous ventilation.

The dead space of the baby is equal to 2 ml/kg body weight. If it is multiplied by 3, it gives the tidal volume. The tidal volume multiplied by the respiratory rate gives the respiratory minute volume of the baby.

Mapleson F System (Fig. 6.7)

In Jackson Rees modification of T-peice system, an open-ended bag is attached to the expiratory tubing thereby converting the system to Mapleson D circuit. Now it is often designated as Mapleson F system. It has some advantages over the T-piece system as stated earlier. Bag movements give the visual impression of the patient's breathing. It provides some degree of continuous positive airway pressure and positive end expiratory pressure. It also provides efficient controlled ventilation by occluding the open end of the reservoir bag and squeezing the bag. The system is equally effective for both spontaneous and controlled ventilation. The system is very simple and offers least resistance as there is no valve in the system. The fresh gas flow should be at least 3 times the predicted minute volume of the patient. The internal volume of the tube between the patient and reservoir bag should exceed the patient's tidal volume; otherwise, reinhalation of the expired gases from the bag may occur. The system is near ideal for pediatric cases but can also be used in adult cases with controlled ventilation by a fresh gas flow ranging from 70 to 100 ml/minute/kg body weight.

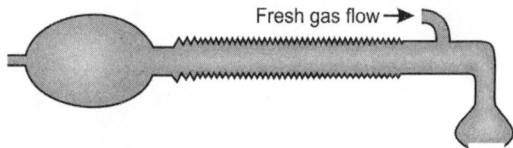

Fig. 6.7: Mapleson F system

Closed Systems

To-and-fro absorption system with Waters' canister can be used in the case of pediatric patients. But in such cases the canister should be of a small size and breathing tube should be of a small diameter. There are possibilities of increasing the dead space, particularly when the soda lime at the patient's end of canister is exhausted. It may increase the risk of inhalation of soda lime dust. The system is somewhat cumbersome as the absorber is placed close to patient's head. In the pediatric anesthetic set, there is provision of attachment of small soda lime canister in the circuit.

Adult circle absorbers can be satisfactorily used in the case of older children above 5 years of age or 20 kg body weight after scaling down the components of breathing system including the absorber and tubes. Light weight plastic tubing and components are often helpful.

PEDIATRIC ANESTHETIC SET (FIG. 6.8)

This set contains various endotracheal anesthetic equipment packed in a box and ready for use in pediatric anesthesia at any time and these include the following:
1. Small face mask for pediatric use.
2. Small (0.5 liter capacity) double ended reservoir bag with adjustable tap at one end.
3. Face mask adaptor.
4. Modified Ayre's T-piece, usually Y-shaped with one expiratory valve.
5. Reservoir adaptor.
6. Small corrugated tube connector.
7. Fresh gas supply tube with tubing mount which fits the anesthetic machine.

54 Fundamentals of Pediatric Anesthesia

8. Endotracheal connector with fresh gas feed inlet.
9. Soda lime canisters usually two in number and in small sizes.
10. Endotracheal tubes for pediatric use.
11. Endotracheal connections.

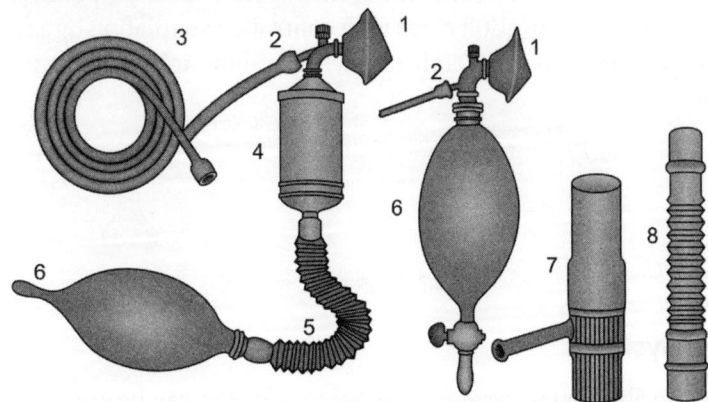

Fig. 6.8: Pediatric anesthetic set [1= Rendel-Baker Soucek face mask, 2 = modified Ayre's T-piece with expiratory valve, 3 = fresh gas inlet tubing with mount, 4 = soda lime canister, 5 = flexible rubber connector, 6 = rat tailed reservoir bag with stop-cock, 7 = endotracheal connector with gas feed inlet, 8 = flexible rubber connector]

All these components are needed for pediatric anesthesia either with semiopen technique or with to-and-fro carbon dioxide absorption technique.

BAIN CIRCUIT (FIG. 6.9)

It is a coaxial breathing attachment introduced by Bain and Spoerel in 1972. It is essentially a Mapleson D system except that fresh gas flow is carried by a tube within the corrugated hose. Its characteristics are mostly similar to those of Mapleson D system. It is used in adult cases but can be efficiently used in pediatric cases when the breathing tubes and the reservoir bags are scaled down. The conventional Bain system for adults can be used in the case of children with over 20 kg body weight.

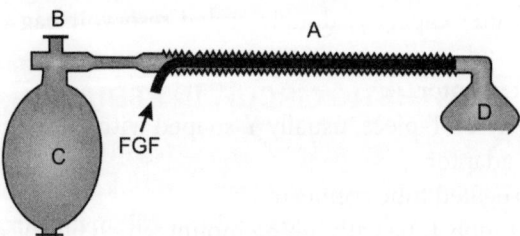

Fig. 6.9: Bain circuit

The Bain circuit consists of 1.8 meter long corrugated plastic tubing of 22 mm diameter. Through this tubing a narrow tube of roughly 7 mm outside diameter is incorporated and it delivers the fresh gas from the anesthetic machine to the patient's end of the circuit. In this system, the fresh gas flow is always through the inner tube and the patient breathes through the annular space or outer tube.

Expiratory gases enter the corrugated hose from the endotracheal tube and flow inside the outer hose and then mostly pass out through the expiratory valve. During inhalation, fresh gas from the inner tube is delivered directly to the patient. Some part of the gas in the corrugated hose near the patient's end is also mixed with fresh gas to go to the patient. For spontaneous ventilation, the fresh gas flow should be at least 2.5 times the respiratory volume; otherwise; significant rebreathing may occur. For an adult, it is roughly 15 liters/minute which is wasteful and uneconomical use of anesthetic gases and vapors. A fresh gas flow of 250 ml/kg/minute may be needed in some cases to prevent rebreathing.

If the fresh gas is allowed to flow directly into the cavity of mask without an angle piece, the dead space of the mask is greatly minimized. Thus, the system becomes more appropriate for use in young children compared to the standard Magill system.

The Bain circuit is simple, light weight and easy to handle. No carbon dioxide absorption is needed. Sterilization of the circuit is easy. Disposable tubing is also available. It causes minimum pull on the endotracheal tube and its attachments. It provides the escape of exhaled gases from the machine end, far away from the operative field and thus reduces the fire hazards. Moreover, the circuit is mostly safe and reliable. It can be used in anesthesia both with controlled and spontaneous ventilation. The circuit may be used both in the case of children and adults, thus, the system may be considered as the universal circuit.

Bain circuit has also got some disadvantages, There may be accidental disconnections and leak of the inner tube at the machine end. A too long inner tube may become occluded by twisting. A transparent outer hose helps to check the inner tube for kinking, wrong connections of the fresh gas hose or any disconnections. For the Bain circuit, a continuous and adequate fresh gas flow must always be provided.

CHOICE OF ANESTHETIC CIRCUIT IN PEDIATRIC ANESTHESIA

1. For children below the age of 5 years or 25 kg body weight, Jackson Rees modification of Ayre's T-piece is the anesthetic circuit of choice.
2. For children above the age of 5 years or 25 kg body weight, adult an-

esthetic circuits may be used with sensible precautions. For controlled ventilation, either the circle or a to-and-fro system with absorber or a ventilator may be used. Bain circuit may also be used confidently.

COMPONENTS OF THE BREATHING ATTACHMENTS

Reservoir Bags (Fig. 6.10)

Reservoir or rebreathing bags should be small in size (0.5 or 1 liter. capacity). The capacity of the bag should never be less than the tidal volume of the patient. The wall of the bag should not be very stiff. It should be soft to allow or maintain a low expiratory pressure. Movements of small bags can be easily observed. Larger bags can be used by hanging the loop of the lower end on a hook and thereby reducing the volume. Capacity may also be reduced by tying the bag around with a string. It should be made of antistatic rubber. A new bag should be cleaned and washed before use otherwise powdered particles may enter the patient's airway.

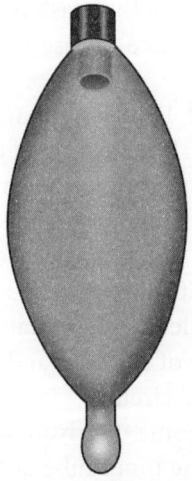

Fig. 6.10: Reservoir bag

A rat-tailed rebreathing bag is used in Jackson Rees modification of Ayre's system of anesthesia. The rat tail may be cut open so that rebreathing becomes minimum as the gas partly escapes to the atmosphere. The open end may have a stop-cock which can be closed or opened according to the need.

Corrugated Rubber Tube

The standard corrugated tube can be used in the case of older children, but it should be scaled down for infants. The tube may also be made of plastic or polyethylene and also be in smooth form. Plastic tubes are light weight and mostly transparent. The tube of smaller diameter is used in pediatrics. These plastic hoses should not be allowed to twist along their long axis; otherwise, resistance will occur.

Expiratory Valves (Fig. 6.11)

The standard Heidbrink valve may offer high resistance for children. Resistance can be reduced by inserting a safety pin inside the valve below the spring or by removing the spring, but this may cause profuse leakage of gases. The fresh gas flow should be high in such cases. A smaller and lighter valve is recommended for pediatric use. The expiratory valve may be replaced by a nonrebreathing Ruben or Ambu E valve.

Face Mask (Figs 6.12 and 6.13)

The ideal pediatric face mask should fit the nose, cheeks and chin for an air-tight seal. It should have low dead space. It should accommodate an oropharyngeal or nasopharyngeal airway during spontaneous or controlled ventilation. It should be made antistatic and nonirritating. It should also be transparent for easy detection of cyanosis or oral secretions or vomitus. The

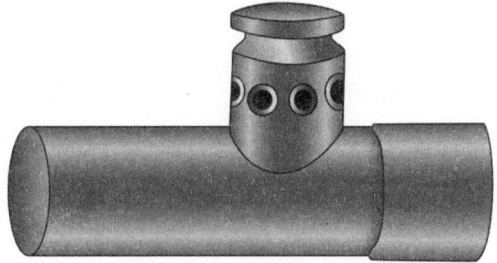

Fig. 6.11: Heidbrink expiratory valve

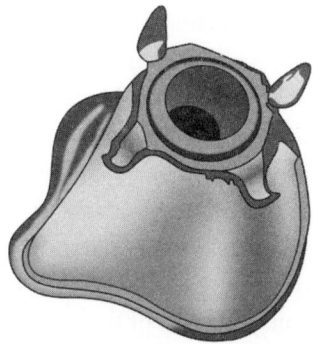

Fig. 6.12: Rendell-Baker-Soucek face mask

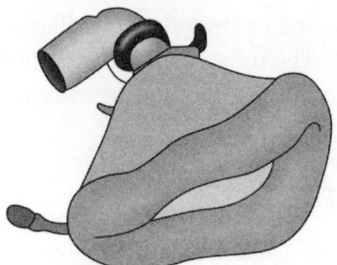

Fig. 6.13: Face mask

pediatric size standard BOC cushioned mask and Rendell-Baker-Soucek mask are in common use.

Pediatric face masks are small face masks with inflatable face pads. These are available in various sizes starting from 0 size. But it has significantly large dead space. Selection of an appropriate face mask is important.

For children under one year of age, a special type of face mask is used. The Rendell-Baker-Soucek face mask is the most popular. It is usually made of rubber or clear plastic. The body is not malleable. It is usually available in 3 different sizes. It has minimum dead space of about 4 ml in size 1 and 8 ml in size 2 when employed with a divided mask adaptor. It adequately fits the contours of the child's face and no special cushioned seal is provided. During positive pressure, ventilation leaks across the bridge of nose or the cleft of the chin can easily occur, if the anesthetist is inattentive.

One should be careful when holding the mask on the face of neonates and infants, so as to avoid digital pressure in the region of the submental triangle; otherwise, it could push the tongue upto the roof of the mouth and cause or aggravate airway obstruction.

Endotracheal Tubes (Figs 6.14A and B)

These tubes should be selected very carefully; otherwise, both the technique of intubation and the tube itself can create hazards. These tubes should be chemically nonirritant to respiratory tract mucosa and should not kink under normal conditions. The tubes can be easily autoclaved. It is better to use sterile disposable endotracheal tubes. All sizes ranging from 2.5 mm (internal diameter) upwards should be available. Endotracheal tubes made of red rubber, portex, latex or plastic PVC are satisfactory for routine use. But red rubber tubes may cause some irritation to the tracheal mucosa. Endotracheal tubes for use in the case of children should never be sterilized in liquid antiseptic solutions as traces of the solution may cause significant irritation of tracheal mucosa in children.

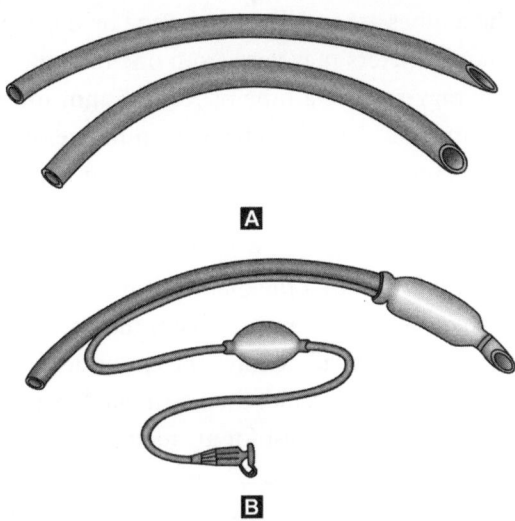

Figs 6.14 A and B: A. Endotracheal tubes (plain); B. Cuffed endotracheal tube

Endotracheal tubes are tested by manufacturers for tissue toxicity either by implant testing or by an in vitro implant testing method. If implant tested, it bears the letters 'IT' and if tested by an in vitro method it bears the marking "Z-79" (a committee of the American National Standard Institute) on the endotracheal tube.

An endotracheal tube is calibrated according to its internal diameter in mm, external diameter in mm and length in cm. It is usually beveled $38 \pm 8°$ off to the left when the tube is held curved up. It helps easy insertion through the vocal cord by a right-handed anesthetist. Endotracheal tube may have a side port or *Murphy* eye near its tip and this may allow ventilation even when the main port is obstructed by tracheal wall, secretions or blood clot.

Plain uncuffed endotracheal tubes should be used for all children below the age of 8 years. Cuffed tubes may cause significant compression of the tracheal mucosa. Endotracheal tubes may be lubricated with sterile water-soluble jelly. Introducers or stylets may cause damage to the airway and actually these are not considered necessary to use in pediatric cases.

The narrowest part of the infant larynx is the cricoid ring. Following endotracheal intubation, a small leak should be heard. If the tube is too tight, it may cause pressure over the mucosa causing edema followed by fibrosis and stenosis. It is said that 1 mm of edema at subglottic level may cause reduction of airway by 60% and thus markedly increase the work of breathing.

The size of the endotracheal tube must always be selected to ensure that a little leak is present. It should be changed down a size if there is no leak. Endotracheal tubes are usually categorized by their internal diameter but their external diameters may vary from one manufacturer to another. A newborn baby may require a tube of 3 to 3.5 mm internal diameter, a premature infant may need even a tube of 2.5 mm size (internal diameter). At 6 months of age, tubes of 4 mm size and at 1 year of age 4.5 mm size are usually needed. For children above 1 year of age, a safe guideline may be accepted as: age in years divided by 4 plus 4.5 equals the internal diameter of the tube in mm. It is said that the diameter of a child's little finger is the same as that of the trachea, but in practice it may not be a much reliable guide. However, it is always safe to have the endotracheal tubes at hand at least one-half size larger and smaller than estimated to allow for individual variability. The most important test for an adequate sized plain tube is the presence of a leak between 20 and 25 cm water peak inflation pressure. This leak can be easily assumed by closing the expiratory valve and then slowly increasing the pressure by gently squeezing the reservoir bag while listening to the sound of air leak over the mouth or larynx with a lightly placed stethoscope. Ischemia of the tracheal mucosa may occur when the pressure from a large-sized endotracheal tube exceeds the capillary pressure of tracheal mucosa. It is about 25 to 35 mmHg in case of adults. Thus, it is recommended that in the case of children the largest possible tube should be intubated that still provides a leak at peak manual ventilation. However, it should also be remembered that decrease in the internal diameter of the endotracheal tube causes increased resistance to breathing and increased work of breathing. Moreover, a small bore endotracheal tube is much prone to occlusion by secretions or blood clot.

The mouth should be packed lightly with sterile roller gauze, preferably soaked with liquid paraffin. This may help stabilization of the tube and absorption of excessive secretions. Neonates, of course, better tolerate a gas tight endotracheal intubation and subglottic complications are not so common in neonates.

The length of the endotracheal tube should also be carefully judged as the length of infant trachea is small and one lung anesthesia may be dangerous for them. The length may be calculated as the age in years divided by 2 plus 12 cm for oral tube and plus 15 cm for nasal tube. The tube should pass 2.5 cm past the vocal cords. It is most important to check that air enters both lungs. Ideally, the tip of the endotracheal tube should lie midway between the cricoid region and the carina.

Various special types of endotracheal tubes are used. Latex, nylon-coil-reinforced, armored tubes are also used.

Polyvinyl chloride (PVC) Magill tubes

These are the most commonly used endotracheal tubes in pediatric anesthesia. These are mostly single use tubes. Originally, these were used only for long-term ventilation. These are nonirritant to tracheal mucosa. These PVC tubes are difficult to see on X-ray films, so a radiopaque line is often incorporated into the walls of the tubes. In cuffed PVC endotracheal tube, the cuff is usually of the high volume low pressure type to minimize tracheal ischemic injury.

RAE Tubes (Figs 6.15A and B)

These are named after their inventors Drs Ring, Adair and Elwyn. The RAE tube is a preformed disposable PVC tube with a bend at the mouth to prevent kinking and a connector at chin level to allow good access for surgery on head and neck. It is available in both oral and nasal versions in different sizes. The length must be checked carefully after its insertion. It may be confmned by X-ray films. The tip of the RAE tube provides two Murphy eyes to provide ventilation even if the tube is advanced too far in one bronchus.

Armored Endotracheal Tubes (Fig. 6. 16)

Latex and silicone reinforced tubers are incompressible and unkinkable. These have the advantage of resistance to collapse or kinking. The tube is floppy, so, stylet is often needed for intubation. As the tube cannot be cut, the position must be checked very carefully after its insertion. It can be used orally, nasally and even through a tracheostomy stoma. A bevel or Murphy eye may not be incorporated in certain designs of the tube. It is usually cuffed but noncuffed types are also available. It is also useful when access is required to the head and neck. These tubes may present some problems

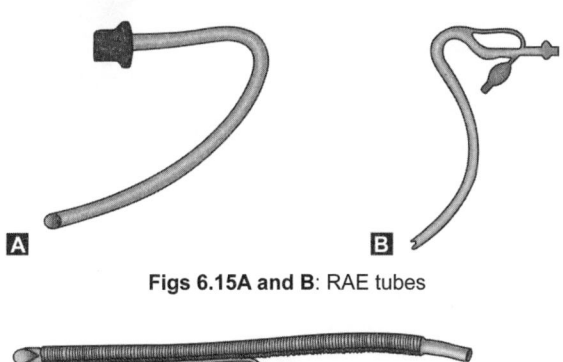

Figs 6.15A and B: RAE tubes

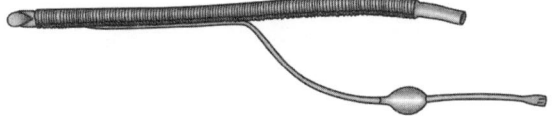

Fig. 6.16: Armored endotracheal tube

such as lumen obstruction difficulty in inflating and deflating, etc. Repeated boiling or autoclaving will soften the spiral and thus collapsing may occur. It may be difficult to pass a, small bore suction catheter down an armored tube due to its corrugations in the inner wall. However, lubricating and rotating the catheter while advancing usually overcomes the problem. These tubes are useful in cases where acute flexion of the neck is expected.

Oxford nonkinking endotracheal tube (Fig. 6. 17)

It is made of red rubber and molded to form a 90° bend inside the mouth. It is meant for orotracheal intubation. The proximal part is thicker to prevent kinking at the junction of endotracheal connection. It may be either cuffed or plain. A special introducer is needed at the time of its use. The tube is useful when the patient is prone or sitting position. But the tube is long and may enter the bronchus. So its position should be carefully checked after its use. This tube is sometimes used for anesthesia for cleft palate surgery.

Cole Tube (Fig. 6. 18)

It is meant for pediatric patients. It is stiff compared with the standard PVC tube. It is used for orotracheal intubation only and not for nasotracheal intubation. The proximal or patient end is of small bore for a length of 2.5 to 4.5 cm. This narrow part is meant for the part from the vocal cord to trachea. The machine end is larger and has a wide bore. Various sizes are available according to the internal diameter of intratracheal part. Cole tube is said to cause less resistance and there is less likelihood of endobronchial

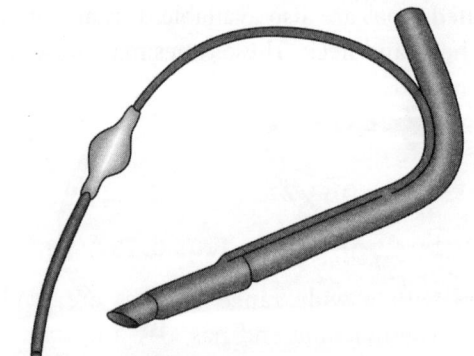

Fig. 6.17: Oxford nonkinking endotracheal tube

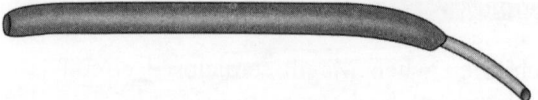

Fig. 6.18: Cole tube

intubation. But it has certain disadvantages. The shouldered part of the tube can cause laryngeal damage. There may be some turbulence through the tube because the narrowing increases the resistance and the work of breathing. The incidence of tube occlusion is high as the narrowed diameter of the tapered tip can make suctioning difficult.

Microlaryngeal tracheal tube

It is specially meant for anesthesia in microlaryngeal surgery. It is available in sizes of 4 mm, 5 mm and 6 mm internal diameter, but the length and cuff size remain the same as those of a standard adult size endotracheal tube. The small internal diameter helps better visualization of the larynx and the large cuff maintains a firm air-tight seal. It is mostly used for adolescents and adults and has little applicability in the case of younger children.

Laser endotracheal tube

An ordinary standard PVC endotracheal tube is not suitable for use in laser surgery. It is prone to ignition due to high energy of laser and high oxygen concentration in anesthesia. Noxious byproducts are also released. Rubber tubes are also prone to ignition but less toxic products are released. Wrapping rubber tubes with metallic tape may help in reducing the danger of ignition. Laser guard endotracheal tubing protector may be used as it is effective against penetration by lasers. It is actually an adhesive laminate of silver foil and sponge material to be wrapped around the PVC or rubber tube. Silicon, which is relatively laser resistant, is impregnated in some laser shield tubes and these can be used in laser surgery. Malleable metal tubes are also used as metal is impervious to laser radiation and its shiny surface reflects laser energy. But these rigid tubes should be intubated very carefully. Cuffs of the laser tubes are also prone to puncture by laser beam. Cuffs should be inflated with saline just to seal the leak. But overinflation with saline can increase the tracheal mucosal pressure and thus cause tracheal ischemic injury. Flexible stainless steel tube is also used. It has a soft silicone tip and provides two cuffs, each with a separate pilot for better safety.

Endotracheal Tube Connectors (Figs 6.19A and B to 6.21)

Plastic connectors with a wide range of sizes are available to fit any endotracheal tube. The machine end has a 15 mm male taper to fit the standard breathing components. A catheter mount is not needed. The connectors should have low resistance. Any curve should be smooth and abrupt angulation is avoided. The internal diameter should not be less than that of the tube.

In older children when Magill semiclosed circuit is used, the conventional metal endotracheal connections can be used. Various sizes are available even for pediatric use. Correct size should be chosen so as to get the wide lumen of the endotracheal tube at the connecting end and snug fitting. The connected ends should be leak-proof, cause minimum reduction of lumen and never be dislodged or disconnected easily. Alcohol is sometimes used on a connector to facilitate insertion of the tube and to make a good union with the tube. Connections may increase the mechanical dead space and it may be significantly excessive for neonates and infants. Magill connections are commonly used.

Magill connections

These are curved connections, one end of which is serrated for the endotracheal tube and the other is meant for connection with the catheter mount. Two types are available, one for oral use and the other for nasal use. Nasal connections have a sharp curve while oral connections are a little longer and more gently curved. Different sizes are also available. Magill connection for pediatric use is also popular.

Rowbatham connections

These are plain right-angled connection. The tapered and serrated end is for the endotracheal tube and the wider end is for connection with the catheter mount. It may cause more resistance to the gas flow due to turbulent gas flow.

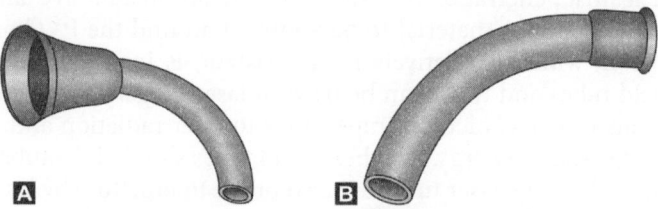

Figs 6.19A and B: Magill connection [A = oral, B = nasal]

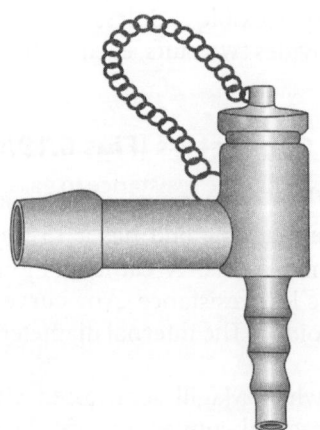

Fig. 6.20: Cobb suction union

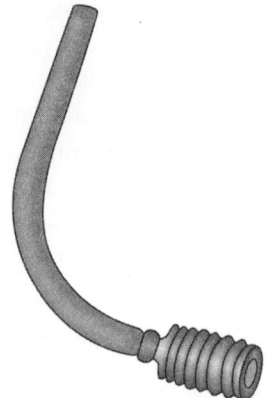

Fig. 6.21: Worcestor connection

Cobb and Magill suction unions

Cobb suction union is a right-angled connection with a removable metal cap in its short projection. Magill suction union is also right-angled but with rubber plug in its short projection. These unions allow endotracheal suction by inserting a suction catheter into the lumen of endotracheal tube.

Worcestor orotracheal connection

This metal connection is longer, particularly at the oral end. It takes a much shortened oral tube and thus it provides a firm basis for Boyle Davis gag for tonsillectomy. The chance of the tube being pressed by the gag is minimal. However, the tube may still kink at the tip of the connection. It is also used in anesthesia for repair of cleft palate.

Catheter mount (Fig. 6.22)

It is made of metal tube and its one end provides a small rubber tube. Its machine end is metallic and it is connected with an expiratory valve. The patient end is connected with the endotracheal tube via a rubber tube. The catheter mount adapts the endotracheal tube with the breathing attachments. It is of standard size with 15 mm male taper to fit the distal end of expiratory valve. The internal diameter of the nozzle of the catheter mount should be wide so that the resistance to gas flow will be less. Recently, plastic catheter mounts have also become available. These are light weight and can be used with full satisfaction.

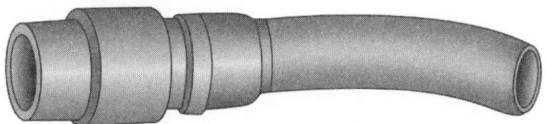

Fig. 6.22: Catheter mount

Laryngoscopes

The anatomy of the neonates and infants requires a different design of laryngoscope. It should have preferably a straight blade to visualize the high anterior larynx and to lift the floppy epiglottis. The design of the blade should be such as to prevent obstruction caused by the large bulky tongue. It should be small, light weight and easy to handle. In pediatric anesthesia, commonly two types of laryngoscope blades are used, one is curved or Macintosh type and the other is straight or Magill type. All other blades are mostly variations on these. The choice of blade is a personal one.

Magill laryngoscope (Figs 6.23 and 6.24)

It consists of a straight metal blade attached to a metal handle. The blade is curved like a half cylinder but flattened at the distal end where there is a bulb for illumination. The tip of the blade lifts the epiglottis forward from behind to expose the laryngeal opening. It relies on direct upward pressure on the epiglottis for vocal cord visualization. It is most commonly used in pediatric cases.

Macintosh laryngoscope (Figs 6.25 and 6.26)

It has a curved blade, flat on one side and ridged on the other side. The blade is inserted into the vallecula anterior to the epiglottis and relies on indirect vallecular traction to lift the epiglottis out of the way. The concavity of the blade fits the tongue. Ordinarily, it is inserted into right side of the patient's

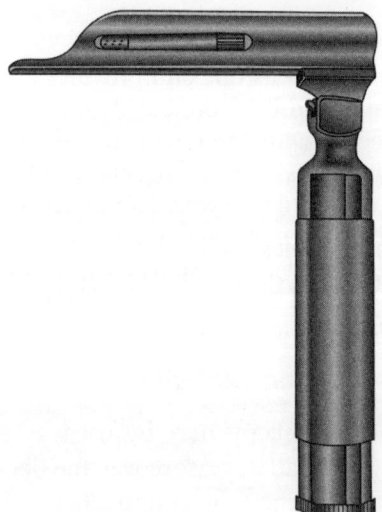

Fig. 6.23: Magill laryngoscope

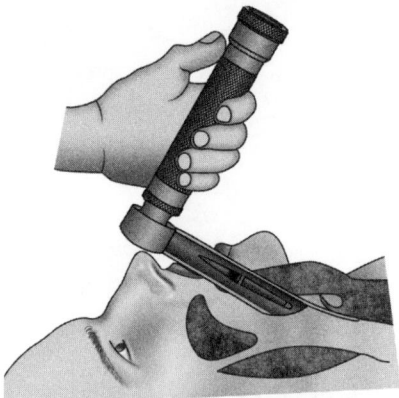

Fig. 6.24: Magill laryngoscope in use

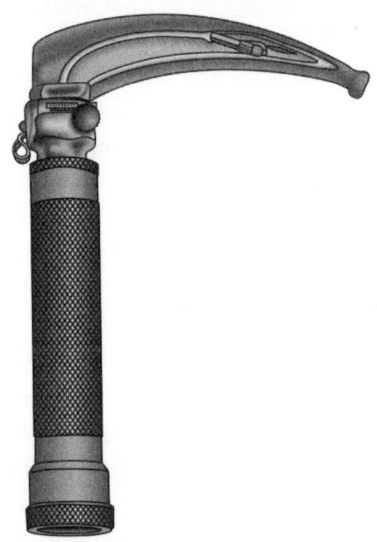

Fig. 6.25: Macintosh laryngoscope

mouth, moving the tongue to the left. However, a blade for the left side is also available for use by left-handed anesthetists. It has got infant, child, medium, adult and large adult sized blades. The blades are interchangeable. Over the age of about 2 years the standard Macintosh curved laryngoscope is mostly satisfactory.

Fiberoptic laryngoscopy and intubation

Flexible fiberoptic bronchoscopy may be used as it permits clear and detailed visualization of the airway. Moreover, the fiberoptic bronchoscope can act as a conduit over which the endotracheal tube can be passed for intubation. This is most sutiable in cases with difficult intubation.

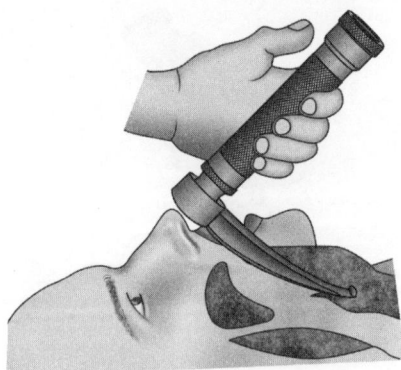

Fig. 6.26: Macintosh laryngoscope in use

The fiberoptic bronchoscope has a light source, a flexible elongated insertion cord and a handle with controls. The child should be premedicated with 0.01 mg/kg glycopyrrolate IV to reduce the secretions. 4% cocaine may be needed to shrink the nasal mucosa. The child should be anesthetized with nitrous oxide, oxygen, and halothane sequence under the face mask. The fiberoptic bronchoscopy should be done followed by endotracheal intubation. The technique needs learned skill and hence requires practice. Moreover, the fiberoptic bronchoscope is an expensive precision instrument and thus needs extra care to handle.

Bullard laryngoscope

It contains a fiberoptic channel which helps to visualize the laryngeal inlet directly. Both infant and adult versions are available. Here the laryngoscopic blade is allowed to slide around the tongue by rotating the handle from the horizontal to the vertical position. Then the blade is elevated against the dorsal surface of the tongue to visualize the glottic opening.

AIRWAYS

Airways are usually curved tubes made of metal or red rubber. When inserted into the mouth, the airways slides over the tongue reaching its proximal end upto the pharynx. Thus, it prevents the tongue falling back against posterior pharyngeal wall and thus provides a reliable clear pharyngeal air passage. There are mainly two types of airways, oropharyngeal and nasopharyngeal.

Oropharyngeal Airway (Figs 6.27 to 6.29)

These are usually made of metal, red rubber or plastic of different types, *Philips airway* (Fig. 6.27) is popularly used. This is a rounded rubber tube with a metal mount flattened on cross section. *Waters' airway* (Fig. 6.28) is made of metal and has two holes in the sides near the pharyngeal end and right or left nipple for attachment of an oxygen catheter or suction line. *Guedal type* (Fig. 6.29) is another standard pharyngeal airway and widely used. It has a central lumen for gas exchange and suctioning. *Connel's airway* is similar to Guedel airway, but it is made of metal and there are holes in the sides near the pharyngeal end. Size of the airway depends on the size of the patient, and various sizes of each type of airway are available.

An airway must be of correct size; otherwise, too small or too large size can aggravate airway obstruction. A too large oral airway may push the epiglottis down into the glottic opening and even precipitate laryngospasm during light anesthesia. It may also protrude from the mouth, making it difficult to fit mask or even impossible. A too small airway may kink the tongne and displace it posteriorly and thus exacerbate airway obstruction. The correct size of the airway can be judged by holding it next to the patient's face. The tip of airway should be just besides the angle of the patient's mandible while the flange should be at the level of lips. However, the position of the airway after its insertion is best determined by getting a free unobstructed breathing.

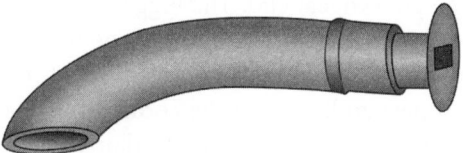

Fig. 6.27: Philips airway

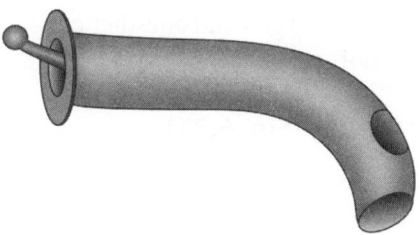

Fig. 6.28: Waters airway

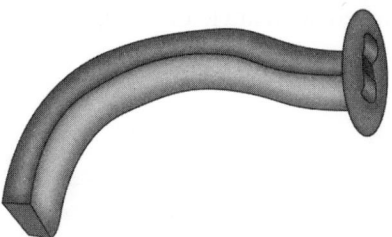

Fig. 6.29: Guedel airway

Nasopharyngeal Airway (Fig. 6.30)

It is used to provide a conduit for gas flow between the tongue and the posterior pharyngeal wall. It is made of soft rubber or PVC. It mostly indicated when the patient is not able to open his mouth or when oropharyngeal airway becomes ineffective. It is better tolerated for prolonged periods and aids nasopharyngeal suction.

The tube extends from the nose upto the pharynx just above the epiglottis and below the base of the tongue. The proper length can be estimated by measuring the distance from the tragus of the ear to the tip of nose and one inch more. It is roughly 30 cm in adults. Magill endotracheal tube of such length may be used satisfactorily as nasopharyngeal airway. However, nasopharyngeal airway is available in sizes 12 to 36 French. A 12 French size is usually meant for full term infant.

Different varieties of nasopharyngeal airway are available. *Bardex airway*, made of soft neoprane rubber, has a large flange at the nasal end and a bevel at the pharyngeal end. *Rusch airway*, made of soft red rubber, has a bevel at pharyngeal end and a firm adjustable flange at the nasal end. *Saklad plastic airway* has a small flange at nasal end with two holes, one on either side near the pharyngeal end. The bigger one faces the midline and acts as a suction catheter and the other, small one is for air passage.

The lubricated tube should be inserted carefully through a nostril in a posterior direction perpendicular to the coronal plane and passed gently along the floor of nasopharynx. It may cause damage to the adenoid tissue and mucosa causing epistaxis or even laryngospasm. The small bore tube may become easily obstructed by mucus, blood or adenoid tissue. It makes possible the insufflation of oxygen and anesthetic gases to a spontaneously breathing patient for short procedures.

Laryngeal Mask Airway (Fig. 6.31)

The laryngeal mask airway was introduced by Brain in 1983 as an alternative to conventional mask anesthesia. Its use in pediatric anesthesia seems to be much advantageous, particularly when intubation presents considerable difficulty. It is essentially a wide-bore endotracheal tube with an oval cushioned mask attached at an angle to the tip. It is to be placed blindly in

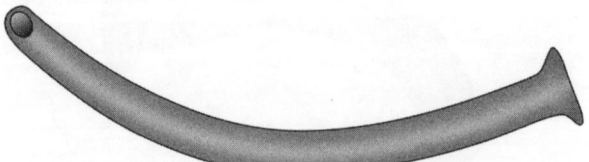

Fig. 6.30: Nasopharyngeal airway

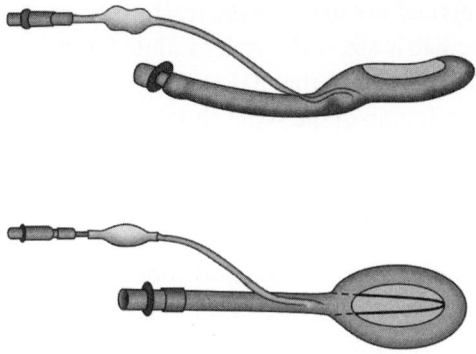

Fig. 6.31: Laryngeal mask airway

such a way that the masked tip is kept over the epiglottis and laryngeal inlet to provide a seal around the supraglottic area.

The child should be anesthetized with nitrous oxide, oxygen and halothane through face mask. Then the mouth should be propped open after extending the head. Then the laryngeal mask airway tube is inserted blindly into pharynx until some resistance is obtained. Then the cuff is inflated and the laryngeal mask airway is observed to ride up slightly. It is then attached to the anesthetic circuit. The proper placement is judged by several smooth unobstructed breaths.

It may be advantageous while holding the face mask for a prolonged period and in case of difficult airways when a conventional oral airway fails to provide adequate gas exchange. But it is only an alternative method of airway management and is not a substitute for endotracheal intubation. It should be borne in mind that it does not protect the airway from pulmonary aspiration and thus needs sensible precautions.

Stylet (Fig. 6.32)

It is an elongated, plastic coated metal rod which fits inside an endotracheal tube. It helps to make the tube more rigid and permits bending (due to its malleability) to facilitate endotracheal placement. It should always be available particularly during difficult intubation. Care should be taken not

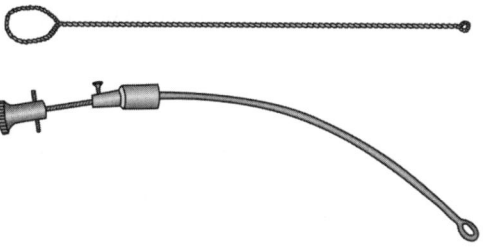

Fig. 6.32: Stylet

to damage the cuffs and not to injure the tracheal mucosa. It is available in a wide variety of pediatric sizes. The stylet should have locking arrangement to fix it at a particular point so that it does not protrude beyond the bevel of endotracheal tube. The tip of the stylet should always be blunt and smooth to reduce the risk of trauma.

Lighted stylet

It is useful for guiding the endotracheal tube into the laryngeal inlet by transillumination. It may be further advantageous in case of a transparent plastic tube.

It is a reusable malleable stylet with a small, battery powered light at its tip. The bulb is highly bonded to the stylet to avoid its breaking off or dislodgement. The smallest endotracheal tube that can be threaded over the stylet has an internal diameter of only 5.5 mm. So its use is much limited to smaller children.

Suction Equipment and Catheter

In pediatric patient care, a relatively low-power vacuum should be used. High pressure vacuum may cause pulmonary atelectasis and damage to the respiratory tract mucosa of neonates, infants and children. A very narrow catheter should also be used for suction. A tight fitting catheter in endotracheal tube may cause significant hypoxia during its use. Some catheters are so designed that by providing its side holes, the tip of catheter remains in the midcavity and does not much contact the tracheal wall. Recommended pediatric endotracheal tubes and sizes of suction catheters are as follows: for premature infant 2.5 to 3 mm endotracheal tube, suction catheter size 5 French; for neonate 3 to 3.5 mm tube and suction catheter size 6 French; for child upto 1 year 3.5 to 4.5 mm tube and catheter 8 French; for child 1 to 2 year. 4 to 4.5 mm tube and catheter 8 French; for child 2 to 6 year. 4.5 mm tube and catheter size 10 French.

ENDOBRONCHIAL ANESTHESIA IN CHILDREN

One-lung anesthesia may sometimes be needed in the case of small infants, particularly with a lung cyst or lober emphysema presented for surgery. During intermittent positive pressure ventilation in such cases the cyst may be preferentially ventilated leading to undue distension and even rupture. The use of a bronchus blocker is technically difficult in these cases, but no doubt, it can efficiently solve the problem. Some anesthetists advocate the use of a plain and soft endotracheal tube for endobronchial intubation, but in such cases the tube should be 1 cm longer than the distance from mouth to carina and the size should be one size smaller than the usual size for the patient. The tube is introduced upto the main stem bronchus and then rotated through 180° to ensure that the orifice does not face the bronchial wall. If the bevel of the tube faces the left, it will be used for left endobronchial intubation and if it faces to right side, it will be meant for right endobronchial intubation.

Bronchoscopy in Children

The problems of anesthesia for bronchoscopy in children are somewhat lessened by the introduction of ventilating bronchoscopes or open bronchoscope with venturi ventilating attachments. A range of bronchoscopes suitable for use in pediatric cases including neonates, infants and children in conjunction with a fiber light source are available. A telescopic attachment, if present, may be much helpful. Each bronchoscope should be fitted with an injector system so that it may be safely used as a ventilating bronchoscope. The injectors meant for pediatric bronchoscopes can safely operate from oxygen pipeline at 60 lb/square inch and are based on 19 s.w.g. injector needles. Nitrous oxide, oxygen blenders can be used in conjunction with a side arm ventilating bronchoscope. Fiberoptic systems are particularly useful when intubation is difficult.

Lung Ventilators

Manual ventilation is largely recommended for most major procedures in pediatric cases and particularly in neonatal anesthesia. For the pediatric patients whose body weight is above 25 kg, a ventilator designed primarily for adult cases, such as Manley, Bird or Blease can be used satisfactorily with some pediatric anesthesia attachments. For neonates, infants and children below 25 kg body weight, specially designed ventilators are needed to produce satisfactory function.

When an adult volume ventilator is being used in the case of pediatric patients, some adjustments should be made to respiratory rate, fresh gas flow, tidal volume and inspired/expired ratio. The pop off valve also needs readjustment for peak inflation pressure. This will convert a volume ventilator to a pressure ventilator. If the pop off valve is not provided in the machine or does not allow any readjustment, the machine should better not be used for small children.

A specially designed pediatric ventilator should have the following capacities:
1. It must enable tidal volumes as small as 10 ml to be delivered.
2. It should provide respiratory rates between 35 and 60 cycles/minute.

3. It must be possible to adjust the inspiratory flow rate within a wide range so that low, mean and peak flow rates can be employed in neonates and small infants.
4. Accurate control of inspired oxygen should be possible. Hazards of oxygen therapy should be borne in mind.
5. It should be possible to employ accurate inspiratory/expiratory ratio.
6. Apparatus should also be capable of delivering gas at high peak pressures, whenever needed clinically. It should have adjustable overpressure valve in the patient circuit.
7. It should have light weight tubing.
8. It should have provision of humidification.
9. It should be provided with reliable alarms for the detection of failures of gas supply, power supply and electronic circuitry.
10. It should incorporate facilities for easy, rapid change over to manual methods so that in adverse situations the child can be ventilated manually at any time.
11. It should have special provisions for intermittent mandatory ventilation (IMV), positive end expiratory pressure (PEEP) and continuous positive airway pressure (CPAP). PEEP may sometimes be needed to prevent airway closure within the normal range of tidal volume. In small infants and children, the closing volume is usually greater than the functional residual capacity of the child. PEEP of 5 cm water pressure is usual. CPAP may be needed to give respiratory support when the child is breathing spontaneously or with intermittent positive pressure ventilation and during weaning.

In recent times, numerous designs of ventilators for pediatric use have became commercially available. One should have a clear understanding of the particular instrument and its clinical implications for using a particular specialized ventilator. The choice of ventilators for pediatric use must be made with adequate skill and care but much depends on personal preference. Typical infant parameters to set ventilator for prolonged intermittent positive pressure ventilation are as follows:

Inspiratory/expiratory ratio is 1 : 1 or 1 : 2.
Respiratory rate is 25 to 50/minute.
Maximum pressure is 30 to 35 cm water pressure.
PEEP is 0 to 5 cm water pressure.
Minute volume 100 to 200 ml/kg body weight.

Sometimes aT-piece occluder is employed in the circuit to provide a satisfactory means of IPPV during pediatric anesthesia. Here in the expiratory limb of the T-piece system a solenoid operated valve is incorporated to provide mechanical occlusion. An electrically operated timing circuit controls the duration of inspiratory flow by opening and closing the solenoid valve. This along with the amount of fresh gas flow from the anesthetic machine determines the tidal volume delivered to the child. At the time of manual ventilation, the solenoid valve should be replaced by an open ended reservoir bag at the end of the expiratory limb. Though the system is very simple and cheap, it is of limited value for use in case of the small infants. These patients need very low flow rates and at such low flow rates most vaporizers are inefficient or inaccurate. On the other hand, the addition of a bag to the expiratory limb allows a much higher inspiratory flow rate with manually controlled ventilation.

Intravenous Needles and Catheters

A wide range of disposable intravenous needles of guaranteed sterility are available. They should have a short bevel and a half inch shaft. They should be trauma-free as far as practicable. A 27 s.w.g. needle is good for fine veins and a 25 s. w.g. needle is mostly used for large veins of the child. Clear needle hubs are desirable for early detection of blood. Needles with a relatively long shaft may be used in older children.

The syringes should be of small capacity preferably with 0.1 ml calibration for accurate measurement of small doses of drugs. Diluted drugs may be administered with a standard 2 ml syringe with 0.2 ml calibrations.

Butterfly (with wings) designed scalp vein needles are popular as these can be inserted into scalp or peripheral veins, and their plastic flanges help to fix them securely in place.

Intravenous catheters are now widely used. Here a flexible catheter is percutaneously introduced into the vein through the needle. After the cannulation the needle is withdrawn. The nonirritant teflon catheters allow them to be curved through a sharp angle and permit them to slide through the skin easily. It is very helpful for long-term use. Disposable three-way-taps should be included in the IV line so that intermittent injections or rapid infusions are possible.

However, complications of pediatric intravenous therapy may include phlebitis, skin slough, septicemia, local abscess, local cellulitis and so on.

Infusion Set

Intravenous solutions are conveyed through the infusion set to needles or venous catheters. Conventional infusion sets with their pinch clamp are not recommended for use in children. The need for accurate measurement of fluid volumes to be administered to the baby makes the use of a Burette type of infusion set mandatory. Burette sets may be of various sizes like 30 ml, 50 ml or 100 ml, and a microfilter must be interposed, particularly in blood transfusion to remove the microemboli. It is also necessary to fit air filters to all infusion apparatus. Conventional cotton wool plugs do not prevent the passage of bacteria and moreover these become useless and inefficient when wet. Millipore filters may be used for all air inlets and included on the side arm of three-way-tap. Conventional glass bottles and rubber sterile disposable tubings are now replaced by PVC containers and tubings. Adequate sensible precautions and care should be taken to decrease contamination, infection and phlebitis.

The density and surface tension of the solution and the venous pressure and the lumen of the needle largely determine the drop size. Continuous vigilance is needed for gravity-fed systems as flow rate may decrease at any time.

Flow Rate Controllers and Infusion Pumps

In pediatric patients, the rates at which the infusion fluid is administered should be regulated carefully. Flow controllers regulate the volume by counting the number of fluid drops administered per unit time through a gravity-fed system. Here the preset rate is compared with the amount delivered and then the controller can compensate the balance and give alarm, if needed. The technique is mostly satisfactory for the fluids of low viscosity and of low specific gravity when administered in a relatively low pressure peripheral vein. It may not be much accurate in case of high specific gravity solutions when given in high pressure central venous sites.

Infusion pumps may also be used to deliver the infusate under pressure at a preset rate. Pressures upto 1000 mmHg may be generated in such systems. Air embolism may occur following use of infusion pumps. Forceful injection of blood through narrow needles or catheters may also cause blood cell damage and hemolysis.

From a practical point of view plastic syringes and three-way taps seem to be very useful for speeding an infusion. An alternative way is to compress a collapsible plastic bottle with a surrounding pneumatic bag. It is not safe for compressed air or extra air pressure to be applied directly to the fluid surface, that is, a head of pressure applied to a sealed bottle by a syringe or hand pump. It can easily cause air embolism. In the presence of vascular shunt, a little intravenous air may cause brain damage.

Spinal Needles (Fig. 6.33)

Traditional cutting-tip spinal needles can be used in the case of pediatric patients for lumbar puncture. Large-bore needles are routinely used for spinal taps to aspirate a large volume of cerebrospinal fluid or to administer subarachnoid chemotherapy. However, small-bore needles

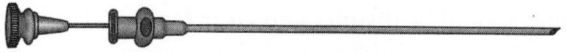

Fig. 6.33: Spinal needle

(22 s.w.g.) should be used for spinal anesthesia. It is said that the incidence of postspinal or postlumbar puncture headache is much less in infants and children. But this may be due to scarcity of such documented reports in children and the inability of infants to verbalize the discomfort or headache. The low incidence of postspinal headache may also be due to the fact that continued cerebrospinal fluid leak in infants is usually absent due to low CSF pressure, a high elastic dura and nonambulation.

Spinal needles should be 25 s.w.g. and short-beveled for neonates and 22 s.w.g. and sharp tipped for infants. Short bevel usually allows the injection of the local anesthetic solution into the narrow subarachnoid space. The needle should be stiff for easy maneuvering, but adequately flexible to allow bending without breakage, if the child struggles. Well-fitted styletted needles may be helpful in such cases. It should be noted that in children the usual distance from the skin to the subarachnoid space ranges from 5 to 10 mm when the spinal tap is done at the level of L_3 and L_4.

A small atraumatic noncutting point spinal needle may be much advantageous for pediatric use as this needle avoids cutting fibers and thus reduces the incidence of postspinal headache, particularly in older children and adolescents. Some needles are provided with the opening laterally and proximally to the needle tip. But it may result in injection of the local anesthetic solution partly in subarachnoid space and partly in epidural space.

Epidural Needle and Catheters (Fig. 6.34)

Epidural block is becoming more common and is useful for more major surgical procedures. A 19-gauge Tuohy needle with a 21-gauge epidural catheter is most popularly used in the case of children.

The epidural needles for pediatric use are mostly similar to those used in the case of adults. A variety of disposable epidural needles with different sizes and lengths are available. Tuohy needle is most convenient and popular. Some modifications should also be borne in mind for its pediatric use. It should have a blunt point to identify the passage through different tissues and loss of resistance. It should have a small terminal needle opening and a well-fitted stylet. Moreover, it should have resistance to kinking and stretching, atraumatic tip design, good length markings and radiopacity.

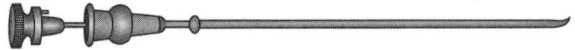

Fig. 6.34: Tuohy needle

The needle hub should be distinct and clear for easy detection of blood or CSF return. In the case of infants and children, stylet may not be needed due to the presence of loose epidural areolar tissue.

A 19-gauge Tuohy needle has a stylet, a winged hand and a short round bevel. The length of the shaft is 5 cm and it is graduated every 0.5 cm. The epidural catheter is a 21-gauge open-ended firm nylon catheter with an atraumatic tip. It is graduated at 2 cm from the tip and thereafter at 1 cm intervals. It is radiopaque. The adult epidural needle and catheter may be used for epidural anesthesia in older children and adolescents. A large number of adult and pediatric epidural sets (disposable) is commercially available.

CHAPTER 7

Monitoring

Routine monitoring of all pediatric cases during anesthesia and in postoperative period is of vital importance as it provides all the information necessary for safe anesthetic care and thus improve the quality of anesthesia. Monitoring is mandatory, particularly in pediatric cases as small children make changes suddenly and without much warning. Careful sensible monitoring can reduce anesthesia morbidity and mortality significantly.

Monitoring literally means warning and its devices measure the physiological variables and indicate the trend of change, so that appropriate therapeutic measures can be taken. These monitoring equipment should function accurately and the information supplied should be reliable. The anesthetist should know the basic principles on which the monitor is based and be able to interpret the information clinically.

Monitoring can be broadly classified as:
a. Direct clinical monitoring by the anesthetist
b. Noninvasive monitoring
c. Invasive monitoring
d. Miscellaneous methods.

DIRECT CLINICAL MONITORING BY THE ANESTHETIST

The presence of a specially trained and well-experienced pediatric anesthetist at all times seems to be most indispensible and vital requirement in anesthetic care of a child. No amount of modern sophisticated and up-to-date monitoring equipment can replace him. He has a specific experience, skill and training to keep a continuous check on the condition of the patient with the full use of his own senses such as looking, feeling and listening. Moreover, he will have to interpret the infotmation supplied by monitoring devices clinically and adopt the necessary measures, whenever needed.

By *looking* one can detect the cyanosis, chest movements, reservoir bag movements, tracheal tug, movements of facial muscles, eyes, even limbs in patients with inadequate relaxation, sweating in cases of hypercarbia, tears in case of light anesthesia, dilated pupils in cases of severe hypotension or cardiac arrest and so on. Operative blood loss is often visually estimated roughly. By listening one can detect the correct position of the endotracheal tube, the nature of lung ventilation, any moist sounds on the chest, heart sounds, any murmur and so on. Any gas leak from the circuit or from the cylinder can be detected by listening. Visual or audible alarms from the monitoring equipment should also be detected accordingly.

Thus, a careful anesthetist should always be alert in the operation theater and never be distracted from the care of his patient.

NONINVASIVE MONITORING

Most pediatric patients undergoing surgery are monitored noninvasively. Nowadays many cardiorespiratory parameters are often easily and safely monitored noninvasively. Common monitoring in pediatric cases includes precordial stethoscopy, electrocardiography, noninvasive blood pressure monitoring, thermometry, continuous pulse oximetry and end-tidal carbon dioxide analysis. All these parameters are most essential to provide adequate patient care during operation and in postanesthetic period as these may protect the patients from anesthetic mishaps and thus reduce the incidence of mortality and morbidity significantly.

Precordial Stethoscopy

Stethoscopy, either precordial or esophageal, seems to be the single most valuable monitoring method for the pediatric patients during anesthesia and it should always be attached before the induction of anesthesia. It provides continuous monitoring of heart sounds for rate, rhythm and intensity and gives an indication of changes in ventilation during anesthesia. It is the simplest aid for continuous monitoring of circulation and ventilation. It is inexpensive and carries little risk. It should be placed on the precordium over the left sternal border at the second or third intercostal space. However, the exact rhythm or qualitative changes of intensity may not be always detected even by the experienced anesthetist and moreover, the type and size of the stethoscope and the length and type of its tubing may affect the quality of sound and its interpretation. The chestpiece should be sufficiently small to sit comfortably on the infant's chest without tilting and should be securely fixed. It provides a single earpiece. The chestpiece should be interchangeable with esophageal catheters.

The use of precordial stethoscope to assess ventilation is also highly limited. Here the bilateral breath sounds cannot be heard and, even the endobronchial intubation may not be detected. It cannot readily distinguish between esophageal and endotracheal intubation. Moist sounds, wheezing, etc. cannot be localized. It can also be displaced by surgeons and their assistants during surgery.

Though the precordial stethoscope has its many limitations, it is still the most important monitoring aid and keeps contact between the patient and anesthetist all the while during operation. It also helps to detect the presence of murmurs, air emboli, laryngospasm, upper airway obstruction and croup.

Esophageal Stethoscope

It is also helpful and popular. The simple variety of esophageal stethoscope is usually a soft catheter with holes in its distal 2 to 3 cm which is covered by cuff. Other varieties are expensive and incorporate ECG probe and/or thermistor probe for electrocardiography and thermometry. Esophageal stethoscopes should be used when the patient is endotracheally intubated. Complications following its use may include esophageal burns from leaking currents, damage of the vocal cord, misplacement or displacement of the probes and so on. In infants, a too large stethoscope may even press the trachea and pulmonary vessels, thus causing ventilatory and circulatory disturbances.

The esophageal stethoscope is indicated when the use of precordial stethoscope is impractical particularly where there is difficult access to the chest. The smallest available esophageal stethoscope is of 12 FG. It should be used with sensible precautions in case of neonates.

Electrocardiogram

Electrocardiogram is an important means for monitoring cardiac parameters of the patient before, during and after anesthesia. It may act as an excellent pulse monitor and provide various information of cardiac irregularities, if present. But it does not give any measure of the efficiency of cardiac contraction or of cardiac output. Abnormal electrocardiographic changes may occur following cardiac inhibition, cardiac excitation, myocardial hypoxia and severe electrolyte imbalances. Bradycardia and tachycardia may occur during anesthesia and thus need early detection with ECG monitoring. It also allows one to differentiate between a normal sinus rhythm and other dysrhythmias like heart block, supraventricular tachycardia and so on. Severe hyperkalemia following massive blood transfusion may produce a characteristic peaked T wave. Hypocalcemia due to citrate intoxication may also prolong the QT interval. Ischemic changes are mostly rare in pediatric patients.

Continuous electrocardiographic tracing provides continuous cardiac monitoring and it is extremely important in all major surgical procedures, particularly during cardiothoracic operations. Standard lead IT monitoring is used widely for routine long-term observation of cardiac rhythm. Lead III should be chosen in cases of right axis deviation as the most pronounced R-wave could be found in this lead.

This method is noninvasive, simple and mostly accurate. But it is not a substitute for other monitors. It should always be used along with monitors which are needed to detect changes in perfusion and blood pressure. The common precautions include the use of large ECG plates rather than needle electrodes, a common earth attached to diathermy plate and the use of high resistance leads.

There are some differences between infants and adults regarding cardiac depolarization, but it is said that these differences have minimum significance in electrocardiography during operation. In infants, the R wave is most pronounced in standard lead III, but in adults it is pronounced in standard lead II tracing.

Noninvasive Blood Pressure Monitoring

There are various methods of indirect noninvasive measurement of blood pressure in neonates, infants and children. This can be done by palpation, auscultation, oscillometry and Doppler ultrasound techniques.

Palpation of the radial pulse while deflating the sphygmomanometer cuff is the commonest method of measuring the systolic blood pressure. But it is mostly inaccurate at low pressures, particularly in case of neonates and infants.

Auscultation of the Korotkoff sounds is simple, reliable and widely used method for measurement of blood pressure. But is seems to be cumbersome for routine use in pediatric anesthesia. In this method, a pneumatic tourniquet or cuff is applied proximal to the point where the radial artery is palpated. The pressure in the cuff is increased to obliterate the arterial pulsation. The cuff is connected to the mercurial manometer. A stethoscope is applied distal to the cuff. When the inflated cuff is gradually released, to level at which the first audible sound appears, it corresponds to the systolic blood pressure level. At the lower point when the sound becomes muffled and dull or just disappears, it indicates the diastolic pressure. While measuring the blood pressure, the arm should be kept at the level of the heart. The cuff should be of adequate size. The width of the cuff should be 2.5 cm for neonates, 6 to 9 cm for children, 12 cm for adult arm and 15 cm for adult leg. If the width of the cuff is smaller than the recommended width, systolic blood pressure reading will become much higher; if it is too wide, reading will be low. The cloth covering the cuff should be one which does not stretch. The pneumatic bag itself should be at least half to encircle the arm and must be placed over the artery. The apparatus should be checked before use, particularly its zero level.

Oscillotonometry is also widely used for measurement of blood pressure in anesthetic practice. It is reliable at low pressure and no stethoscopy is needed. It provides a double cuff, one upper small occluding cuff that overlaps a lower and longer sensing cuff, is attached to the oscillotonometer. The cuffs are inflated above the anticipated systolic pressure and then a slow leak is allowed mechanically. Then the system gives the pressure waves arriving at the lower cuff to be displayed as oscillations of the needle. In this technique, measurement of systolic pressure is more accurate than that of diastolic pressure.

In recent times, an automated method of oscillotonometry has become much popular. Here the machine automatically inflates the cuff at preset time intervals. It is helpful for measurement of heart rate, systolic and diastolic pressure as the cuff deflates. Some models suitable for pediatric use are also available.

Arterial pressure can also be measured by *Doppler ultrasound technique.* An ultrasound emitter and receiver surrounded by an inflatable cuff are placed over the brachial artery. Movement of the vessel walls generates a signal which can be noted in the machine. Both the systolic and diastolic pressures are displayed. The machine is, no doubt, very expensive, but reliable and accurate even at low pressures. It is very helpful in pediatric cases.

Hazards of automated cuffs include possibility of electric shock, damage of nerves due to over inflation and so on. These monitors are said to be less accurate in measuring diastolic pressures than the systolic pressures. In neonates and infants, automated cuffs with long inflation times and short intervals between measurements should be avoided; otherwise, perfusion of the limb may suffer.

Peripheral Perfusion

Peripheral perfusion should be observed frequently during anesthesia in pediatric cases. Warm, dry and pink skin of the extremities denotes adequate perfusion while cold and white extremities indicate inadequacy. Cold periphery usually occurs in hypovolemia and shock. The core to peripheral temperature gradient also indicates the nature of peripheral perfusion. Nasopharyngeal or esophageal temperature is taken as core temperature and peripheral temperature is taken at great toe. The gradient increases in presence of vasoconstriction and low cardiac output. It decreases gradually as vasodilatation occurs and cardiac output increases.

Urinary Output

It essentially indicates the renal perfusion and thereby adequacy of circulation or perfusion of vital organs. It should be at least 0.5 to 1 ml/kg/hour. Measurement of urine volume should be done in cases of major surgery, major vascular surgery, shocked patients, cardiac surgery and so on.

Pulse Oximetry

In recent years, pulse oximetry is widely used in the case of infants and children during anesthesia. It measures the arterial oxygen saturation of the patient. Here light of known intensity and a given wavelength is allowed to shine through a tissue such as the nailbed of a finger or toe, the lobe of pinna of the ear or even the tongue and the pulse oximeter analyses the changes in the transmission of light through any pulsating arterial vascular lead and computers the oxygen saturation of the arterial blood. The probe of the pulse oximeter includes two narrow band light emitting bodies functioning at wavelengths in the red and infrared part of the spectrum. As only two wavelengths are used in pulse oximeter, it can distinguish only two forms of pigments such as reduced and oxyhemoglobin. Thus, pulse oximeter is affected by dyes like methylene blue, nail polish, carboxyhemoglobin and methemoglobin, ambient light and so on. Fetal hemoglobin has no effect on its accuracy. The effect of ambient light interference can be avoided by covering the oximeter probe with an opaque cover. Low flow states and motion artifact may interfere with the accuracy of measurement of arterial oxygen saturation. It is said that all oximeters are accurate only between 70 and 100% saturation.

It provides early evidence of impending oxyhemoglobin desaturation before hypoxemia-induced changes in vital signs. It is useful in guiding the FiO_2 selection and thereby helps in reducing the risk of hypoxemia in premature neonates.

Pulse oximetry is an essential monitoring aid to detect hypoxia well before the appearance of visible cyanosis. It is of great help in a wide variety of problems during pediatric anesthesia. In neonates and infants, the neonatal oximeter probe can be placed on the fleshy part of the hypothenar eminence of the hand and the lateral aspect of the foot to provide adequate waveform.

Hazards of pulse oximeter may include risk of electrical shock and burn injury. All oximeters should be electrically isolated.

Transcutaneous PaO_2 and $PaCO_2$ Measurement

Here transcutaneous electrode provides a continuous, noninvasive measurement of arterial oxygen and carbon dioxide tension. It is more accurate in the case of children where the skin is rather thin.

End-tidal Carbon Dioxide Estimation

Estimation of carbon dioxide concentration in expired gases is needed in certain clinical conditions such as detection of air, fat or pulmonary embolism and malignant hyperpyrexia. Routine intraoperative monitoring particularly in carotid artery surgery may also be needed. End-tidal carbon dioxide fairly correlates with $PaCO_2$.

Capnometry is the measurement and numerical display of expired carbon dioxide. Capnography is the measurement and graphic display of expired carbon dioxide. When the graphic display is calibrated, capnography includes capnometry.

These provide various types of information about the patient and the function of the artificial airway, breathing system and the ventilator. These may help in detection of critical incidents, breathing system leaks and rebreathing. These are also helpful in assessment of ventilation.

In this device, the principle of infrared absorption spectrophotometry is used. The electronic circuitry gives a direct read out or immediate recording to indicate the carbon dioxide level in expired gases. It may be incorporated into the breathing system during anesthesia. Respiratory gas may also be measured by mass spectrometry, acoustic spectroscopy or Raman scattering.

Respiratory gas for analysis may be aspirated from the airway or analyzed when it flows through a sensor inserted into any location of the breathing circuit.

Simple carbon dioxide analyzers are also available. Here the end expiratory sample of the gas is collected for analysis. The sampling probe is introduced into the catheter mount of the gas delivery system. Endotracheal tubes may have a pilot tube specifically designed for sampling end tidal gas.

In the case of infants and children, these devices of capnography usually provide accurate measurements. When the sampling catheter is obstructed, it is necessary to change tubes or clear the secretions back into the trachea. Aspirating capnography can also be done in spontaneously breathing nonintubated children. Here the sampling catheter should be placed and taped adjacent to the external nares. Due to large dead space of the face mask and high fresh gas flows, there may be wide difference between arterial and end tidal carbon dioxide values, but the method may be helpful in monitoring respiratory trends and detecting respiratory obstruction.

In the case of infants and children with acyanotic congenital heart disease, end tidal carbon dioxide may closely approximate arterial carbon dioxide, but in cases with cyanotic heart diseases it may not reliably estimate arterial carbon dioxide tension due to significant venous admixture.

Thermometry

Thermometry during anesthesia should be routinely used, particularly in the case of neonates, infants and children. It is of particular importance to detect hypothermia which readily occurs in children during prolonged anesthesia and surgery involving large body cavities and also to detect malignant hyperthermia.

General anesthesia usually inhibits body metabolism and depresses the thermoregulatory center in the hypothalamus. Heat loss is potentiated in prolonged anesthesia and exposure of large surface area of tissues. The use of wet packs, cold blood transfusion and dry inspired gases exaggerate the problems. Small children are very prone to heat loss as their surface area is much larger in proportion to body weight than that in the case of adults.

The thermoregulatory mechanism usually keeps the central body temperature within about $0.2°$ C of accepted normal of about $37°$ C. Body temperature is recorded with the help of various thermometers such as mercury-in-glass, thermistors, thermocouples, infrared thermometers, temperature sensitive liquid crystals, etc. Thermocouples which measure a temperature-dependent bimetal electrical potential are most popularly used in anesthetic practice.

Generally speaking, there are two types of temperature values, surface or peripheral temperature and core or central or internal temperature. There are different temperature monitoring sites and they have their own physiological and practical significances as different tissues may have different temperature.

Surface temperature is usually taken in axilla or groin. It is not always reliable. It may give different values at different locations. It may vary with peripheral blood flow, sweating, radiation and conduction of heat to and from surroundings. During measurement of surface temperature, external thermal influences like drafts, sweating and others should be avoided. Measurements should be taken after allowing some time to attain an equilibrium with room temperature.

Axillary temperature is very useful clinical thermometry. It is most commonly used site for temperature measurement in pediatric cases. But it does not correlate well with central temperature and is considerably less than the central temperature.

Internal temperature can be measured at different sites like sublingual, nasopharyngeal, esophageal and tympanic.

Sublingual temperature may vary widely in salivation or after drinking and eating. Nasopharyngeal site often gives a good reliable measure of core temperature. It closely approximates the temperature of carotid vessels or hypothalamic temperature. The probe should be placed in the nasopharynx posterior to soft palate. The site is less subjected to trauma but the nasal probe may cause epistaxis. Nasopharyngeal temperature may reflect the temperature of respiratory gases and may give inaccurate readings in presence of gas leak around the endotracheal tube.

Rectal probe is often used for measurement of core temperature in children. The temperature may vary due to insulation of feces, cool blood returning from legs, the influence of an open abdominal cavity, etc. Heat bearing organisms in the rectum may elevate the temperature. The site is, no doubt, wide away from heart and central nervous system and has no thermal significance of its own. But it usually reads similar to or a little higher than other core temperatures.

Esophageal temperature is more reliable core temperature as it approximates the cardiac temperature. It is widely used during induced hypothermia. The electrode or probe is positioned in mid or lower third of esophagus. It is usually incorporated into esophageal stethoscopes and placed in the distal third of the esophagus at the point of maximum audible heart sounds. In infants and children, the respiratory gas temperature may influence the esophageal temperature during anesthesia due to minimum thermal insulation between tracheobronchial tract and esophagus. Care should be taken; otherwise, the actual site may be deflected and it may even enter the stomach.

The tympanic temperature is so far best core temperature as it provides a reasonable approximation of hypothalamic temperature. The site is usually dry and mostly clean. It is convenient, reliable and relatively easy and it causes less embarrassment and discomfort to the patients. However, the delicate membrane can be easily damaged by aural thermistors. Thus the probes should be soft and flexible as far as practicable. After placement of the probe the aural canal should be blocked with cotton wool to prevent cooling of the probe by ambient air movement.

Body temperature can be measured using a variety of thermometers. Most clinically used thermometers are reasonably reliable and accurate. The electrical thermometers and thermocouples are also available. Different thermistor probes are also available for different sites. The instrument contains glass sensitizing tips for skin temperature and needles for measurement of subcutaneous or muscle temperature. The battery powered thermocouple is more portable and easy to handle. Before using them, the instrumental error, if any, should be predetermined. Sometimes, it may be needed to measure the temperature of the inspired gases when an efficient humidifier is used, in order to prevent thermal burns to the respiratory tract.

INVASIVE MONITORING

In recent years, invasive monitoring in pediatric anesthesia practice has rapidly expanded. Monitoring equipment are sophisticated and complex and mostly needed for operations on the heart and lungs and central nervous systems. Common invasive monitoring examples in the case of pediatric patient include arterial cannulation for direct blood pressure measurement and central venous pressure or pulmonary artery pressure measurements.

Direct Intra-arterial Blood Pressure Monitoring

Direct intra-arterial blood pressure monitoring is somewhat restricted in pediatric cases due to the narrow, small size of arteries. In recent years, high quality narrow gauge arterial cannulas have become available and thus are now widely practiced in pediatrics. However, they should only be used with sensible precautions and risk-to-benefit ratio should always be considered.

A suitable peripheral artery such as radial or temporal is catheterized. Other arteries may include the ulnar, brachial, axillary, dorsalis pedis, posterior tibial and even the umbilical artery in newborn. Size of the cannula is important. Ideally, it can be easily inserted, samples can be easily withdrawn and there will be risk of vessel thrombosis. Usual recommendations are 24 gauge for infants less than 3 kg, 22 gauge for infants weighing 3 to 10 kg and 20 gauge for others. Teflon catheters are mostly used. Polyurethane is less rigid and thus seems to be less traumatic.

An electronic pressure transducer is introduced in the artery. Heparinized normal saline solution is used to maintain the arterial line patent. The catheter is passed as centrally as possible. The insertion of the catheter may be either percutaneous or through a surgical cut down. The positioning of the transducer needs careful attention. Conventionally, the reference point of the transducer is at the level of right atrium.

When the cannula is properly placed, it should be adequately fixed, otherwise dislodgement or disconnection may occur. The pressure change signal passes from the transducer and it is processed to have a continuous recording of both systolic and diastolic pressures, and mean arterial pressure displayed digitally on a calibrated paper.

Contraindications of intra-arterial monitoring include infected skin at the site of insertion, inadequate collateral blood flow with the risk of distal ischemia and coagulopathy. Complications of short-term cannulation are relatively minor and infrequent. But long-term cannulation carries risks of morbidity such as arterial wall damage, thrombosis, embolism, disconnection, hemorrhage, sepsis, tissue necrosis and so on.

The intra-arterial cannula may be connected with a manometer to record the blood pressure. Blood clot in the cannula may give faulty results. Air bubbles, kinking of the catheter and arterial spasm may cause dumping of the system.

Central Venous Pressure Monitoring

Central venous pressure reflects the pressure of the right atrium. Central vein should be one that is not separated from the right atrium by a venous valve. The neck veins and arm veins are popularly used for cannulation. The basilic vein in the cubital fossa, the subclavian vein and the internal jugular vein can also be utilized. The femoral and other leg veins are not suitable due to risk of venous thrombosis and pulmonary embolism. In newborn, umbilical vein may be utilized.

The central venous pressure usually varies with age. In general, the normal accepted value ranges from 3 to 12 cm water pressure for most healthy infants and children.

Indications of central venous cannulation include measuring the central venous pressure for administration of irritant drugs, for long-term parenteral nutrition, for frequent blood sampling and for removing air from right ventricle in case of venous air embolism. Contraindications to central venous cannulation are sepsis at the site of insertion, coagulopathy and so on.

Central venous catheters may vary in size, length, ratio of internal to external diameter, material composition, stiffness and number of lumens. Proper selection should be made on the basis of size and weight of the child and the purpose of cannulation. The teflon, silastic or polyurethane catheters are widely used.

A long catheter is passed intravenously so that its tip remains in one of the great veins near to right atrium. Confirmation of its correct position is obtained by noting the fluctuations with respiration. The other end is connected to an infusion set through a three-way tap. The third limb of the tap is usually connected with a simple water or saline manometer. Ordinarily, the infusion runs in the usual way through the tap and the manometer is kept out of the circuit. During measurement of CVP, the tap is turned to connect with the manometer and the infusion set is kept out of the circuit. A zero point is ascertained beforehand by leveling with the manubrium sternum of the child. During recording the height of water column is measured in centimeters from the zero point. Thus, it gives the CVP, 'plus' when it is above or 'minus' when it is below the zero level.

Complications may include pneumothorax, infection, malposition, fluid overload by continuous infusion, perforation of great veins or even heart, air embolism, thrombosis, thromboembolism, injury to nerve plexus and so on. Catheter occlusion, kinking, leaking or thrombus may also occur.

Measurement of central venous pressure is useful in various situations such as major surgery, cardiothoracic surgery, neurosurgery, pheochromocytoma surgery, shocked and critically ill patients and for frequent blood gas analysis.

Pulmonary Artery Pressure Monitoring

Pulmonary artery pressure can be measured and monitored with the help of balloon tipped, flow directed catheter (swan-ganz). It can quantify, monitor and modify the hemodynamic status of the patient during therapeutic applications. Its use in pediatric cases is limited and depends on the clinical situation considering the risk-benefit ratio.

Pulmonary artery catheter may be indicated to monitor pulmonary artery pressure. It is used in cardiac surgery for management of preload and afterload with fluids or drugs and for assessment of cardiac output. It is also used for measurement of CVP and monitoring oxygen carrying capacity of blood. It is also used for electrocardiogram by incorporating the bipolar electrical lead wires.

An intracardiac or extracardiac defect may result in faulty catheter course, incorrect interpretation of data or a high risk of emboli. It should not be used in presence of thrombocytopenia coagulopathy, local sepsis and so on. Pre-existing conduction defect may be worsened following the passage of catheter.

Pulmonary artery catheter may be inserted through the internal jugular vein, subclavian vein, the femoral or basilic vein. The internal jugular and femoral routes are most commonly used.

The pulmonary artery floatation catheter should be inserted in the same way as a standard central venous catheter. But the port of entry should be large and often dilatation of the vein is needed. After inflation of the balloon, the catheter is advanced slowly to reach the pulmonary artery through right ventricle. Further advancement will lead the tip of catheter into a branch of pulmonary artery where pulmonary artery wedge pressure can be detected. The correct placement of the catheter may be established by use of the pressure transducer to display waveforms as in the case of adults. In the case of small children, the fluoroscopy may be much helpful.

A chest radiograph should be performed after every insertion to detect the exact position of catheter and to exclude pneumothorax.

Complications of pulmonary artery catheterization may include thrombophlebitis, injury to nerve artery or vein, air embolism, perforation, hydrothorax, hemothorax, cardiac dysrhythmias, balloon rupture, kinking or knotting of the catheter and so on.

MISCELLANEOUS METHODS

Neuromuscular Function Monitoring

General anesthesia usually involves the use of muscle relaxant drugs and thus the patient's neuromuscular function should always be monitored and assessed. The patient should not have any residual block at the time of recovery from anesthesia. Incomplete recovery from muscle relaxants increases the anesthetic morbidity and mortality in pediatric patients.

Clinical assessment is no doubt most important, but these criteria are mostly imprecise and frequently misunderstood. In infants, the diaphragm is the major muscle of respiration responsible for tidal volume respiration. It is resistant to neuromuscular block relative to the neck and the abdominal intercostal muscles which are most important for coughing, swallowing and supporting the airway. Thus, it may so happen that the child may not protect his airway at one time of recovery though his tidal volume is within normal limits.

Common clinical parameters used to assess recovery from neuromuscular block are head lift for 5 seconds, sustained hand grip, no nystagmus or diplopia, wide opening of the eyes, normal voice, tongue protrusion, coordinating swallowing, negative inspiratory effort at least 32 cm water pressure (55 cm H_2O in adults) against an obstructed airway, vital capacity more than 15 ml/kg, lifting both legs, sustained arm lift for at least 45 seconds and so on. All these give some idea of adequacy of neuromuscular transmission. However, the pediatric patients pose difficulty in application of volitional parameter and many times are unable to follow commands. Thus, the response to stimulation of motor nerve must be assessed to evaluate recovery from neuromuscular blocking drugs as the method is independent of patient's effort.

Nerve stimulator is applied to peripheral motor nerve and the state of the patient's neuromuscular function is assessed by way of supramaximal stimulation of the motor nerve. Usually, the ulnar nerve at the wrist, the common peroneal nerve at the lateral side of the knee or the facial nerve in front of the ear (observation of the orbicularis oculi muscle) is employed for this purpose. When the ulnar nerve at the wrist or elbow is stimulated by the nerve stimulator, the constriction of fingers (adductor pollicis and flexor digitorum muscles) is observed, palpated or recorded as electrical activity through electromyography (EMG). The electrical impulse may be given as single shock or high frequency tetanic stimulation or as trains of low frequencies. Electrical stimulus should be adequate for a given period of time. When applied over the skin a current upto 50 mA may be applied for 0.2–1.0 minute and this may need a voltage ranging from 50 to 300 V. This type of stimulation usually does not cause any adverse cardiac effects. The method is helpful as it indicates the amount or the degree of neuromuscular block and type of block, either depolarization or nondepolarization, but it needs careful interpretation. Electromyography (EMG) measures the compound action potential generated by the summation of the individual action potentials of contracting muscle fibers and thus serves as a good method to quantify the motor response to nerve stimulation.

Blood Gas Analysis

Monitoring of PaO_2 $PaCO_2$, oxygen saturation, oxygen content and pH is particularly indicated in major thoracic and vascular surgery, neurosurgery, one lung anesthesia and induced hypothermia. These parameters are accurately assessed by arterial blood gas analysis. The sites for arterial catheterization most commonly used are radial and femoral artery, but axillary, brachial, ulnar, temporal or dorsalis pedis artery can also be used. Modern automated blood gas analyzers are unique for blood gas measurements. Here microelectrode systems are used and only small quantity of heparinized blood of about 0.2 ml is needed. Results are obtained within 2 to 3 mintues. A blood gas machine usually provides various variables such as pH, $PaCO_2$, PaO_2, HCO_3, total CO_2, standard bicarbonate, base excess, standard base excess, oxygen saturation, hemoglobin percentage and temperature measurement.

The data of blood gases should be interpreted very carefully.

Blood Loss Measurement

Blood loss measurement during anesthesia and surgery is of vital importance as it dictates the intravenous fluid therapy and blood transfusion in exact amounts; otherwise, too much or too low fluid or blood administration may be hazardous. Blood losses of upto 10% of blood volume are more or less tolerated well and may be replaced by an appropriate volume of crystalloid solution. Blood loss exceeding 10% of blood volume in children during surgery should always be replaced by whole blood.

Various methods can be adopted to determine the exact amount of operative blood loss.

1. **Subjective assessment:** The experienced anesthetist may be able to make an approximate estimation of the blood loss from visual observation. It is mostly unreliable and there may be individual variations. However, the method may be helpful as a guide of preliminary blood transfusion therapy when no other methods are feasible or available.
2. **Patient weighing:** In this method, the patient is weighed before and after operation to note the difference. This may amount to the blood and fluid loss. But the method is not reliable and may have inaccuracies due to drain, infusion, urinary output, surgical excision of tissues and so on. The method needs a large weighing table. Here it is assumed that 1 g equals to 1 ml of blood.
3. **Gravimetric method:** The method is very simple but very useful and practical to determine the blood loss, particularly in children. The pre-weighed mops, towels and swabs are used during operation and these are again weighed after contamination with blood. The difference in weight in grams gives the amount of blood loss in ml. One ml of blood weighs approximately 1 g. The method is said to be accurate within 10% of actual loss. Mops or swabs should be weighed promptly to avoid evaporative loss. The surgeon should be asked not to use other linens or water and not to contaminate in gowns.
4. **Volumetric method:** Here the blood is sucked through the suction apparatus and collected in a calibrated jar. The volume of blood in the jar roughly gives the amount of blood loss. A small amount of defoaming agent may be added to avoid error due to foaming. It may have some inaccuracies, but gives a rough idea about blood loss.
5. **Gravimetric-volumetric method:** In this method, both swab weighing and measuring the volume in the suction bottle are adopted. It seems to be a simple and more or less reliable method of blood loss measurement.
6. **Colorimetric method:** It is more accurate method. Swabs, gowns, and drapes are washed with a known volume of fluid and the hemoglobin content measured colorimetrically. Blood loss in ml equals the colorimeter reading × vol (ml) of washing fluid divided by (200 × patient's Hb g%).

    Technical errors may occur due to chemical changes in hematin, presence of fat interfering with optical density, incomplete extraction of blood from clot and contamination of bile. The method can only be used at the end of operation.

7. Automatic blood loss meter: It may be of value as it gives a continuous estimation of blood loss. It works on the principle of electrolyte conductivity. All blood contaminated sponges, towels, mops and other linens are taken in a water bath and the change in the conductance of the solution is detected. The method is reliable and able to detect even a small amount of blood loss.

CHAPTER 8

Anesthetic Pharmacology

Pharmacokinetics in the case of neonates, infants and children differ widely from that in the case of adults because of reduced protein binding, larger volume of distribution, immature renal and hepatic functions and small fat stores. The response to drugs in children depends upon the absorption, distribution, metabolism and excretion of the drug concerned. Salient features may be enumerated as follows:

1. In infants absorption of drugs from the gastrointestinal tract is usually slow and may be erratic.
2. Peripheral circulation is mostly unstable and thus pharmacokinetics of drugs parenterally used may be unpredictable.
3. Kidneys are immature. Infants change their hydration rapidly and thus there is always chance of qualitative changes in the distribution of the drug. Renal excretion of drugs may be slow in infants and children.
4. Liver is partly immature in neonates. But it seems to be the center of protein production and drug detoxication. In the case of neonate, there may be quantitative and qualitative variations in plasma protein with a reduction in plasma albumin, and more drug may remain active due to less protein binding. Some drugs are metabolized slowly in the liver and thus there is increased risk of toxicity.
5. Liver microsomal enzymes are also immature in the case of children. It is said that halothane related hepatic damage is rare in children for this reason.
6. Central nervous system: In newborn, neurones are usually complete but myelination is incomplete. However, the major part of body fat is within the central nervous system. This implies that lipid-soluble drugs reach and concentrate more easily and rapidly compared to adults. Blood-brain barrier is more permeable in neonates and thus barbiturates and opioids should be given with extreme caution. Some drugs like sulfonamides, and salicylates may displace bilirubin from

its bonds with plasma albumin, and bilirubin can cross the blood-brain barrier and produce neurotoxic effects (kernicterus). Antibiotics also cross the barrier more easily.
7. The immature central nervous system and high metabolic rate in children may be the major factors, for increasing the minimum alveolar concentration of the inhalational volatile anesthetic agents in children.
8. Relatively large extracellular space in infants may necessitate modification of the dose of drugs like muscle relaxants accordingly.
9. Basal metabolic rate is high in infants, so safe dose of a drug should be determined taking sensible precautions. Drugs with a wider margin of safety should be advised. It is said that at about the age of 18 months and above, the metabolic rate is roughly proportional to the body surface area. Thus, the metabolic rate per kg body weight decreases as the body weight increases. Some doctors advocate the use of surface area as a basis of safe dose calculation. But in clinical practice, the dose of a drug is estimated on the basis of body weight and it is widely accepted.
10. Genetically induced variations of drug response may be found in the case of infants and children with serious consequences. They may include hemoglobinopathies, abnormal or deficient pseudocholinesterase, hyperkalemia or hyperpyrexia (malignant). The defective pseudocholinesterase may lead to prolonged apnea following suxamethonium.
11. Drug interactions in pediatric anesthesia are not uncommon. Steroid and anesthetics may cause hypotension. Phenothiazines and anesthetics may cause hypotension and anesthetic potentiation. Curare and some antibiotics like streptomycin, neomycin, kanamycin, etc. may cause intensive relaxation. Curare and diazepam have additive effect. Curare and diuretics may cause profound relaxation by reducing potassium level.
12. It is evident that children show wide variations in response to various anesthetic drugs and allied agents. Thus, the proper dose of a drug should be estimated and the route of administration should be judged with sensible precautions. Over and above, constant vigilance is mandatory.

This chapter essentially deals with the basic pharmacological aspects of commonly used drugs in pediatric anesthesia, such as inhalational agents, intravenous agents, muscle relaxants, narcotics, antiemetics, benzodiazepines and so on in a brief and concise manner. Entire pharmacology related to this subject is not within the scope of this presentation.

INHALATIONAL AGENTS

There is rapid uptake of inhalational anesthetic agents by the lung in infants and young children in comparison to adults. This is mostly due to high level of alveolar ventilation in relation to functional residual capacity (FRC), greater cardiac output and a greater portion going to vessel-rich tissues. The uptake is less in congenital anomalies like Fallot's tetralogy with pulmonary ischemia, airway obstruction and high ventilation perfusion ratio. Effects are stronger with the use of soluble anesthetic agents. Excretion of inhalational anesthetic agents is also rapid in infants provided there is no ventilatory depression.

The minimum alveolar concentration (MAC) of inhalational anesthetics is higher in infants than that in older children and adults. MAC for anesthesia is greater than MAC required for cardiorespiratory depression. Therefore, the margin for safety is significantly reduced. Thus, great care and adequate monitoring are needed during their use in the case of children.

An ideal inhalational anesthetic agent should have low blood gas solubility, high potency and volatility, noninflammable nature and no serious side effects. It should have resistance to biotransformation, as some metabolites are harmful.

Nitrous Oxide

It is a true anesthetic gas as its saturated vapor pressure is above ambient pressure and thus it exists as liquid under pressure only. It is a nonirritant sweet smelling gas and provides a smooth and rapid induction of anesthesia due to its low blood-gas solubility. But it is a very weak anesthetic agent when used alone with oxygen. Thus, it is used as a carrier gas and a supplement for most inhalational anesthetics. It is a good analgesic. It may cause mild depression of cardiovascular system, but it is usually not a problem in routine clinical use. Nitrous oxide has mild depressant effects on systemic hemodynamics, particularly in sedated children. It does not cause elevation in pulmonary artery pressure and pulmonary vascular resistance as in the case of adults. Muscle relaxation is minimal. Nausea and vomiting are rare. It rapidly crosses the placenta and there may be rapid uptake by the fetus, but it does not adversely affect the fetus in normal conditions. 'Diffusion hypoxia' may occur in early postoperative period. It can be prevented by adequate oxygenation during the initial phase of recovery from nitrous oxide anesthesia.

Following nitrous oxide anesthesia, there may be an increase in the volume of air-containing spaces. It should be kept in mind in case of lesions of lung like pneumothorax and congenital lobar pneumonia. Expansion of the gut in diaphragmatic hernia, exomphalos or gastroschisis may cause cardiorespiratory embarrassment due to diaphragmatic splinting. In necrotizing enterocolitis, the gas within the gut may also worsen the clinical condition of the baby.

Diethyl Ether

It is a colorless, pungent volatile liquid. It is relatively soluble in blood and thus provides a slow induction and recovery. It is very potent but its high flammability limits its use in modern anesthesia. However, it is safe, reliable and cheap and widely used in developing countries. It can be used by open drop method, in air-ether draw over technique or through a Boyle anesthetic apparatus in a closed or semiclosed system. Vapor strengths upto 20% are needed for induction, 3 to 5% for maintenance of light anesthesia and upto 10% for deep anesthesia.

Ether at first induces analgesia, then excitement and lastly anesthesia. It causes overall depression of cerebral cortex, medulla and spinal cord. It may cause mild myocardial depression but the effect is somewhat counteracted by sympathetic stimulation. Heart rate and blood pressure are increased initially, but remain more or less unaltered later. Respiration may be increased a little, but is depressed in toxic doses. It may cause excessive salivation and bronchial secretion. It dilates the bronchial musculature. Nausea and vomiting are common. It produces excellent muscular relaxation and potentiates the nondepolarizing muscle relaxants. Both liver and kidney functions are depressed, but permanent damage does not occur. It may cause hyperglycemia by mobilizing liver glycogen. The drug is mostly (about 85–90%) excreted unchanged by lungs and the rest is metabolized in liver. Ether does not cause sensitization of the myocardium to catecholamines, so it is safe to use adrenaline with local anesthetic agents.

Halothane

It is colorless and has a sweet, pleasant smell. It is noninflammable in air and oxygen in the concentrations used in anesthetic practice. It is safe to use with soda lime. It is a potent anesthetic agent (MAC 0.75). It is delivered through specially designed flow and temperature controlled vaporizers.

It is nonirritant and well-tolerated and provides a smooth rapid induction of anesthesia. Salivary and bronchial secretions are less and there is a decrease in bronchomotor tone. It produces a dose-related fall in blood pressure due to myocardial depression and vasodilation. It sensitizes the myocardium to circulating catecholamines causing occasional arrhythmias. Halothane causes bradycardia which can be readily reversed by atropine. It potentiates the nondepolarizing muscle relaxants. The incidence of nausea and vomiting is little. It depresses the gastrointestinal motility. There may be postoperative shivering in the early recovery period.

Halothane is metabolized in liver in significant amounts, about 20% by oxidative pathways and the end products are excreted in urine. Halothane itself is not hepatotoxic but may be associated with nonspecific hepatotoxic damage. It may be due to its reductive metabolic pathway with intermediate hepatotoxic metabolites. Liver damage may occur following repeated halothane administration. So at least a 3-month period should be kept between repeat halothane anesthesia. But halothane induced hepatic failure is rare in children.

Enflurane

It is clear and colorless with a pleasant ethereal smell. It is noninflammable and compatible with soda lime. It is half as potent as halothane and its MAC value is 1.68. It is a stable compound and only about 2% is metabolized in liver to nonvolatile compounds which are excreted in urine.

It produces a rapid and smooth induction of anesthesia. It is nonirritant and does not increase salivary and tracheobronchial secretions. It may cause depression of the cardiovascular and respiratory systems rather more than halothane. But arrhythmias are uncommon and there is less sensitization of the heart to catecholamines. Hepatotoxicity following enflurane anesthesia is rare. It produces dose-dependent depression of neuromuscular transmission and potentiates the nondepolarizing muscle relaxants.

Isoflurane

It is fluorinated chlorinated ether and is an isomer of enflurane. It is a potent anesthetic agent, its MAC value is 1.15. It is noninflammable. It is more soluble in blood and produces a rapid induction and recovery. But it is irritant and may cause breath holding, coughing and even bronchospasm. It can produce respiratory and myocardial depression. Isoflurane causes vasodilation and reflex tachycardia in anesthetic doses. But it depresses the heart less than halothane. It potentiates the neuromuscular blocking agents. Negligible amount (about 0.2 %) is metabolized in liver and heptotoxicity after its use is unlikely.

Sevoflurane

It is a potent volatile anesthetic agent. It is mostly nonirritant and well-tolerated by most children. Its MAC value is 1.9. It provides very rapid induction and recovery, mostly due to its low blood/gas solubility. During induction, sudden apnea can occur. Excretion of sevoflurane is entirely through lungs.

INTRAVENOUS INDUCTION AGENTS

These drugs are widely used for inducing loss of consciousness in children. An ideal intravenous induction agent should be stable in solution, preferably, be water-soluble, nonirritant, safe and without any serious side effects, particularly on cardiovascular and respiratory systems. It should have rapid onset of action and produce a rapid recovery with little hangover effect. Thiopentone is most popular IV induction agent in children. Ketamine and diazepam can also be used successfully. Methohexitone, etomidate, propofol, propanidid, althesin are all useful drugs but are not much suitable for pediatric practice as these may cause severe pain on injection.

Thiopentone Sodium

It is most commonly used IV induction agent even in infants and children of all ages. It is a yellowish-white power which is soluble in water. It is given as 2.5 mg/kg body weight and provides a smooth rapid induction. It is not painful on injection, but care should be taken to avoid extravasation around the veins and intra-arterial injection. In pediatric cases, the correct dose on weight basis should be given slowly. Its metabolism is rather slow, about 10 to 15%/hour; thus, some hangover after its administration is most likely. It causes peripheral vasodilation, direct myocardial depression and transient respiratory depression depending upon the rate of injection and the amount of the dose. It may produce a mild degree of bronchoconstriction. It may be associated with histamine release. Anaphylactic reactions are rare. There is a reduction of skeletal muscle tone while increasing central depression.

The drug is contraindicated in cases of porphyria, airway obstruction, fixed cardiac output states, severe shock, adrenocortical insufficiency and so on. The drug should never be used in places where no resuscitative measures are available.

Methohexitone

It was used as an alternative to thiopentone in a dose of 1.5 mg/kg body weight in 1% solution. It provides a pleasant rapid induction of anesthesia. But it is associated with excitatory central nervous system phenomena such as hiccups and abnormal muscle movements. It also produces pain along the course of injected vein. It can be minimized by prior injection of a small dose of lignocaine (1 mg/ml of 2% lignocaine). The drug should not be used in children with epilepsy as it may initiate convulsion. Recovery following methohexitone is also rapid. The drug has been also used by rectal route in a dose of 25 mg/kg body weight. It is contraindicated in cases of porphyria.

Ketamine Hydrochloride

It is a derivative of phencyclidine and produces dissociation that is intense analgesia with only superficial sleep. It can be used as induction agent and also as sole anesthetic agent. Ketamine is used in a dose of 2 mg/kg IV to produce sleep within 30 to 60 seconds lasting for 5 to 10 minutes. Repeated doses may be given to get a longer effect. Ketamine 10 mg/kg IM provides surgical anesthesia within 2 to 8 minutes and lasts for 10 to 20 minutes. It can also be given as continuous infusion in a dose of 50 µg/kg/minute for production of analgesia.

Ketamine does not depress the cardiovascular and respiratory systems. Mild tachycardia and rise of blood pressure may occur. It may cause hypertonus, salivation, nausea and vomiting, emergence delirium and hallucinations. But emergence disturbances are uncommon in children. It may increase metabolic rate.

Ketamine is indicated as sole anesthetic agent for minor surgery in children. It is helpful for inducing anesthesia in poor risk cases due to stimulating effect on cardiovascular system. It is also useful for repeated anesthesia in small children such as burn dressing, radiotherapy, etc. The drug should not be used in patients with hypertension, pheochromocytoma, raised intracranial pressure, penetrating eye injury or psychiatric disorder.

Diazepam

It is benzodiazepine tranquillizer and provides anxiolysis, sedation, hypnosis, amnesia and mild muscle relaxation. It is used as premedicant, as an induction agent and as sole anesthetic agent for cardioversion and cardiac catheterization in children. For premedication, it is used in a dose of 0.25 mg/kg IM. It can also be used orally in doses of 0.4 mg/kg. The dose as inducing agent is usually large and ranges from 0.3 to 0.5 mg/kg body weight. With IM route, the absorption is slow, erratic and often incomplete. The injectable solution is irritant and painful and may cause thrombosis following IV injection.

Induction of anesthesia and recovery following diazepam are considerably slow. So it is not much used in pediatric anesthesia. However, it does not cause depression of respiratory and cardiovascular system. It potentiates the effects of nondepolarizing muscle relaxants.

Midazolam

It is a new water-soluble benzodiazepine. It causes sedation, anxiolysis, and anesthesia depending upon the dose. It is used in premedication in a dose 0.07 to 0.08 mg/kg IM. For induction of anesthesia, 0.3 mg/kg may be needed IV. But it has a slower induction time than thiopentone. However, it has a more rapid onset of action than diazepam and a quicker recovery. It does not cause pain on injection. The drug should be injected slowly and the accurate dose should be given. It gives rise to more anterograde amnesia than diazepam. The drug is also indicated for sedation during endoscopy and dentistry.

Etomidate

This is imidazole derivative and a very potent drug. It is used in doses of 0.2 to 0.3 mg/kg IV. Onset of action is rapid, 10 to 65 seconds of injection depending on the rate of injection and the amount of dose. Recovery is also rapid with no residual drowsiness. There is usually no respiratory and cardiovascular depression. Histamine release is absent. But its common disadvantages include pain on injection, myoclonic movements, hiccup, coughing, nausea, and vomiting, and so on.

Etomidate by infusion is contraindicated as it is associated with depression of adrenocortical secretion. A single dose usually lasts 5 to 6 minutes. It is metabolized in the liver and the breakdown products are excreted through kidneys.

Propofol

Propofol is available as 1% and 2% solutions in a lipid emulsion. It is insoluble in water. The anesthetic dose ranges from 2 to 4 mg/kg/body weight. It causes depression of cerebral activity. Intracranial pressure is reduced. It is anticonvulsant. It may sometimes cause apnea during induction. It is a potent intravenous anesthetic agent and produces sleep in one arm-brain circulation time. Induction of anesthesia is usually smooth. But pain along the vein and mild involuntary movements may occur. Recovery is mostly rapid and pleasant. Mild respiratory and cardiovascular depression may be found. Incidence of nausea and vomiting is low. Propofol is rapidly redistributed and it is metabolized by the liver and does not accumulate. Thus, the drug seems to be suitable for continuous infusion. Hypersensitivity reaction following its use is rare.

NEUROLEPTANALGESIA/NEUROLEPTANESTHESIA

In this technique, a combination of potent tranquillizer like droperidol and a short-acting potent analgesic like fentanyl is used to make the patient tranquil and pain-free. It is indicated mostly in procedures performed under local anesthesia. The neuroleptanalgesia essentially needs some cooperation from the patients and thus it is not much helpful in children. However, in older children it can be tried.

In neuroleptanesthesia also a combination of droperidol and phenoperidine is used to supplement nitrous oxide with or without muscle relaxants. The technique is easy and mostly safe even in children of all ages. This technique is said to maintain the cardiovascular stability and adequate tissue perfusion due to alpha blocking effects of droperidol.

Fentanyl is a potent analgesic; 0.05 mg fentanyl has the analgesic potency of 10 mg morphine or 100 mg pethidine. It may cause respiratory depression, myosis, nausea and vomiting. Effects on cardiovascular system is minimal. In children, it may cause bradycardia and a mild fall in blood pressure. Postoperative muscle rigidity may be found in some cases.

Phenoperidine is also a potent drug; 1 mg phenoperidine is equianalgesic to 100 mg pethidine. The drug causes profound respiratory depression. It has little effect on cardiovascular system in clinical doses. It can be given IV, IM or orally.

Droperidol is a neuroleptic drug of the butyrophenone series. It causes mental detachment, absence of voluntary movements, mild alpha blocking effect and inhibition of chemoreceptor trigger zone which controls nausea and vomiting. It usually does not cause respiratory and cardiovascular depression. It may cause extrapyramidal dyskinesia, particularly in large doses.

Phenoperidine and *droperidal* combination is most popular both for neuroleptanalgesia and neuroleptanesthesia. In neuroleptanalgesia where nitrous oxide is not being used, droperidol 0.2 mg/kg and phenoperidine 0.05 to 0.1 mg/kg with increments of 0.025 mg/kg body weight are mostly satisfactory. But in neuroleptanesthesia where nitrous oxide is being used, phenoperidine 0.025 mg/kg and droperidol 0.2 mg/kg may be successfully given.

OPIOIDS AND RELATED DRUGS

Morphine

Morphine is the time-honored narcotic analgesic and still the drug by which other analgesics are compared. It causes analgesia by elevating the pain threshold at spinal and thalamic levels and diminishing the emotional factor of the limbic systems. It causes nausea and vomiting by stimulating chemoreceptor trigger zone in the medulla. It causes direct depression of medullary respiratory center. There is mild hypotension due to reduction in vasoconstriction tone and histamine release. Other features include myosis, cough suppression, increase in smooth muscle tone, reduced gastrointestinal motility and addiction.

Morphine may be used in preoperative sedation but in modern anesthesia there is little indication for narcotic premedication. However, it is indicated in presence of pain. It is also indicated for children with cyanotic congenital heart disease preoperatively. Neonates are sensitive to morphine mostly due to the permeability to blood-brain barrier. Morphine is also used to control the postoperative pain. Usual dose in pediatrics is 0.1 mg/kg IM. Morphine crosses the placental barrier and there may be profound respiratory depression of the neonates.

The correct dose of the narcotics should always be evaluated and one should be careful to avoid the risk of respiratory depression. When administered IM or IV peak analgesia occurs in 90 minutes and 20 minutes respectively and duration of effect is roughly 4 hours.

Pethidine

Pethidine hydrochloride is a synthetic narcotic analgesic agent. It is widely used in premedication and for postoperative analgesia. It is also used during anesthesia to supplement analgesia. Usual pediatric dose ranges from 1 to 1.5 mg/kg body weight IM or IV.

It is a potent analgesic, about one-tenth as powerful as morphine. It relieves all types of pain, particularly those related with plain muscle spasm, except biliary colic. It has atropine like actions causing dry mouth, dilated pupils, etc. It is reported not to release histamine in significant amounts. It may cause depression of respiration and cardiovascular system. Usual side effects may include sweating, hypotension, nausea, vomiting, vertigo, and so on. Pethidine passes through placental barrier and blood-brain barrier significantly. Narcotics are better avoided in children less than 6 months of age due to the unpredictable response in this age group.

Pentazocine

It is benzomorphan derivative. It was introduced as nonnarcotic analgesic but also shares properties with narcotic analgesics. It is one-fourth to one-third as potent as morphine. It causes analgesia, sedation and respiratory depression. Cardiovascular changes are little. Nausea and vomiting may occur. It may produce dysphoria. It crosses the placenta to lesser extent. It is less cumulative and mostly metabolized in the body. Usual dose in children is 1 mg/kg body weight orally or intramuscularly. It can be used IV in a dose ranging from 0.25 to 0.04 mg/kg.

Naloxone Hydrochloride

Naloxone, a derivative of oxymorphone, is a narcotic antagonist. All the effects of opioids such as respiratory depression, sedation and hypotension are reversed. It is also an antagonist to the narcotic effects of pentazocine unlike nalorphine or levallorphan. Naloxone is used in a dose of 0.01 mg/kg IV in children. It has a rapid onset of reaction within 1 minute of IV injection and duration of effect is roughly 30 minutes. Naloxone is the drug of choice in opioid analgesic induced depression in the neonate.

ANTICHOLINERGIC DRUGS

Atropine Sulfate

It is a parasympatholytic anticholinergic drug. It is widely used in premedication. It causes marked drying of secretions and inhibition of salivation and may reduce the coughing and respiratory tract irritation caused by inhalational anesthetics. It protects the patient against the vagal overactivity produced by anesthetic drugs like halothane, visceral traction or endotracheal intubation. Atropine causes tachycardia, dilated pupils, central nervous system effects (sedation or excitation), dilatation of the vessels of face, inhibition of sweating and thereby rise of body temperature, particularly in children. It is a mild antiemetic. It reduces the tone and peristalsis of the gut and urinary tract. Usual dose in children is 0.02 mg/kg body weight IM or IV.

In the reversal of neuromuscular block caused by nondepolarizing muscle relaxants, atropine sulfate is given prior to or with neostigmine to antagonize its muscarinic effects.

Atropine should be avoided in premedication in presence of pyrexia, thyrotoxicosis, in cardiovascular disease and in children with glaucoma.

Hyoscine Hydrobromide

It is an alternative anticholinergic drug with better antisalivary and drying effects, but weaker vagolytic effects on heart. It is depressant of central nervous system causing drowsiness, sedation, sleep and amnesia. It is a mild respiratory stimulant and may counteract the depressant action of morphine. Mydriasis is briefer than that with atropine. It can cause restlessness and disorientation, particularly in the aged. It possesses good antiemetic property. Hyoscine can be given subcutaneously, IM or IV. In children, the dose is 0.015 mg/kg body weight orally or IM.

Glycopyrrolate

It is a synthetic quarternary ammonium compound and does not cross the blood-brain barrier. So, it does not cause any central nervous system stimulation. It has profound antisialogogue activity. It causes less tachycardia than atropine when given intravenously.

Glycopyrrolate can be used in pediatric premedication in a dose of 1 µg/kg body weight IM. It can also be given by oral or IV route. For decurarization, a dose of 0.2 mg is given IV along with each 1 mg neostigmine. It can be given before or with neostigmine.

ANTIEMETIC DRUGS

Promethazine

It is a phenothiazine group of drug. It has sedative, antihistaminic and anticholinergic effects. It potentiates the effect of hypnotics, narcotics and anesthetic drugs. It reduces the incidence of postanesthetic nausea and vomiting due to its action on chemoreceptor trigger zone. Mild tachycardia may occur, but blood pressure usually remains unchanged. While used alone, it is said to increase the sensitivity of pain (antanalgesic). Bronchial tone may be depressed. It may produce extrapyramidal side effects. It is widely used in premedication. It can be given orally, IM and IV. The pediatric dose is usually 1 mg/kg body weight.

Trimeprazine

It is a phenothiazine derivative, widely used in pediatric premedication by oral route. The drug is a potent central sedative, powerful antihistaminic, antiemetic and a good spasmolytic and antipruritic agent. It has no significant effect on cardiovascular system. It may have some anticholinergic activity. It may potentiate the sedative and anesthetic drugs. The usual dose in pediatric premedication is 1 mg/kg IM or 3 to 4 mg/kg orally.

Prochlorperazine

Prochlorperazine, a phenothiazine derivative is a potent and effective antiemetic agent. It has less sedative effects than other phenothiazines. It has weak antihistaminic and spasmolytic actions. Cardiovascular effects are negligible. The drug can be given 2.5 to 5 mg orally in children. It can also be given by IM route.

Metoclopramide

Metoclopramide, a derivative of procainamide, is a potent antiemetic drug. It increases the rate of gastric emptying, relaxes the pylorus, dilates the duodenal bulb and causes some increase in peristalsis of the gut. It controls nausea and vomiting, acting both centrally and locally. The drug does not potentiate the narcotic or anesthetic agents. No respiratory depression occurs in usual clinical doses. It does not prolong anesthesia awakening time. Overdose may cause drowsiness, restlessness, dystonic muscle movements and extrapyramidal effects.

MUSCLE RELAXANTS

Soon after the introduction of muscle relaxants in adult anesthetic practice in 1940, their use in infants and children also started. But the practice did not become much popular as muscle relaxants were thought to be dangerous in pediatric patients as these might cause difficulty in re-establishing spontaneous respiration. However, the advent of neostigmine as curare antagonist in 1942 by Koppany, advanced monitoring devices of neuromuscular block, effective measures for prolonged ventilation and pioneer research trials on children proved the potentiality and safety of muscle relaxants in pediatric anesthesia.

Muscle relaxants are traditionally classified into two groups, the depolarizing and nondepolarizing drugs. Of the depolarizing group, suxamethonium is the only muscle relaxant in common use. Of the nondepolarizing agents, gallamine, tubocurarine, pancuronium, vecuronium and atracurium are being widely used. Alcuronium, metocurine and fazadinum are not much popular. The newer muscle relaxants like mivacurium, doxacurium and pipecuronium are still under clinical trial and seem to be useful in modern anesthetic practice. However, the drugs have their own merits and demerits and these should be evaluated for the individual child on the basis of risk-benefit ratio.

Newborn and infants are in some respects different from adults in addition to their small size. There are some basic differences between the effects of neuromuscular blocking drugs in newborn and adult and there is wide variation in response to drugs depending on absorption, distribution, metabolism and excretion of the drug concerned. It seems better to understand the various factors affecting the sensitivity of muscle relaxants in children.

1. Maturation of neuromuscular transmission: It is usually said that the neonate is mostly sensitive to nondepolarizing drugs due to myasthenic characteristics. There is no doubt that during the first few months following birth, the end plates of the newborn undergo some changes. At birth, the muscle fibers are sensitive to acetylcholine throughout their length, only after a few weeks the normal adult end plate sensitivity develops. Moreover, the end plate potentials are

greater in amplitude, but are less frequent in neonates than in adults. However, it is now thought that the so-called increased sensitivity of nondepolarizers is most probably due to poor respiratory reserve and dependence on diaphragm rather than the myasthenic response of normal neuromuscular function. Moreover, due to shorter elimination half-life and greater clearance of the drugs like tubocurarine, repeat doses are often needed.

Thus, following neonatal period or at most 6 months of age the child usually behaves as an adult on his body weight basis. So, for surgical relaxation a scaled down adult dose can be used judiciously and confidently. Residual paralysis or difficulty in reversal at the end of anesthesia is mostly associated with acid-base imbalance, electrolyte imbalance, or hypothermia. Correction of these usually restores the muscle activity to normal. Routine monitoring of neuromuscular transmission with a nerve stimulator is always recommended.

Infants are said to be resistant to depolarizing muscle relaxants. The dose of suxamethonium is approximately twice the adult dose, that is about 2 mg/kg. This is mostly related to distribution of drug in the relatively larger extracellular space, smaller body mass and greater muscle blood flow in children. Pseudocholinesterase level is usually low in early childhood.

2. Dosage based on body weight/surface area: It is said that on the basis of a body weight/dose relationship, the infants are resistant to depolarizing drugs but are as sensitive as adults to curare. But on the basis of surface area/dose relationship, the infant shows a sensitivity similar to adult towards suxamethonium, but increased sensitivity towards curare. Considerable overdose may result, if curare is calculated on the basis of body surface area.

3. Potentiation by inhalational drugs: Interaction of nondepolarizing muscle relaxants with inhalational agents is well known. Halothane and other volatile anesthetic agents potentiate the action of tubocurarine and this should be taken into account in assessing the effect of nondepolarizing muscle relaxants in infants.

4. Variation in protein binding: After intravenous injection into the circulation, all drugs are bound to plasma proteins to a certain extent. Tubocurarine mostly binds to gammaglobulin, alcuranium to albumin, gallamine to beta and gammaglobulin and pancuronium to globulin and albumin. The availability of free drug to reach the end plate is also dependent on the qualitative affinity of plasma protein. The qualitative binding is said to increase with age, so that more drug is bound per molecule of protein and that might cause decreasing sensitivity of tubocurarine with increasing age.

Depolarizing Muscle Relaxants

Suxamethonium

It is excellent for providing quick and reliable intubating condition including 'crash' induction where speed of induction is of prime importance. The drug acts by holding the ion channel open and thus prevents repolarization. Usual dose in children is 2 mg/kg body weight. It has rapid onset of action and endotracheal intubation can be done satisfactorily within 60 seconds. Duration of clinical relaxation is brief, ranging from 3 to 5 minutes, because of its rapid hydrolysis by plasma pseudocholinesterase. Duration of effect may be roughly 10 minutes.

Side effects of suxamethonium

i. Intragastric pressure is usually less in infants and there may even be fall following administration of suxamethonium. Older children mayhave some rise of intragastric pressure and it may be due to more intense muscular fasciculations.
ii. There may be transient rise of *intraocular pressure*. It is partly due to contraction of extraocular muscle and partly due to increase in arterial and venous pressure.
iii. Cardiovascular effects—Transient bradycardia is common. It is entirely parasymapthomimetic and can be prevented and treated with IV atropine.
iv. In younger age group, the incidence of muscle *fasciculations* and *myalgia* is less in comparison to older age group. But there is no correlation between them.
v. Prolonged action—Deficiency or abnormality of the enzyme pseudocholinesterase will lead to prolongation of its effects. *Dual block* may also occur following repeated administration. Lack of muscle fasciculations and the early tendency for the neuromuscular block to change to a phase II block with its associated characteristics (tetanic fade, posttetanic facilitation and reversal with anticholinesterase drug) is said to be the myasthenic characteristics of newborn.
vi. In normal children, the degree of *potassium efflux* is less than that in adults.
vii. Suxamethonium is notorious for initiating *malignant hyperpyrexia* in susceptible children. Masseter spasm may be the early sign.
viii. Muscle damage may occur and there is a marked rise of serum creatine phosphokinase (CPK) level. There may be myoglobinuria.
ix. Muscle *hypertonus* may be seen in cases of mytonia congenita.

Nondepolarizing Muscle Relaxants

1. The doses of nondepolarizing muscle relaxants in children are as follows:
   - Tubocurarine 0.5 to 0.6 mg/kg body weight (0.1 mg/kg)
   - Gallamine 1.5 to 2 mg/kg body weight (0.5 mg/kg)
   - Pancuronium 0.08 to 0.1 mg/kg body weight (0.015 mg/kg)
   - Vecuronium 0.08 to 0.1 mg/kg body weight (0.015 mg/kg)
   - Atracurium 0.3 to 0.6 mg/kg body weight (0.15 mg/kg).

   The bolus or the intubating dose and the maintenance dose in brackets are shown. The dose in children above 6 months of age should be calculated according to body weight. It is more or less same as in adult, but should be scaled down and titrated against the need of the child. Neonates and the infants below 6 months should get less amount as they are sensitive to nondepolarizing muscle relaxants. The maintenance or top-up dose should be restricted to one-tenth of the intubating dose in the case of neonates and one-third to one-sixth in the case of older children. Relaxant drugs should be well-diluted to prevent inadvertent overdoses, as for example, pancuronium and vecuronium upto 0.02 mg/ml, tubocurarine 1 mg/ml and suxamethonium 2.5 mg/ml.

2. The duration of effect and clinical relaxation of muscle relaxants commonly used in children are as follows:

	Duration of effect	Duration of clinical relaxation
Tubocurarine	30 to 60 minutes	20 to 30 minutes
Gallamine	20 to 40 minutes	20 to 30 minutes
Pancuronium	45 to 120 minutes	30 minutes
Vecuronium	30 to 45 minutes	15 minutes
Atracurium	20 to 40 minutes	20 minutes

Duration of clinical relaxation is the time till recovery of neuromuscular transmission by twitch height to a level of 25% of control twitch. Total duration of effect is the time till the recovery upto 90% of twitch height. Suxamethonium, the depolarizing agent is, no doubt, short-acting, 3 to 5 minutes, and till now it seems to have no alternative so far as its rapid onset of action and short duration of effect are concerned. Next are intermediate acting. Amongst the nondepolarizers, vecuronium and atracurium provide 15 to 20 minutes of clinical relaxation. The others are long-acting, clinical relaxation ranging from 20 to 30 minutes. In the case of pancuronium, the total duration of effect may last for 120 minutes, but the period of clinical relaxation is 30 minutes on average.

3. The common side effects of nondepolarizing muscle relaxants are as follows:

	Histamine release	Ganglion block	Vagal block	Sympathomimetic effect
Tubocurarine	++	++		
Gallamine			++	
Pancuronium	–	–	+	+
Atracurium	+	–	–	–
Vecuronium	–	–	–	–

Vecuronium lacks any serious side effects such as histamine release, ganglion blockade, vagal blockade and sympathomimetic effect. Tubocurarine causes histamine release and ganglion blockade. Gallamine causes vagal blockade. Pancuronium causes vagal block and sympathomimetic effect and atracurium causes mild histamine release.

Gallamine

It is a potent synthetic nondepolarizing muscle relaxant. Its pediatric use is much limited as it causes tachycardia. Tachycardia may be detrimental in presence of pre-existing tachycardia and in certain cardiac diseases. But it may by useful in prevention of oculocardiac reflex during strabismus surgery in children. Gallamine is almost entirely excreted by kidneys.

Tubocurarine

It is a potent muscle relaxant and provides excellent intubating condition. It has ganglion blocking effect and can release histamine. But it produces less hypotension in children than in adults. Neuromuscular block is more prolonged in younger children. Reversal is excellent following atropine (0.02 to 0.04 mg/kg) and neostigmine (0.05 to 0.08 mg/kg) depending on the original dose and the time of reversal. Excretion is through both biliary and renal routes.

Alcuronium

It is a potent muscle relaxant. A dose of 0.03 mg/kg body weight IV produces excellent intubating condition in about 60 seconds. Duration of effect ranges from 20 to 40 minutes and that of clinical relaxation is about 20 minutes. Mild histamine release may occur. In children, mild tachycardia and rise of blood pressure may occur, but in adults hypertensive response is mostly absent. Reversal of myoneural block is easy with atropine and neostigmine.

Fazadinium

The usual intubating dose in 1 mg/kg body weight IV. Duration of effect is about 60 minutes and that of clinical relaxation is about 20 minutes. It produces profound muscular relaxation within 2 to 3 minutes. Mild tachycardia may occur due to its vagal blocking effect. It is not much popular in clinical anesthesia.

Pancuronium

It is a long-acting nondepolarizing muscle relaxant and is more potent than curare. Intubation time is somewhat prolonged, about 90 seconds. Tachycardia and mild rise of arterial blood pressure may occur. Tachycardia may be disadvantageous in children who normally have rapid heart rate. It is excreted by both biliary and renal routes.

Vecuronium

It is a useful relaxant in the case of children in doses of 0.1 mg/kg body weight, but with intermediate duration of action. It provides satisfactory clinical relaxation for about 15 minutes and can be easily reversed. Smaller doses of neostigmine are needed for reversal and even spontaneous recovery may occur. It can be used in infusion technique. It does not cause histamine release and lacks serious side effects.

Rocuronium

This is a steroid-based nondepolarizing muscle relaxant. The usual dose is 0.5 mg/kg/body weight for endotracheal intubation. It can be used in infusion and the rate may vary according to response. The duration of action ranges from 25 to 40 minutes.

The drug has minimal adverse effects on cardiovascular system. Complete respiratory paralysis occurs within 2 minutes. Rocuronium provides satisfactory intubating condition within 60 seconds, if given a larger dosage of 0.8 to 1 mg/kg. It can be reversed successfully 15 minutes after an intubating dose. The drug is metabolized in liver and excreted mainly by kidneys. Histamine release is negligible. Its neuromuscular block is potentiated by antibiotics, particularly aminoglycosides. The effect is related to prejunctional and postjunctional membrane stabilization.

Atracurium

It is potent muscle relaxant and unique in the sense that it is not dependent on liver, kidney and enzymatic breakdown for its elimination. It is self-destroyed by Hofmann degradation at normal body pH and temperature. It is also broken down by ester hydrolysis. It is not cumulative and can be used in infusion technique. The drug provides short duration of action and fast recovery. Mild histamine release can occur, but major side effects are rare.

Cisatracurium

It is a new potent neuromuscular blocking agent and resembles atracurium. It has an ED_{95} of 0.05 mg/kg. The usual dose is 0.1 mg/kg to achieve good intubating condition. The duration of action following a single dose ranges from 20 to 30 minutes. Complete respiratory paralysis occurs within 1.5 to 2 minutes. It has minimal adverse effects on cardiovascular system. The drug may be useful in patients with hepatorenal failure as it is metabolized by Hoffmann degradation which is spontaneous and occurs at normal body pH and temperature. Side effects are usually minimal. Metabolites include laudanosine and a monoquarternary acrylate. It does not cause histamine release. It does not accumulate in the body to a significant degree. It can be used through infusion technique.

ANTAGONISM OF MUSCLE RELAXANTS

The goal of recovery from the effect of neuromuscular blocking agents is primarily to restore the ability of the child to breathe adequately, cough efficiently, swallow and protect the airway. Neostigmine in combination with either atropine or glycopyrrolate is used to reverse the nondepolarizing neuromuscular block. The doses of drugs are roughly as follows: neostigmine 0.05 to 0.08 mg/kg; atropine 0.02 to 0.04 mg/kg; glycopyrrolate 0.004 mg/kg. The dose of neostigmine depends on the amount of the initial dose of muscle relaxants and the time interval between the last dose and the time of reversal. However, children require smaller doses of neostigmine as compared to adults. The more intense the paralysis, the slower is the effect of an anticholinesterase. Adequate reversal should be assessed through the neuromuscular monitor and also clinically. A child crying loudly with good strong movements is mostly safe. Clinical criteria for assessing recovery from neuromuscular block are: (1) Head lift for at least 5 seconds, (2) sustained hand grip, (3) sustained arm lift, (4) lifting both legs, (5) wide open eyes, (6) absence of nystagmus and/or diplopia, (7) normal voice/crying, (8) coordinated swallowing, (9) tongue protrusion, (10) vital capacity more than 15 ml/kg, and (11) negative inspiratory force of a magnitude more than 32 cm water pressure (55 cm water pressure in the case of adults).

For monitoring of neuromuscular block, a nerve stimulator can be used. It provides a small stimulating current to a nerve at predetermined intervals and records the response of distal muscle groups. Usually, a train of four stimuli is used where four supramaximal electrical impulses at 0.5 seconds intervals are given to record the twitch response. The number of twitches denotes the level of block as no twitch means 100% block, 1 twitch means 90% block, 2 twitches mean 80% block and 3 twitches denote 75% block. Use of accelerometer makes the assessment better, as it can measure the amplitude of twitches. Tetanic response can also be used. Fade during tetany indicates the presence of residual block and absence of fade indicates adequate reversal of block.

Neostigmine

It is an anticholinestase drug widely used as an antagonist to nondepolarizing muscle relaxants. It acts by decreasing the breakdown of released acetlylcholine and thereby prolonging the lifetime to acetylcholine at the neuromuscular junction, so that it can compete with the relaxant for occupation of the nicotinic receptors. However, its muscarinic effects such as bradycardia, hypotension, profuse salivary, bronchial secretions, bronchospasm, stimulation of smooth muscles, particularly of hollow viscera, etc. should be obtunded by prior administration of antimuscarinic agents such as atropine or glycopyrrolate. Atropine and neostigmine may be given in combined form safely. When the drugs are given separately, atropine should be given first, when tachycardia will occur. One should wait for 5 minutes to obtain the antisialogogue effect, then give neostigmine gently. Overdose of the drugs should always be avoided. Neostigmine is also used in the treatment of myasthenia gravis.

LOCAL ANESTHETIC DRUGS

Lignocaine

Lignocaine is the standard local anesthetic and most commonly used for regional anesthesia in children. The onset time is rather slow and the duration of analgesia is usually short, less than 1 hour. However, addition of adrenaline may prolong the effect. It is available in a wide range of concentrations from 0.05 to 4% solutions. The maximum safe dose of plain lignocaine is 3 mg/kg and that of lignocaine with adrenaline is 7 mg/kg. The drug is relatively less toxic. The drug is also effective in the treatment of cardiac dysrhythmias. It is also being used in the management of neonatal convulsion.

Bupivacaine

The drug is being widely used as a local anesthetic and is said to be more potent than lignocaine. Bupivacaine has increased lipid solubility and protein binding compared with lignocaine and this leads to prolonged duration of action. Adrenaline may be added as it can decrease absorption and increase the quality of block. It is available as 0.75%, 0.5%, and 0.25% solutions. Bupivacaine can be used for nerve blocks and epidural analgesia. Bupivacaine causes sensory block more efficiently than motor block. It is not recommended for intravenous regional anesthesia as it is relatively more toxic on the heart in an overdose. Maximum safe dose of bupivacaine is 2 mg/kg and with adrenaline it is 2.5 mg/kg.

CHAPTER 9

Preanesthetic Assessment

It is a mandatory that the anesthetists should visit his child patient to assess fitness for anesthesia and surgery and to develop a good relationship with the patient. It also helps to allay preoperative fear, anxiety, tension and uncertainty through proper reassurance, careful explanation and an adequate sympathetic attitude. It may be necessary to discuss about the illness with the parents of the patients and give them a simple and factual explanations about the problems of the patients. The free visiting by parents may be advantageous and the child may not feel bored due to separation from his parents. But the parents should not pass on their fears and anxieties to their children. The anesthetist should gain confidence to the children and parents.

The psychological state of the child may influence the outcome of surgical procedures. Fear makes the child noncooperative, causes resistance to anesthesia and may lead to postoperative reaction and even psychotic episodes. Clinically, fear causes tachycardia and tachypnea. It may increase the metabolic rate and secretion of catecholamines. Hence, fear should always be alleviated as far as practicable either by proper reassurance or by pharmacological approach (by giving anxiolytic drugs).

Beside the psychological considerations, preanesthetic assessment should be done with adequate history taking, physical examination and special investigations. This assessment should determine the operative risk, if any. It will also enable the anesthetist to choose the proper anesthetic agents and techniques, and to take sensible precautions for better and safe anesthesia.

HISTORY

Relevant history of the presenting illness should always be taken. Previous medical history is also of great interest and direct questions should be asked to parents, particularly in respect of jaundice, renal disease, respiratory disease and cardiovascular disease. Enquiries should be made of any congenital defect; presence of one congenital anomaly may be associated with others. Drug allergy, if any, should also be noted. A familial history of some hereditary conditions such as malignant hyperpyrexia, dystrophia, myotonica, porphyria, cholinesterase abnormalities and so on should be sought for, as these imply anesthetic problems and need proper investigations.

Drug history has certain anesthetic implications. Children receiving steroid therapy may suffer from iatrogenic adrenocortical insufficiency. Certain antibiotics like streptomycin, neomycin, kanamycin, polymixin, and tetracycline may potentiate the nondepolarizing muscle relaxants. Sedatives and tranquillizers often potentiate the effects of anesthetic drugs. Diuretics may produce hypokalemia and this may lead to arrhythmias, potentiation of the effects of muscle relaxants and precipitation of digitalis toxicity. Suxamethonium may cause severe ventricular arrhythmias in digitalized child.

Previous anesthesia record, if any, should be thoroughly examined. It may help to detect any anesthetic complication like postoperative nausea and vomiting, jaundice, efficacy of previous anesthetics, any difficulty in intubation, etc. Very often children need repeat anesthesia and in such cases halothane should not be repeated within 3 months of halothane anesthesia.

PHYSICAL EXAMINATION

The clinical assessment should include name, age and body weight of the child. These are most important as drugs should be calculated as per body weight and various equipment such as endotracheal tube, etc. specific to the child need to be prepared. The average weight of a child is calculated as (age in years + 2) multiplied by 3 kg.

A full physical examination should be done and must be documented in records before subjecting the child to anesthesia and surgery. It should include general condition, color of the child, nutrition, hydration and all the systems, particularly cardiovascular system and respiratory system.

A normal healthy child should have normally 15 g of hemoglobin per 100 ml of blood. Anemic patient may pose various problems during anesthesia. A lower limit of 80% hemoglobin concentration is a basic guideline of demarcation between operability and nonoperability. But the sound decision should only be made considering the individual situation and evaluation. Sensible precautions should be taken when anesthesia is undertaken in anemic patients and hypoxia and hypotension should be avoided at all costs. Often the nutritional state of the child may parallel the hemoglobin level. In elective surgery, drug treatment of anemia may be helpful. But in semiurgent cases, preoperative blood transfusion is indicated, particularly for all major operations, when the Hb content is below 10 g%. The amount of blood to be given is calculated as normal blood volume × Hb rise required, divided by Hb of blood given. Hb of whole blood is taken as 10 g% and that of packed cell 20 g%. Blood volume, upto 1 year of age ranges from 90 to 100 ml/kg, between 1 to 2 years of age 80 ml/kg and above 2 years of age, it is 75 ml/kg body weight.

Jaundice indicates liver dysfunction. Hypoxia, hypercarbia, hypotension and hepatotoxic drugs and anesthetic agents should be avoided in such cases. *Cyanosis* implies hypoxemia and there may be congenital cyanotic heart disease. *Edema* may be found in case of severe anemia, cardiac failure or in renal failure. Dehydration means fluid deficiency in the body and it should always be corrected as far as practicable before subjecting the patient to anesthesia and surgery.

Particular attention should be paid to detect any anatomical characteristics which make endotracheal intubation difficult. The teeth should be examined, there may be damaged or loose teeth. Full opening of mouth and extension of cervical spine should be confirmed. Receding lower jaw with obtuse mandibular angles, protruding incisors with relative overgrowth of premaxilla, and long high-arched palate with a long narrow mouth may pose difficulty in intubation. Treacher Collins syndrome and Pierre-Robin syndrome may be associated with difficult intubation.

All vital signs such as pulse, respiration, blood pressure and body temperature should be recorded. In case of pyrexia, there may be an infection and operation should be postponed, if possible.

The child may have congenital cardiac defects. Growth retardation and anemia may be related to cardiac disease. Cyanosis, finger and toe clubbing may also be associated. Some children with severe heart disease may have lung infection. In case of cardiac failure, there are edema, increased venous pressure and large liver and heart size. In infants, the normal liver may be palpable upto 3 cm below the right costal margin decreasing to less than 1 cm at about 5 years of age. Thus, careful check must be made for circulatory problems, cardiac enlargement, murmurs or heart failure. Veins should be inspected for suitable venepuncture sites.

Tachycardia is common in children and premature beats, paroxysmal tachycardia of supraventricular origin and heart block are the common arrhythmias in small children. Sinus arrhythmia is common in older children. Hypertension is not common in children, but if present, its exact cause should be judged. This may be due to renal disease, coarctation, patent ductus arteriosus, pheochromocytoma, thyrotoxicosis, and rarely essential hypertension.

RESPIRATORY SYSTEM

Usual complications are cough, dyspnea and expectoration. In the case of upper respiratory tract infection, there may be purulent secretions and pyrexia. In such cases, operation should better be postponed, as there is increased risk of laryngospasm, bronchospasm, bleeding and bacteremia.

In case of common cold, elective operation should be avoided as it increases the risk of postoperative lung complications. In urgent cases, it may have to be done under antibiotic cover.

The presence of bronchospasm carries a significant risk. The patient should be adequately treated before anesthesia. Certain drugs like opiates, thiopentone and beta blockers should be avoided in such cases as these may precipitate bronchospasm.

A careful examination of ventilation is essential as insufficient air movement may be associated with many disease conditions. Signs of an obstructed airway should be looked for very carefully for its early detection. The existence of minor ventilatory impairment in the preoperative period may become a major hazard during the course of anesthesia and in postoperative period.

OTHER SYSTEMS

A healthy child presented for surgery may not be needed to undertake all full examinations of other systems, but in presence of pre-existing impairment of systems like central nervous system, urinary or hepatic system, the relevant thorough examinations should be made and recorded. Meningocele, myelomeningocele, hydrocephalus, etc. are common among infants and children and thus assessment of central nervous system is essential in such cases. Impairment of renal function or hepatic function may be present in children. Preoperative recognition of such malfunctions is important so that the proper precautions can be taken during anesthesia. Because of poor vitamin K absorption in obstructive jaundice, vitamin K should be given IM preoperatively to lower the prolonged prothrombin time. In the case of neonates, vitamin K should always be given intramuscularly in preoperative period as immature hepatic enzymes may not synthesize it.

Children with mental subnormality and epilepsy need special attention. Epileptic children may occasionally be on a course of steroid therapy.

ROUTINE INVESTIGATIONS

Urine analysis should be carried out for acidity, specific gravity, albumin and glucose. Occasionally suspected diabetes mellitus may be detected.

Full blood count and hemoglobin estimation should also be done. Total count, differential count, blood group, bleeding time and clotting time should be done. Hb estimation will reveal previously undiagnosed anemia and also provide an indication of the amount of blood needed to be transfused.

SPECIAL INVESTIGATIONS

Urea and Serum Electrolytes

It may be needed in the case of children receiving diuretics, antihypertensives or digoxin or in the case of patients with dehydration, metabolic diseases, etc.

- Chest X-ray: It is indicated in the case of children with cardiac and/or pulmonary diseases.
- Cervical X-ray: It may be needed in some cases with anticipated difficult intubation.
- ECG: It is indicated particularly in cardiac cases.
- Acid-base status: Arterial blood gas analysis should be done in major thoracic and vascular surgery. These measurement essentially imply the respiratory assessment of the patient.
- Liver function test: These are needed in the cases with pre-existing liver diseases.

Investigations like respiratory function tests, blood gas analysis, thyroid function tests and so on are required only when these are specially indicated. Sophisticated pulmonary and cardiac function tests are not practicable in the case of all pediatric patients.

Considering all these preoperative studies, the anesthetist should identify the risk, if any. If there is any risk or problem, this should be quantified and tackled with great care as far as practicable before subjecting the patient to anesthesia and surgery.

Calculation of children's body weight on average
Neonate : 3 kg
4 months of age: 6 kg
1–8 years of age : 2 x age + 9 kg
8–13 years of age : 3 x age kg

CHAPTER 10
Preanesthetic Preparation and Premedication

PREANESTHETIC PREPARATION

Adequate reassurance, explanations and a good rapport between the anesthetist and child are essential to allay preoperative fear, anxiety and tension. Older children may express a preference for either inhalation or intravenous induction and this should be accepted, if not otherwise impossible. Parents should also be consulted.

The child should be fit for anesthesia. Presence of upper respiratory tract infection may be a contraindication to anesthesia in elective cases. Presence of pyrexia mostly indicates infection and thus the exact etiology should be known and treated accordingly before subjecting the patient to anesthesia.

Food should be restricted for at least 4 hours before induction of anesthesia. Children under 1 year of age may be given a drink of clear fluid like 5% dextrose solution 10 ml/kg body weight 4 hours preoperatively. Normal human breast milk passes through stomach more rapidly than does any other formula. Thus the child requires at least 4 hours of fasting after a breast milk feeding. In children of 1 to 5 years, milk 10 ml/kg body weight may be allowed. No solid food is allowed after midnight. But the emptying time of the stomach may be delayed by emotion, fear or in presence of peritoneal irritation for more than 12 hours. Therefore, a Ryles tube preferably be passed into the stomach and the gastric contents and secretions aspirated, particularly in suspected cases. In emergency cases, operation should be delayed, if possible allowing the stomach to empty. In dire emergency, gastric aspiration should be done. Prolonged preanesthetic fasting may lead to hypoglycemia, ketosis, fluid deficit and electrolyte and acid-base imbalance. Normal blood glucose level in infants is approximately 40 mg/100 ml. In cases of hypoglycemia, the child may look pale, become restless and sweating. There may be headache, convulsion and even coma. It may occur in preoperative or in postoperative period. To prevent hypoglycemia, all children should have glucose containing fluid infusion during surgery.

In case of neonates, vitamin K 1 mg should be given intramuscularly in the preoperative period as immature hepatic enzymes may not synthesize it.

The degree of dehydration and electrolyte imbalance, if any, should be carefully assessed and adequately treated in the preoperative period. Peripheral veins should be inspected with regard to intravenous induction and the establishment of intravenous infusion. In cases of inaccessible veins, a cut down technique should be adopted even in the preoperative period.

Urinary bladder should be emptied, particularly in case of children before sending the patient to operation theater. This is to prevent him voiding urine during induction of anesthesia and to promote surgical access to the pelvis. Full bladder causes distress, restlessness and discomfort to the child under premedication or when operated under local anesthesia.

Artificial limbs, artificial eyes and shoes should be taken off. Care should be taken about the loose teeth and these may be removed, if necessary. No tight clothing, no lipstick or nail varnish are allowed. Adequate oral hygiene should be maintained. OT dress should be given. Patient should have an identification label around his wrist or neck.

Patient's consent to surgical treatment is absolutely essential. In case of children, parents or guardian must sign and consent to anesthesia and surgery. Absence of written consent of anesthesia and operation is an absolute indication of postponement of operation.

Night sedation may be helpful, particularly for older children to promote adequate sleep in the night before the day of operation. Several hypnotic drugs such as phenobarbitone, diazepam, trimeprazime, etc. are in common use. These drugs should be given orally.

No routine preparation is needed in extreme emergencies, such as cases with rupture of major vessels, cases with acute upper airway obstruction and in surgery on patients trapped and immobile.

PREMEDICATION

Preanesthetic medication or premedication is indicated to facilitate the induction and maintenance of safe anesthesia and also to bring a smooth recovery from anesthesia.

Main Objectives

The main objectives in patient premedication are as follows:
a. To allay preoperative fear, anxiety and tension.

b. To reduce salivary secretions and secretions of respiratory tract.
c. To provide a degree of vagal block.
d. To protect the patient against the toxic effects of anesthesia.
e. To provide analgesia and thus to potentiate the anesthetic drugs.
f. To reduce the incidences of postoperative complications such as restlessness, nausea, vomiting, etc.

The ideal premedication should be anxiolytic, sedative, amnesic, antisialogogue and vagolytic. It should not adversely affect the body and always be safe and easy to administer. It should not affect the vital centers like the cardiovascular, respiratory and central nervous system. It should facilitate smooth induction of anesthesia and prevent postoperative complications.

Many premedicant drugs have been tried, but no single drug or a combination of drugs possesses all the above mentioned attributes. It is very difficult to prescribe premedication in children as most sedatives and analgesics can easily depress the vital centers. Drug dosages should be estimated on body weight basis accurately. Even a mild overdosage may adversely affect the body. Actually, the premedication should depend on individual patient, the anesthetist's preference and the operation to be performed.

To decrease the fear, anxiety and tension psychological approach seems to be the best method. A well-conducted preoperative visit by a kindly, friendly and honest anesthetist is always helpful. Attention of parents' fears may sometimes be needed.

Various drugs like barbiturates, narcotics, tranquillizers and anticholinergic drugs are used for premedication in the case of infants and children. All have their own merits and demerits and these should be balanced on the basis of risk-benefit ratio. The drugs should be prescribed on a dose for weight basis.

Method of administration should be well-accepted by the child. Children usually dislike injection. *Oral* method is usually well-tolerated, but is unpredictable as it may be vomited out or have unreliable absorption. It should be given at least 90 minutes before induction of anesthesia. *Intramuscular route* provides a reliable effects, but the child may have fear of needles. It should be given at least 45 minutes preoperatively. *Intravenous* route is usually meant for administration of anticholinergics. Narcotics should better be avoided by IV injection in premedication of infants. It is given about 5 minutes before induction of anesthesia. Rectal route is not popular as it is unpredictable due to unreliable absorption of the medicine.

Premedication is not always a routine requirement. Even without premedication, the child may be anesthetized depending upon the individual patient. This is mostly indicated in minor surgery and for day stay procedures. However, routine premedication is recommended as follows: In case of neonates and smaller children only atropine and in case of older children, atropine and sedation are indicated.

Drug sensitivity is greatly increased under certain conditions such as adrenocortical insufficiency, pituitary insufficiency, hepatic or renal dysfunction, myasthenia gravis and so on. Porphyria needs special consideration, because if barbiturates are prescribed in these cases, there may be abdominal pain, vomiting, hematuria, paralysis, and even respiratory arrest.

Besides conventional premedicant drugs certain other drugs are often used in premedication. Hydrocortisone may be needed in the case of children receiving steroid therapy to prevent iatrogenic adrenocortical insufficiency during surgery. Bronchodilator drugs are indicated in asthmatic children to prevent bronchospasm during anesthesia. Ranitidine and metoclopramide may be given to prevent acid aspiration syndrome. Prochlorperazine may be indicated to reduce the incidence of nausea and vomiting. Antibiotics are often used for prevention of infection, particularly for infective endocarditis in children with heart valve lesions.

Sedatives

Barbiturates like quinalbarbitone, phenobarbitone, pentobarbitone, and secobarbitone were used in pediatric premedication for a long time. These usually produce sleep in a child. But sometimes particularly in presence of pain, the child may be restless and uncontrollable. These drugs can be given by either oral or IM route.

Diazepam (0.2 mg/kg body weight) can be used in premedication of infants and children by oral route. It is mostly satisfactory and does not cause respiratory depression or vomiting. But it has poor antisialogogue and no analgesic actions. Trimeprazine tartrate (2 to 4 mg/kg body weight) is much popular in a pediatric premedication. It is a phenothiazine derivative with marked antihistaminic, antiemetic and antisialogogue actions. Promethazine, another phenothiazine derivative, is also widely used either alone or in combination with an analgesic. Promethazine has antihistaminic, sedative and antisialogogue properties. But it has antianalgesic action. It can be given IM or orally in a dose of 1 mg/kg body weight. Trichlorethyl phosphate (trichlophos) is also used in premedication for infants and children. It can be given orally in a dose of 70 mg/kg body weight. It is a good sedative and usually does not cause respiratory and cardiovascular depression. Sedatives are not usually needed in premedication of neonates as they are presumed not be anxious and fearful and the drugs may adversely affect the babies.

Analgesics

These are used in premedication for their sedative and analgesic actions. These are also useful as an adjunct to the anesthetic drugs. They prevent pain and awareness during operation. Morphine is, no doubt, a very potent analgesic, but it may cause respiratory depression and vomiting.

Pethidine, pentazocine and fentanyl are also used. However, premedication with narcotic analgesics is not much popular now, unless there is pain in the preoperative period. Narcotics must not be used in the case of infants less than 6 months of age. Pentazocine is a good analgesic, but it has hallucinogenic effects in conscious subjects.

Anticholinergic Drugs

Amongst anticholinergic drugs, atropine, hyoscine and glycopyrrolate are being widely used in pediatric premedication. These are used for drying of secretions, for their antisalivary and vagolytic action. *Atropine sulfate* is the time honored drug and it is used in a dose of 0.02 mg/kg IM. Atropine is not routinely used, but its use is mandatory when vagotonic drugs like suxamethonium, cyclopropane or halothane are used. It also protects the patient against vagal overactivity caused by visceral traction or endotracheal intubation. During squint surgery atropine should be used to obtund the oculocardiac reflex. Side effects of atropine include tachycardia, dysrhythmia, rise of body temperature, diminished sweating, increased basal metabolic rate and so on. Routine preoperative use of anticholinergic drugs may mask hypoxemia with its accompanying bradycardia. However, routine use of pulse oximetry largely eliminates this problem.

Hyoscine is another anticholinergic agent with better drying effect but weaker vagolytic effect on the heart. As it crosses blood-brain barrier, it produces marked sedation and amnesia. It is antianalgesic. It is used in a dose of 0.015 mg/kg body weight intramuscularly.

Glycopyrrolate is also an anticholinergic drug recently introduced. It is used in a dose of 0.004 mg/kg body weight IM. It has no action on central nervous system, a few cardiovascular effects and an intense antisialogogue effect.

An anticholinergic drug is not usually needed in the case of newborn as vagal tone is low in such cases. Moreover, plugging of the small airways with dry inspissated mucus may occur. But in infants the vagal tone is high and they need atropinization before anesthesia and surgery.

Common drugs and doses in pediatric premedication
Atropine sulfate: 0.02 mg/kg IM
Hyoscine: 0.015 mg/kg IM
Glycopyrrolate: 0.004 mg/kg IM
Pethidine: 1 mg/kg IM
Morphine: 0.1 to 0.2 mg/kg
Pentazocine: 0.2 mg/kg IM
Fentanyl: 0.001 mg/kg IM
Trimeprazine tartrate: 3 mg/kg orally
Diazepam: 0.2 mg/kg orally
Promethazine: 1 mg/kg orally
Trichlorethyl phosphate: 70 mg/kg orally
Pentobarbitone: 2 mg/kg IM or orally
Secobarbitone: 2 mg/kg IM or orally

CHAPTER
11

Anesthetic Management

Anesthetic management of pediatric patients needs meticulous attention and care. A smooth and safe management of anesthesia mostly dictates the outcome of the surgical procedures. Before induction of anesthesia several prerequisites are essential:
1. The child patient should be thoroughly examined. Preanesthetic assessment is most vital.
2. The pediatric anesthetist should understand the psychology of the patient. He should have a good rapport with the child to gain his confidence. Psychological management prior to anesthesia and surgery is most important to allay the preoperative fear, anxiety and tension.
3. The patient should be adequately prepared for anesthesia. Proper premedication in accurate doses and in optimum time schedule should be given. The route of administration may be according to the choice of the patient, if not otherwise contraindicated.
4. The anesthetic room should be quiet and pleasing to the child. All noise and conversations should be forbidden routinely.
5. The anesthetic machine, other equipment and circuit, the suction apparatus, etc. should be well-checked.
6. Monitoring equipment should also be checked.
7. The drugs should be labelled and diluted as needed.
8. A skilled and dedicated assistant is always helpful during the conduct of anesthesia.

INDUCTION OF ANESTHESIA

Methods of induction include intravenous, inhalational, intramuscular and rarely rectally. It seems better to explain the procedures truthfully but unnecessary alarming details should be avoided. It is often helpful to meet the child's special requests or choice of induction technique. The child may be allowed to bring his favorite toy or a similar thing in the operation theater. If not otherwise contraindicated, the parents may accompany the child and reassure the child as far as practicable. But the parents must not show their emotional reactions and disturb the child with their own fear and anxieties.

Intravenous Induction

A very fine needle (preferably 27 s.w.g.) with a sharp bevel should be used. The usual sites of venepuncture are dorsum of the hand, medial aspect of ankle, lateral aspect of foot and scalp veins in infants. The veins in antecubital fossa should better be avoided for the risk of accidental intra-arterial injection. The risk seems to be higher in the case of children due to close proximity of vessels. If the child is already on IV infusion, it may be used for injecting induction agents provided it is running correctly.

Thiopentone sodium is most commonly used. The dose ranges from 2.5 to 4 mg/kg body weight in a 2.5% solution and it provides a smooth and rapid induction. Adequate care is mandatory to prevent extravasation and intra-arterial injection. Methohexitone is also useful (1.5 mg/kg) but it can cause pain during injection. Etomidate and propofol can also be used, but these also produce pain during injection.

At the time of IV induction, some muscle relaxants are used. The doses of commonly used muscle relaxants are as follows: Suxamethonium 2 mg/kg; d-tubocurarine 0.8 mg/kg; pancuronium 0.1 mg/kg; vecuronium 0.1 mg/kg; atracurium 0.5 mg/kg; gallamine 2 mg/kg.

The doses of other common intravenous drug are morphine 0.125 mg/kg, pentazocine 0.25 mg/kg and fentanyl 0.001 mg/kg.

The intravenous induction of anesthesia is mostly pleasant provided the needle prick is done in the first attempt. But the method may not be possible when the venous access is either difficult or nonavailable.

Inhalational Induction

This method of induction is mostly chosen in neonates and in the very small child, when the venous access is either difficult or unavailable and when the child prefers the technique. It may be pleasant, smooth and rapid in experienced hands.

In this method Boyle anesthetic machine with suitable circuit for pediatric anesthesia such as Rees modification of Ayre's T-piece system should be used. Rendell-Baker-Soucek face mask of appropriate size is mostly satisfactory to minimize the dead space. Sometimes Guedel oropharyngeal airway may be needed to get a clear patent airway. The drugs and equipment for rapid endotracheal intubation such as suxamethonium atropine, laryngoscope, endotracheal tubes, suction catheters, etc. should be kept ready at hand.

Halothane is most commonly used and it provides a smooth and rapid induction. Nitrous oxide and oxygen mixture or oxygen alone is used as the carrier gas. The minimum alveolar concentration of anesthetic drugs is usually higher in the case of the children compared to adults. The MAC of halothane is said to be more than 1% in children, but only about 0.8% in adults. The child should have atropine in premedication. In higher doses of halothane, cardiovascular depression may occur.

Nitrous oxide, oxygen and diethyl ether mixture is used for induction. But ether is much irritant to respiratory tract and its stage of excitement is notorious. Nausea and vomiting can also occur. It is now not much popular in modern anesthesia.

Cyclopropane 50% with oxygen provides pleasant and very quick induction. But the drug is not used due to its potential dangers. It causes excessive salivation and respiratory secretions and occasional bradycardia, so prior administration of atropine is essential. It is highly inflammable and much expensive.

Enflurane and isoflurane can also be used in induction. But induction is said to be less smooth. Isoflurane may cause breath holding, coughing and spasm. Overdose of enflurane may cause electroencephalographic changes of epileptiform nature; thus, the dose should be adjusted accordingly.

Methoxyflurane was also being used for induction. But it is not much popular now because of its nephrotoxic effects. However, methoxyflurane induced renal dysfunction is unlikely in children unless a very large dose is given.

Following induction with inhalational agents, endotracheal intubation can be done. However, a relaxant IV may sometimes be needed to get a better intubating condition.

Intramuscular Induction

In this method, ketamine hydrochloride may be used for induction, particularly when the venous access is difficult. In such inductions, ketamine is used in large doses and thus may be associated with prolonged recovery.

Rectal Induction

The method is not much popular possibly due to uncertain absorption with residual depot in the gut, large doses needed and adverse emotional impact. Thiopentone is used for basal narcosis. The dose is 1 g/22 kg (50 lb) given in 5 to 10%-solution by rectal route. Methohexitone can also be used in the rectal route in a dose of 25 mg/kg. Sleep usually comes within 15 minutes.

Mask Anesthesia

Here the child is on spontaneous ventilation. Induction of anesthesia is by inhalational technique and no muscle relaxant is used.

During mask anesthesia the usual equipment for endotracheal intubation such as laryngoscope, endotracheal tubes, suction apparatus and suxamethonium should be kept ready for use, whenever needed. The face mask should fit the contour of the face and minimize the dead space. The Rendell-Baker-Soucek mask is mostly satisfactory for infants and small children. An oropharyngeal airway of suitable size may be needed in some cases, where there is obstruction due to relatively large tongue and adenoid hypertrophy in older children. The mask should be held gently, otherwise the soft laryngeal cartilages and tracheal rings may be compressed by the fingers during mask anesthesia. Care should be taken at the time of positive pressure ventilation; otherwise, large amounts of gases and vapors may enter the stomach causing undue distension of stomach. In such cases, a lubricated Ryles tube may have to be passed into the stomach to aspirate the gases; otherwise, a distended stomach may lead to emergence regurgitation and hamper the breathing of the child.

ENDOTRACHEAL INTUBATION

Endotracheal intubation provides free unobstructed airway, thereby a patent clear airway is guaranteed. It gives best protection against dangers of full stomach. Aspiration of blood, mucus or vomits into lungs is prevented. Ventilation can be controlled or assisted, whenever needed. It is mostly safe, but some hazards such as trauma, reflex disturbances (bronchospasm, cardiac arrhythmia, etc.), disconnection, obstruction and infection are present. However, these hazards can be overcome by adequate care and attention.

Endotracheal intubation and ventilation are mostly indicated in prolonged surgery, intracranial or thoracic operations, operations of the head and neck, operations in the oral cavity, in abnormal positions (prone, sitting or kidney position), in patients with airway or ventilatory problems and where muscle relaxants are to be used. It is also indicated to prevent aspiration of vomitus.

Endotracheal intubation in the case of child is usually difficult in comparison to an adult due to the anatomical and physiological differences. Before intubation, the child must be preoxygenated with 100% oxygen; otherwise, the child will rapidly become hypoxic. In smaller neonates and in small infants with low general condition, an awake intubation may be used where no induction of anesthesia is needed prior to intubation. These patients usually tolerate well the awake (conscious) intubation technique. A high ventilating pressure should not be used before intubation; otherwise, overdistension of stomach will occur.

Preoxygenation

Preoxygenation is important before administration of the induction agent. It is needed to replace air in the functional residual capacity of the lungs with 100% oxygen. This provides a reservoir of oxygen during apnea, if any, during endotracheal intubation. This helps the anesthetist to enable safe endotracheal intubation even without resorting to hand inflation by bag and mask. Hand inflation in the case of children increases the risk of aspiration and regurgitation. Preoxygenation should always be done by application of a close fitting face mask and delivery of 100% inspired oxygen through a proper anesthetic machine for a minimum period of 4 to 5 minutes.

Laryngoscopy

Before laryngoscopy, the teeth should be examined carefully as the children may have loose deciduous teeth. The head of the child should be correctly positioned, in the 'sniffing' position and supported by low head ring. A straight-bladed laryngoscope is passed under to lift the floppy and large epiglottis and expose the larynx. As the larynx is high and anterior in children in comparison to adults, a gentle cricoid pressure by a skilled assistant may sometimes be helpful. A curved blade (Macintosh type) of appropriate size may also be used. But on occasions visualization of glottis in infants and small children may not be easy.

For infants, a neutral head position is vital. The shoulders should be flat on the table surface with moderate extension of the head on the neck, the occiput resting on the same flat surface. Laryngoscope blade should be short and straight to facilitate the view.

Intubation

The correct size of the endotracheal tube should be determined. An ideal tube must be such as to slip through the cricoid ring without effort and large enough to fit it snugly. The size of the tube should be as follows:

Preterm baby: 2.5 mm i.d.
At term: 3 mm to 3.5 mm i.d.
At 6 months: 4 mm i.d.
At 1 year: 4.5 i.d.

Above 1 year of age: $\frac{\text{age in years}}{4} + 4.5$ mm i.d.

At the time of intubation, several tubes of different sizes should be kept, at least half a size larger and half a size smaller, besides the proper predetermined size. It should be noted that the narrowest part of the larynx in infants is at the level of the cricoid ring. Much pressure at that part may cause trauma and thereby subglottic edema. Cuffed tubes are not usually recommended in infants, as these may limit the internal diameter of the tube and increase the resistance and turbulence. Plain red rubber or portex tubes are mostly satisfactory. The length of the endotracheal tube should be: Age in years divided by 2 plus 12 cm in the case of orotracheal tube and plus 15 cm in the case of nasotracheal tube. The endotracheal tube should pass 2.5 cm into the trachea up midway between cricoid and carina. A leak must be present around the tube when positive pressure is applied to the circuit; otherwise, the tube is changed for a smaller size.

The mouth should be lightly packed with sterile rollar gauze soaked with sterile water. This may help the endotracheal tube to stabilize and to absorb excessive secretions. The endotracheal tube must be firmly fixed to the cheeks of the child with stripes of nonallergenic adhesive tape. A bite block may be needed to prevent kinking. Adequate care should be taken to prevent pressure caused by anesthetic hoses, etc. on the child's face or head. Endotracheal connections should have a lumen at least equal to internal diameter of the tube and must be firmly inserted; otherwise, turbulence, resistance and disconnection, etc. may occur.

Ventilation must be checked to ensure that all areas of both lungs are inflating after intubation. Positioning of the head and neck is also important. Extension of the neck may move the tip of the endotracheal tube proximally in the trachea and the flexion may advance the tip. This should be borne in mind during positioning.

The endotracheal tube is connected with Jackson Rees modification of Ayre's T-piece system by means of a Magill connection and then with Boyle anesthetic machine to provide fresh gas flow. Care should be taken to provide least resistance to flow and avoid airflow turbulence.

MAINTENANCE OF ANESTHESIA

Following induction, general anesthesia is usually maintained with oxygen and nitrous oxide mixture, supplemented with some volatile anesthetic agents like halothane, enflurane or isoflurane. Some analgesic drugs like pethidine or pentazocine should also be given IV. These drugs can be used safely while the child is ventilated. In the case of neonates and spontaneously breathing infants, special care should be taken.

Controlled ventilation of the lungs with the mixture of oxygen and nitrous oxide may also be used. Intermittent doses of analgesic drugs and muscle relaxants like pancuronium, vecuronium or atracurium, etc. may also allow the optimum maintenance of anesthesia. The technique is mostly satisfactory as it ensures good oxygenation, eliminates work of breathing, provides adequate muscle relaxation and allows a rapid return of reflexes at the end of anesthesia.

Jackson Rees modification of Ayre's T-piece can be used most satisfactorily with a fresh gas flow 2.5 to 3 times the respiratory minute volume of the child and a minimum flow of 3 liters per minute. Manual ventilation is recommended in the case of neonates and infants.

Manual ventilation by an experienced hand may sometimes be superior to mechanical ventilation. However, mechanical techniques can provide predictable and constant ventilation over time. The preset ventilators can be effectively used in most cases. But the use of ventilators requires specialized skill, experience and monitoring. The choice of breathing circuit, type of ventilator, and appropriate ventilator settings are most important. Though manual ventilation is strongly advocated in the case of most neonates and small children, mechanical ventilation is preferred for some specific cases and under certain conditions.

Muscle relaxants should be used in incremental doses equal to one-tenth of the initial dose, whenever needed. Small doses of analgesic drugs such as pethidine 1 mg/kg, pentazocine 0.25 mg/kg, morphine 125 µg/kg or fentanyl 1 µg/kg may be given intravenously to exclude awareness and pain.

During maintenance of anesthesia, adequate monitoring of vital signs is essential. Pulse, respiration, blood pressure and body temperature should be monitored. Stethoscope, precordial or esophageal should be applied to monitor heart and breath sounds. A thermistor probe (axillary, esophageal or rectal) is also needed. In selected cases, electrocardiogram, central venous pressure or blood gas monitoring may also be needed.

An intravenous infusion must be started either preoperatively or just after induction of anesthesia. Half strength Hartmann solution in 5% dextrose solution is mostly satisfactory for IV infusion in the intraoperative period. The amount of fluid will depend on preexisting dehydration, maintenance fluid and the fluid (blood) loss during surgery. If the blood loss exceeds 10% approximately, blood should be replaced. Fluid management needs much attention as either dehydration or overhydration badly affects the physiology of the child. A fluid chart-intake and output should be maintained.

Dextrose 4% in 0.18% saline is also used widely as maintenance fluid in all children except neonates. An approximate guide can be taken as: first 10 kg body weight 100 ml/kg/ 24 hours; second 10 kg body weight 50 ml/kg/24 hours. Potassium may be given 2 mmol/100 ml provided urine output is adequate.

RECOVERY

Whenever the anesthesia is maintained with volatile anesthetic agents, at the end of surgery, these should be gradually discontinued and the child should be fully oxygenated till recovery, when extubation should be done with great care.

Antagonism of Muscle Relaxants

To reverse the effects of nondepolarizing muscle relaxants, neostigmine in combination with atropine or glycopyrrolate is given. It should be noted that neostigmine is needed in relatively smaller doses for children. Adequate reversal should be detected by a neuromuscular monitor and also by clinical assessment.

Clinical criteria for assessing recovery from neuromuscular block are as follows:
1. Head lift, lifting both legs
2. Sustained hand grip/arm lift
3. Wide open eyes, absence of nystagmus/diplopia
4. Normal voice
5. Tongue protrusion
6. Vital capacity more than 15 mg/kg
7. Negative inspiratory force of a magnitude more than 32 cm H_2O (55 cm H_2O in adults).

Extubation

Endotracheal extubation in children should be done very carefully as they are very prone to laryngeal spasm, particularly when extubated under light plane of anesthesia. Extubation should be done either when the child is fully awake or deeply anesthetized. Before extubation, all the facilities of oxygenation, ventilation and reintubation should be available. Extubation should never be attempted when the child is coughing or straining on the tube. However, in certain conditions such as in the case of infants, in emergency cases and in cases with difficult intubation the child should be fully awake before extubation is done.

Before extubation, the blood pressure, heart rate and heart rhythm should be well within normal limits. The respiratory rate and tidal volume should also be adequate. Gastric contents should be aspirated as far as practicable through a Ryles' tube. It reduces the risk of postoperative nausea and vomiting and thereby aspiration pneumonitis. It also helps in better ventilation as the intra-abdominal pressure is reduced. The oropharynx should be suctioned, and oral packs must be removed before extubation. In some cases even tracheobronchial suctioning through a small bore catheter may be needed to clear out excessive secretions, if any.

Special note

1. Bain circuit, a coaxial modification of Mapleson D system can be used satisfactorily in pediatric cases. A minimum fresh gas flow of 2.5 to 3 liter/minute with an additional 100 ml/kg/minute is usually recommended. Higher flow rates 2 to 3 times the minute volume of ventilation are needed during spontaneous breathing to clear carbon dioxide. Capnography is helpful to adjust fresh gas flow and minute ventilation. In this system, fresh gas flows through a tube that lies inside the expiratory tube through which warm expired air flows. These systems waste large volumes of gases and vapors, because they depend on large total flows to clear carbon dioxide.
2. A pediatric circle system can be used safely in most children. Fresh gas flow rate should be adequate and carefully judged. The system should include a small bore delivery system tubing, a 0.5 to 1 liter rebreathing bag and pediatric bellows for mechanical ventilator.
3. Various potent volatile anesthetic agents such as halothane, enflurane, isoflurane, desflurane and sevoflurane can be used. These can provide amnesia, analgesia, control of autonomic nervous system reflexes and muscle relaxation. Enflurane is not suitable in the case of children as it is somewhat pungent, with bad odor and can cause convulsions. Desflurane is also not much used as it can cause excitement, breath holding, coughing and even laryngospasm. Halothane is most commonly used in pediatric anesthesia. It is nonirritant and causes less breath holding, coughing or laryngospasm. Isoflurane can also be used. Sevoflurane has a pleasant odor and may cause minimum airway irritation. MAC values of halothane, isoflurane and sevoflurane are increased in infants compared to adult values.
4. Halothane is myocardial depressant and may cause hypotension and bradycardia. Isoflurane tends to reduce peripheral vascular resistance and to maintain or increase heart rate. Cardiovascular stability is expected with the use of isoflurane. Sevoflurane also maintains the stability of blood pressure and heart rate.
5. Halothane and isoflurane provide rapid anesthetic induction and recovery. Inhalational induction with sevoflurane is also rapid. It has acceptable odor and low solubility, blood-gas partition coefficient being 0.6.

SPECIAL CONSIDERATIONS IN THE CASE OF NEONATES AND SMALL INFANTS

1. Neonates are very prone to become hypothermic, so adequate precautions should be taken. The neonate should be brought to operation theater while still in a heated incubator. The operation theater should be at an ambient temperature of 25°C. The baby should be placed on a warming blanket. A thermostatically controlled water blanket is mostly satisfactory. The central body temperature should always be monitored by either an esophageal or a rectal probe. It is better to warm all fluids to be used IV or for skin preparations. The gases should be humidified.
2. Neonates are must susceptible to infection. Thus, adequate cleanliness and sterility must be maintained.
3. All neonates should be given vitamin K preoperatively to prevent undue hemorrhage.
4. Narcotics should not be used preoperatively.
5. IV fluids should be given with sensible precautions. Accurate measurement of all IV fluids even those given with drugs should be done and intake-output chart should be maintained.
6. Hypoglycemia may occur, particularly on pronged fasting. Monitoring of blood sugar level at frequent intervals is essential.
7. Premature babies may suffer from apneic episodes. These babies should be monitored very carefully. Assisted ventilation and oxygenation may be needed even in preoperative period and postoperatively.
8. Premature babies are always at risk of high inspired oxygen which may cause retrolental fibroplasia and pulmonary oxygen toxicity. High inspired oxygen and high inflation pressure may cause focal air trapping, cyst formation and even fibrosis. Thus, in the case of neonates inspired oxygen concentration must be kept minimum as far as practicable.
9. Neonates should be premedicated with atropine sulfate as they have copious secretions and the vagus nerve is very active in neonates.
10. All neonates should be endotracheally intubated to protect the tracheobronchial tree and to allow controlled ventilation of the lungs.
11. Awake intubation may be attempted in certain cases such as:
    a. In cases of difficult intubation
    b. When ventilation with a face mask is difficult
    c. When the anesthetist is not much skilled in neonatal practice
    d. In emergency cases where aspiration is apprehended
    e. In moribund cases.
12. Induction with inhalation method (nitrous oxide + oxygen + halothane) is also satisfactory.

13. Intravenous induction may be needed in certain cases. Satisfactory muscle relaxation can be achieved by using muscle relaxants. The sensitivity of neonates to nondepolarizing relaxants should be borne in mind. Neonates are resistant to depolarizing relaxants and usually need larger dose than adults on body weight basis.
14. The endotracheal tube should be of adequate size. A proper tube is one that passes the glottis easily and allows a slight leak during positive pressure ventilation. The endotracheal tubes must be in sterile condition and the sterility must be maintained at the time of insertion. The endotracheal tube should be passed 2 cm below the vocal cords. The length of trachea in newborn is usually 4 cm. Air entry to all areas of the lung fields should be checked before taping the tube firmly in place. A soft rubber bite block may be needed in some cases.
15. Laryngoscopy and intubation must be atraumatic. The neonatal larynx is placed anteriorly and higher in the neck. The epiglottis is large, floppy and V-shaped. Thus, a laryngoscope with a straight blade such as Magill laryngoscope is most satisfactory for easy visualization of laryngeal inlet.
16. A throat pack is necessary as the plain endotracheal tubes (noncuffed) are to be used in neonates.
17. The Jackson Rees modification of Ayre's T-piece is the most suitable circuit for neonates. Once the endotracheal tube is correctly positioned, it is connected with the anesthesia circuit and manual ventilation is continued with nitrous oxide and oxygen.
18. Manual ventilation is mostly safe as little changes in compliance can be detected early and adjustments can be made accordingly to maintain ventilation.
19. Anesthesia can be maintained with nitrous oxide and oxygen supplemented with volatile anesthetics like halothane or enflurane. Intermittent doses of narcotics and muscle relaxants can also be used.
20. Monitoring of pulse, respiration, blood pressure and body temperature is essential.
21. An intravenous infusion must be established, preferably by cannulating the vein on the scalp, dorsum of the hand or foot or the long saphenous vein at the ankle. Overload should be avoided by very careful control of IV infusions. Syringe pumps and controlled infusion are essential.
22. At the end of anesthesia adequate decurarization with neostigmine and atropine must be done.
23. The throat pack should be removed and extubation should be done gently. Oxygenation by face mask should be done for few minutes. Apneic spells should be monitored very closely, particularly in preterm babies. The risk of such apnea is said to be increased during the first 15 hours following operation.

24. Head and the body of the baby are to be covered adequately to warm before sending him to recovery room.

DIFFICULT INTUBATION

Some children may pose the problem of difficult intubation. Common causes are as follows:

Congenital Causes

a. Pierre-Robin syndrome: Hypoplastic mandible, retrognathos, glossoptosis, bulky tongue, small epiglottis, high-arched palate usually with cleft and small mouth orifice.
b. Treacher Collins syndrome: Receding chin, obtuse angled mandible, high arched palate with or without cleft, abnormal maxillae, coloboma of eyelid or iris, deafness, choanal atresia and micrognathia.
c. Huge cystic hygroma of the neck.
d. Others: Gargoylism, achondroplasia and Marfan's syndrome.

Anatomical Causes

a. A short muscular neck with full set of teeth.
b. Receding lower jaw with obtuse-angled mandilble.
c. Prominent upper incisor teeth, protruded or relative overgrowth of premaxilla.
d. Long high arched palate and long narrow mouth.

Acquired Causes

a. Restriction of jaw movement: Trismus, fibrosis of temporomandibular joint, etc.
b. Restriction of neck movement.
c. Neck instability: Cervical spine injury.
d. Swelling of the neck: Trauma, burns and Ludwig's angina.
e. Huge bleeding following intraoral operation and posttonsillectomy.
f. Neck contracture: Postburns.
g. Laryngeal causes: Edema, tumor and stenosis.
h. Tracheal causes: Tumor.
i. Intraoral tumor.

Management

1. The child should be preoperatively assessed to recognize the potentially difficulty intubation and plans should be made accordingly to overcome the problem.

2. Awake intubation may be tried with or without local analgesia.
3. No intravenous inducing agent and muscle relaxant should be used.
4. Induction may be done with inhalation method using nitrous oxide, oxygen and halothane. Spontaneous ventilation is maintained. Then laryngoscopy is performed to visualize the glottis. External manipulation of larynx may be helpful. Thus, an experienced assistant must be present at the time of induction. An IV infusion should be established and atropine sulfate 0.02 mg/kg should be administered.
5. The use of fiberoptic laryngoscope is much limited in pediatric cases, as it cannot pass through small size endotracheal tubes.
6. Laryngeal mask airway is often helpful in such cases.
7. Blind nasotracheal intubation. Several suitable nasotracheal tubes should be kept ready for use. The size and patency of the nares should be judged. IV barbiturates and muscle relaxants must not be used. Inhalation induction with nitrous oxide, oxygen and halothane/ether is done. When the child is in deeper plane of anesthesia, the head should be positioned slightly extended as in the sniffing position. The lubricated endotracheal tube is passed through the nostril and advanced gradually, listening at the end of the tube for maximal breath sounds. It may go in following directions such as:
   a. Larynx: This is the desired location and here the breath sounds are well-heard.
   b. Esophagus: No breath sounds are heard. The tube should be withdrawn a little and then reinserted after extending the head maximally.
   c. Right or left of larynx: Obvious bulge over the neck. The tube should be withdrawn a little, then rotated towards midline and then reintroduced.
   d. In the vallecula or anterior commissure: The tube should be withdrawn a little, then reintroduced after slight flexion of the patient's head.
   e. At the site of adducted vocal cords. There is usually cough. It should be held up cautiously till the opening of vocal cords during inspiration and then reintroduced gently. Rotation of the tube may help entering the tip into the larynx at some point.

   If this is unsuccessful, the maneuver may be repeated using the other nostril. Sometimes a second tube is passed to the other nostril to block the esophagus. External pressure to the neck may direct the glottis towards the tip of the tube. The technique of blind nasal intubation largely depends on the experience and skill of the anesthetist.

8. Mask anesthesia with volatile anesthetics may be adopted, if not otherwise contraindicated. Spontaneous ventilation should always be maintained.
9. Regional analgesia may be given, if the situation permits.
10. Tracheostomy and transtracheal intubation may have to be done in extreme cases.

Minimum monitoring of the pediatric patients during perioperative period
1. Electrocardiogram (to know the cardiac rhythm)
2. Blood pressure
3. Body temperature
4. Precordial or esophageal stethoscope
5. Pulse oximeter
6. Capnography

CHAPTER 12

Postanesthetic Care and Complications

The postanesthetic recovery period is the most vulnerable period for children following anesthesia and its course is different from that for adults. These children need vigilance and adequate monitoring to prevent many complications.

These children, particularly the neonates should be taken to a separate room, better called recovery room. Here all sorts of drugs, resuscitative measures and monitoring equipment are provided. Well-trained nurses will take care of the children. This special unit provides special care and adequate sterility is maintained to protect the children from infection.

TRANSPORT TO RECOVERY ROOM

It is most important as many complications like aspiration, airway obstruction, etc. can occur during that period. Thus, the children should not be sent without some trained expert attendant. In critical cases, anesthetist himself should accompany the child during transport. Pediatric patients should be transported on stretcher with raised guard rails or safety straps to prevent the children from falling off. All patients must be placed in a lateral position during transport.

During transport skin, color, respiratory movements and pulse signals should always be monitored. Adequate care for the IV line should be taken. Following major thoracic, abdominal or neurosurgery, the child may need special attention. The intubated child may need assisted or even controlled ventilation during transport. The child should be covered adequately; otherwise, hypothermia may occur.

POSTANESTHETIC RECOVERY SCORE

It is an objective type of evaluation of children to have a uniform documented system for discharge. The modified Aldrete score system is most popular and it is based upon the evaluation of activity, respiration, blood pressure, consciousness and color as follows: (International anesthesia clinics, 1993).

1. Major activity : Active motion, voluntary or on command: 2
   Weak motion, voluntary or on command : 1
   No motion: 0
2. Respiration : Coughs, cries: 2
   Maintains good respiration: 1
   Needs airway maintenance: 0
3. Blood pressure : ± 20 mmHg of preanesthetic level: 2
   ± 20–50 mmHg of preanesthetic level: 1
   ± 50 mmHg of preanesthetic level: 0
4. Consciousness : Fully awake: 2
   Responds to stimuli: 1
   No response: 0
5. Color : Pink: 2
   Pale: 1
   Cyanotic: 0

Here total score is maximum 10. However, a simplified scoring system is also available. It evaluates the consciousness, airway and movements as follows:

1. Consciousness : Awake: 2
   Responding to stimuli: 1
   Not responding: 0
2. Airway : Coughs/cries: 2
   Maintains good airway: 1
   Airway needs maintenance: 0
3. Movement : Purposeful limb movements: 2
   Nonpurposeful limb movements: 1
   No movements: 0

Here the total score is maximum 6. The anesthetist should evaluate the child carefully before discharging from the recovery room. The evaluation must be documented in postoperative visits by the anesthetist.

In the recovery room, vital signs such as pulse, respiration, blood pressure and body temperature should be monitored. Fluid therapy should also be judged according to the need of the child. In critical cases, electrocardiogram, blood gas studies and pulse oximetry may be needed. In cases of respiratory insufficiency, reintubation may have to be done and artificial ventilation may be needed in the recovery room. The neonates, particularly the preterm babies should be kept in warm, oxygen-enriched incubator. Recovery should take place in a calm and quiet area with minimum tactile and auditory stimulation.

In the recovery room every child should be given humidified oxygen through a face mask or through nasal catheters. Before transferring the child to the care of nurses, it should be ensured that the child maintains his airway well.

A child with a oropharyngeal airway still needs the care of the anesthetist. Postoperative orders regarding analgesics, IV therapy and respiratory therapy must be carefully judged and documented.

Children are often anxious and fearful as they are separated from their parents. It seems helpful to allow parents to visit their child as soon as he awakes. It may reduce the anxiety considerably. But care should be taken that the parents do not transmit their own anxieties to their child. Anxious children may show tachycardia, rise of blood pressure and restlessness and may not cooperative well in the most stressful recovery period. An unfamiliar environment with many unknown persons in the room may upset the child further. Thus, a preoperative visit, reassurance and sympathetic attitude of all concerned with patient care, are most vital.

POSTOPERATIVE ANALGESIA

Postoperative pain is common and it is physically and psychologically harmful to the child. So pain should always be alleviated by analgesic drugs. Extreme caution should be taken during ordering the analgesics for children, particularly infants weighing less than 5 kg. Intraoperative narcotics, local or regional analgesia can extend their action in the postoperative period, if given at appropriate time. Narcotics should not be given to neonates and small infants less than 6 months unless ventilated. Common analgesic drugs with their dosages are as follows:
- Codeine phosphate 1 mg/kg body weight IM 4 to 6 hourly
- Pethidine hydrochloride 1 mg/kg body weight IM 6 to 4 hourly
- Morphine sulfate 0.1 to 0.2 mg/kg body weight IM 4 to 6 hourly
- Papaveratum 0.2 mg/kg body weight IM 4 to 6 hourly
- Paracetamol 12 mg/kg body weight orally 6 hourly
- Pentazocine 0.25 mg/kg body weight IM 4 hourly.

POSTOPERATIVE SEDATION

Postoperative sedation is needed to make the child calm and quiet and to treat restlessness. Undue restlessness can interfere with surgical dressing and wounds and make the child noncooperative. Certain drugs are useful for sedation. These are as follows:
- Diazepam 0.2 to 0.4 mg/kg body weight
- Trimeprazine 2 to 4 mg/kg body weight.

Fluid Management

This is adequately dealt with in a separate chapter. However, the volume and type of fluid requirement should be judged carefully considering all aspects like preexisting dehydration before operation, period of preoperative fasting, maintenance fluid needed, blood loss and alterations of body temperature, if any. It should be remembered that the reestablishment of oral intake may be delayed following long surgical procedures.

Infants frequently develop either hypoglycemia or hyperglycemia and thus blood glucose estimations may be needed. Electrolytes should also be provided in fluid therapy. The adequacy of fluid replacement should be judged all the while by monitoring the cardiovascular indices and urinary output. Whenever blood loss amounts to 10% of the estimated blood volume of the child or greater, blood transfusion is needed. In such cases, all sensible precautions should be taken to minimize the hazards of blood transfusion.

For infants and small children, the rate of infusion should be accurately controlled. A minidrop administration set (60 drops equal to 1 ml) with an infusion pump is much helpful in such cases. Careful aseptic technique should be adopted during venepuncture and insertion of intravenous cannula. Intake-output chart should be maintained.

Normally, glucose 5%, half or tripple strength with normal saline is given. Ringer lactate is also satisfactory as its electrolyte concentrations are mostly similar to those in extracellular fluid. In critical cases, serum electrolytes should be estimated and blood gas analysis may have to be done to detect any abnormalities.

Airway and Ventilation

The child should be in lateral position. Mouth and pharynx should be clear. In presence of secretions, proper suction is needed. In early postoperative period, oxygenation must be provided by means of a nasal catheter or by a face mask.

In some cases with respiratory insufficiency, the patient may need reintubation and positive pressure ventilation in the recovery room. Then the exact cause of respiratory insufficiency should be sought for and managed accordingly.

For prolonged positive pressure ventilation, a lung ventilator may be needed, particularly in the case of older children. Manual ventilation is recommended for neonates and small infants. Following lengthy operative procedures, such as cardiothoracic surgery, neurosurgery, etc. adequate respiratory measurements and blood gas analysis may have to be done. Water seal drain in cases of cardiothoracic surgery should be watched carefully, whether it is working correctly, or not.

Management of Body Temperature

Continuous monitoring of body temperature with a thermistor probe is essential even in the recovery room. The temperature should be monitored either in esophagus or the rectum. Rectal temperature is more or less satisfactory in infants and children. Axillary temperature can also be taken in older children. It may also reflect the core temperature provided the tip of the probe is close to axillary artery and the child's arm is adducted.

Hyperthermia can occur in children, when the operation is done in hot ambient temperature in a nonairconditioned operation theater. Pyrexial reactions due to infection or blood transfusion reaction should also be borne in mind. Rarely, it may be due to malignant hyperpyrexia syndrome.

Hypothermia is common in neonates, infants and children following operation in an airconditioned theater. Infants lose heat rapidly in cool ambient temperature due to relatively larger surface area in comparison to body weight, lack of subcutaneous fat, immature heat regulating center and so on. The baby should be kept well-covered and warm all the time; otherwise, hypothermia can increase the risk of postoperative morbidity.

COMMON POSTANESTHETIC COMPLICATIONS

Airway Obstruction

Airway obstruction may occur in early postoperative period. This may be due to resedation from the effects of residual anesthetic agents and analgesics, laryngospasm, foreign bodies, secretions, posttonsillectomy hemorrhage, expanding cervical hematoma and so on. Fall back of the tongue in an unconscious or semiconscious children is the most common cause of airway obstruction.

Most cases may resolve with simple techniques like opening of mouth and providing chin lift or jaw thrust or placing the child in lateral position. An appropriate oral or nasopharyngeal airway may also help. Secretions should be sucked out carefully. In some cases reintubation may be needed. Posttonsillectomy hemorrhage or cervical hematoma may need direct surgical intervention.

Hypoxemia

Mild hypoxemia is common and it often complicates recovery from anesthesia for various reasons. Pulse oximetry is essential in recovery room. Controlled oxygen therapy should be given in all major surgical cases. Oxygen mask may also be applied till the child is well awake. Children with preexisting upper respiratory tract infection should receive special attention, as they are prone to develop hypoxemia suddenly.

Specific anesthesia and surgery related causes of hypoxemia may include airway obstruction, ventilatory depression, bronchospasm, pneumothorax, congestive cardiac failure due to excessive fluid overload and so on. Management should be according to the cause of hypoxemia.

Ventilatory Depression

It may be caused by various factors such as pain, overdose of narcotics and anesthetics, inadequate decurarization, overdose of muscle relaxants, hypothermia, bronchopulmonary problems due to secretions and so on. Careful examination is needed. Radiographs may be helpful to detect areas of lung collapse, if any. Endotracheal or bronchial suction is very beneficial in case of excessive secretions. Whatever might be the cause, the child should be ventilated properly with 100% oxygen till the ventilatory adequacy regains. Neuromuscular block should be judged and in presence of the block, adequate decurarization is needed. For pain, analgesics in proper doses should be prescribed.

Laryngospasm

Laryngospasm may occur during recovery particularly following improperly timed extubation. It may also occur following endoscopy or following use of a large-bored endotracheal tube in a light plane of anesthesia. Ventilation with oxygen via a face mask should be done and positive pressure maintained using Jackson Rees modification of Ayre's T-piece. Reintubation may be needed and in such cases suxamethonium 1 mg/kg IV is beneficial. Undue delay should not be made; otherwise, cyanosis will occur.

Laryngospasm should be differentiated from upper airway obstruction caused by soft tissues like fall back of tongue. In such upper airway obstruction, there is absence of breath sounds in spite of respiratory efforts. Placing the child in lateral position or insertion of oral or nasal airway may help to relieve the obstruction.

Postintubation Croup

It is postintubation laryngeal edema, common among infants and children. 1 mm of edema in neonates may decrease cross section area of larynx by 65%. It is mostly due to trauma of larynx, particularly at the level of cricoid. Cricoid cartilage prevents any external expansion when edema occurs. The other factors responsible may be tight fitting endotracheal tube, coughing with the endotracheal tube in place, changing the patient's head position, duration of intubation and neck surgery. It may be aggravated in presence of anemia, hypoxia and hypotension. Its incidence is high in children with Down's syndrome.

Proper precaution should be taken to avoid such an incidence. The incidence may be decreased by giving 0.2 to 0.4 mg/kg dexamethasone prior to intubation in susceptible children. If the stridor develops, the child should be set upright in bed and cool humidified mist inhalation should be provided. Adrenaline should be administered by aerosol. Usually, 0.25 to 0.5 ml of adrenaline 1 in 200 solution, diluted in 3 to 5 ml normal saline is aerosolized using a nebulizer and administered by inhalation. The use of corticosteroids in the treatment of croup is controversial. Dexamethasone topical spray and 4 mg IV every 4 hours may be tried. Antibiotics should be given. Tracheostomy may have to be done in extreme cases. Further endotracheal intubation is not usually recommended.

Postoperative Pain

Pain is the most common problem experienced by children in the recovery period. Children of all ages including newborn and premature babies experience pain. Management of postoperative pain may be started even in the operation theater. Intravenous narcotic analgesics or regional blocks may be provided before the child awakens. Use of caudal, epidural or spinal narcotics is not recommended in pediatric cases. Intravenous fentanyl 0.5 to 1.0 µg/kg body weight or morphine 0.5 to 0.1 mg/kg or pethidine 1 mg/kg are mostly satisfactory to treat postoperative pain in older children. Narcotics are better avoided in children below 6 months of age, unless ventilated.

Postanesthetic Restlessness

It is a common problem in the immediate postoperative period. The factors responsible may be pain, hypoxemia, drug effect and the child's psychological make-up. Barbiturates, hyoscine or promethazine may increase the incidence of restlessness when given without an analgesic, particularly in presence of pain. Prolonged hypoglycemia may also cause restlessness. Restlessness causes tachycardia, tachypnea, hypotension, cyanosis, pallor, sweating and low oxygen tension in arterial blood.

Restlessness largely depends on the temperament of the child. After emergence from anesthesia, if the child does not see the parents and known faces in an unfamiliar environment, he may become restless.

It is always wise to diagnose the specific cause and treat accordingly. A preoperative visit is always stressed for better understanding of the child's psychology. Proper and adequate premedication should always be chosen and a postoperative analgesic may have to be given, if postoperative pain is anticipated. In all cases, hypoxemia should be ruled out and oxygen should always be given in postoperative period. Postoperative sedation may be attempted with sedative drugs like diazepam or trimeprazine.

Postoperative Shivering/Rigidity

It is common during recovery from anesthesia, particularly following halothane anesthesia. It may also occur following administration of cyclopropane, ether or thiopentone. Shivering increases metabolic rate and oxygen consumption. There may be increased ventilation and increased production of carbon dioxide. Demand hypoxia will occur. The child needs general supportive measures and adequate oxygenation. Shivering can be abolished by IV injection of methylphenidate hydrochloride 0.15 to 0.04 mg/kg body weight.

Postanesthetic Convulsion

The child may be a known epileptic. Stress of surgery, fever or hypoxia may precipitate convulsion in such patients. Hypoglycemia, cerebral hypoxia and hyperpyrexia may also cause it. Overdose of ether or enflurane and toxicity of local anesthetic drugs may also cause convulsion.

Thus, hypoxia, eletrolyte imbalance and hypoglycemia should be prevented. Body temperature should be maintained normal as far as practicable. In a known epileptic, proper treatment and prevention should be done by administering anticonvulsant drugs IM before and after surgery.

Management should include proper maintenance of airway, oxygenation and intermittent positive pressure ventilation (IPPV), whenever needed. Symptomatic treatment with IV diazepam is mostly satisfactory. Underlying causes should be detected and treated accordingly.

Nausea and Vomiting

Postanesthetic nausea and vomiting are common. Vomiting carries the risk of aspiration pneumonitis and, if continued for prolonged period, it may cause hypovolemia, hyponatremia and dehydration. Various factors responsible for vomiting include age, history of motion sickness, type of surgery, anesthetic technique, anesthetic drugs, full stomach and the skill of the anesthetist. Powerful analgesics may have emetic side effects. Ether may cause vomiting. Swallowing of posttonsillectomy bleeding, positive pressure ventilation following extubation, bucking, introduction of Ryles' tube, etc. may also initiate vomiting. Pain may also cause nausea and vomiting. Certain surgical procedures like repair of strabismus, middle and inner ear surgery, tonsillectomy, etc. are usually associated with postoperative nausea and vomiting.

Thus, proper preparation of the patient to keep the stomach empty as far as practicable is essential. In premedication, morphine or pethidine should be avoided. Phenothiazines may help to reduce the incidence of emesis. Hypoxia, hypotension and drugs like diethyl ether should also be avoided. Some patients may need antiemetic treatment by drugs like phenothiazine or metoclopramide. Ondansetron may also be prescribed.

Hypotension

Postoperative hypotension is a common feature and it is mostly due to operative blood loss, inadequate fluid replacement, blood transfusion and phenothiazine drugs and so on. Blood pressure should be monitored continuously during and after operation and maintained within physiological limits. Intravenous line should always be provided at the time of operation. Blood transfusion may be needed in major surgery.

Fluid and volume replacement should be adequate. Plasma, blood or plasma substitutes may be needed. Atropine may have to be given when hypotension is associated with slow heart rates. Vasopressors, steroids, alpha blocking drugs may be indicated in selective cases. Underlying causes should be detected and treated accordingly.

Persistent Sedation

Prolonged unconsciousness after general anesthesia may occur due to residual sedation from anesthetic medications such as long-acting sedatives (promethazine, droperidol, lorazepam, diazepam, etc.) and inhalation anesthetics. Following a standard typical anesthetic course, complete arousal usually occurs within 30 minutes. Profound residual muscular paralysis may mimic unconsciousness. The child exhausted preoperatively or whose normal sleep routine is interrupted as in an operation at night, may often be difficult to recover from general anesthesia. Physiological derangements such as hypoxia, hypercarbia, severe hypotension, hypoglycemia, hyperglycemia, hypothermia, hyponatremia, acid-base defect, operative trauma of the brain, etc. can cause persistent sedation. Prolonged anesthesia, preexisting cerebral edema, liver failure, kidney failure, meningitis, encephalities, etc. may cause recovery to be difficult.

Proper diagnosis is most vital in such cases. Attention should be given to the timing and dose of all preoperative and intraoperative medications those may account for undue sedation. All vital signs should be carefully checked. Evaluation of ventilation, heart rate and rhythm, blood pressure, pupillary size, response to stimuli (verbal or firm tactile), paresis, etc. should be done. Laboratory investigations should include blood examination, blood gas studies, blood urea, sugar and electrolytes, chest and skull X-rays, cerebrospinal fluid examinations and so on.

Management should be done with proper care of the airway, mouth and eyes, maintenance of adequate ventilation, oxygenation and IPPV whenever needed, general supportive measures and maintenance of nutrition, fluid electrolyte and acid-base balance. Normal body temperature should be maintained. Further treatment will be according to the underlying cause.

Postoperative Pyrexia

Mild rise of body temperature is common in postoperative period due to metabolic response to injury. But fever or pyrexia may occur due to intercurrent infection (wound infection, bronchopulmonary infection, urinary tract infection), sepsis, blood product or drug reaction and inadvertent overwarming of the child during operation. Any rigor or convulsion may increase the body temperature. Atropine or hyoscine may induce fever particularly in children. Incidental diseases like malaria, kala-azar, influenza, etc. should be borne in mind. Very rarely malignant hyperpyrexia syndrome can also occur.

Pyrexia may cause tachycardia, increased cardiac output and increased oxygen consumption, and may even lead to cardiac failure. Management includes bed rest, antipyretics, cooling, fluids and oxygenation, whenever needed. Broad-spectrum antibiotics are needed to combat infection. Causative factors should be detected and specific drugs should be used as far as practicable.

Inadvertent Hypothermia

Inadvertent hypothermia during routine operations can occur in children, particularly in small infants and neonates, specially in prematures. Hypothermia depresses ventilation and prolongs the recovery from anesthetic drugs. It decreases oxygen metabolism, depresses the myocardium directly, and precipitates characteristic arrhythmias like bradycardia, premature ventricular contractions, ventricular tachycardia and ventricular fibrillations. It may render the most drugs ineffective by interfering in uptake or metabolism of these drugs. The effects of these drugs are often more apparent during regaining of the normal body temperature. It is said that about 90% of heat loss in infants is from conduction, convection and radiation and only 10% is from evaporation via skin and lungs, inspired air and excreta. Thus, the baby should always be kept warm.

Monitoring of body temperature during surgery and anesthesia and in postoperative period is of vital importance. The ambient temperature of the operation theater and recovery room should be adjusted to 25°C or a little higher. A heating blanket set may be provided. The infrared heater may also be used. The infant may be placed in a warmed incubator at the end of anesthesia and then returned to recovery room. Hypothermia, if it occurs, should be treated with rewarming, oxygenation, IPPV and other supportive measures. Passive rewarming using fluid warmers, warming blankets and increased environmental temperature is usually satisfactory to prevent major heat loss.

Hypoglycemia

Hypoglycemia may occur rapidly in children due to immature liver and glycogen stores and a high metabolic rate. Prolonged preoperative fasting may also cause it. It is always a serious risk, particularly in the early postoperative period when sedation may mask its clinical features. Blood glucose should always be monitored during and after anesthesia. Fluids as 5% or 10% dextrose solution should be given during surgery. It is always sensible to allow the babies milk feeds upto 6 hours before anesthesia and to give them a sugar containing drink 4 hours prior to surgery.

Minor Complications

1. *Sore throat*: It may be due to trauma to the pharynx during intubation, from the passage of a nasogastric tube or the insertion of the throat pack. Irritation of the larynx by an endotracheal tube is also a common cause of sore throat. Sore throat may also occur even in absence of endotracheal intubation. The drying effect of unhumidified anesthetic gases and a preoperative antisialogogue may also cause sore throat. However, it is usually of short duration and the patient becomes symptom-free within 48 hours.
2. *Ocular complications*: Damage to the eyes and corneal abrasions may occur and these are mostly due to carelessness on the part of anesthetist concerned.
3. *Trauma to teeth*: It usually occurs during laryngoscopy, particularly when the intubation becomes difficult. Loose teeth are mostly prone to damage. Proper preoperative examination should be done and adequate precautions should be taken.
4. *Thrombophlebitis* is common.
5. *Postoperative parotid swelling*.
6. *Suxamethonium pains*: Muscle pain following the administration of suxamethonium is unusual in young children.
7. *Emergence delirium or excitement* and other psychic phenomena following ketamine anesthesia are less common in children. These may be reduced further by premedication with diazepam. Patient should be kept in a calm, quiet recovery room and have a undisturbed recovery period.

Emergence delirium may be due to various causes such as use of anticholinergic drugs, particularly atropine, benzodiazepines, ketamine and the sole use of potent inhalation anesthetics. Pain may also be a factor. Midazolam may cause disorientation, dysphoria, agitation, restlessness, etc.

Abnormal behavior due to hypoxemia or pain should be differentiated judiciously. Appropriate analgesic may be given to relieve pain. Pulse oximetry is always helpful in excluding hypoxemia. Flumazenil may be needed to reverse the effects of midazolam and diazepam.

CHAPTER 13

Anesthesia for ENT Surgery

Anesthesia for ear, nose and throat surgery in infants and children may require special skill and management mostly due to basic anatomical differences in this age group in comparison to adult care. Problems increase manifold particularly during airway management. Carful clinical assessment and proper radiological evaluation may prove usful. This chapter outlines the pathophysiology, diagnosis and anesthetic management of the common ENT conditions in children.

ANESTHESIA FOR TONSILLECTOMY

Anesthesia for tonsillectomy may pose various problems during and after anesthesia. Tonsillectomy is still common in ENT surgery. Most operations are elective and the mortality and even morbidity are often related to anesthesia and surgery as well. The basic principles of anesthesia are mostly similar to those for other branches of surgery. But it has its certain own problems and anesthetic requirements.

The problems related to it may be enumerated as follows:
1. Patients are usually of pediatric age group.
2. Airway obstruction may be there due to enlarged tonsils.
3. Operation is inside the mouth.
4. Aspiration of blood may occur.
5. Blood loss may be upto 4.5 ml/kg body weight.
6. Cardiac arrhythmia is common due to laryngeal and pharyngeal stimuli. It may be accentuated by hypoxia, hypercarbia and halothane anesthesia.
7. Sharing the airway with the surgeon.
8. Intubation may be difficult due to acute infection or extreme lymphoid hypertrophy.
9. Risk of bleeding postoperatively.
10. There may be bleeding diathesis. Child may have history of recent salicylate ingestion.

These patients should have adequate preanesthetic evaluation. History and physical examination are most important. Children in these age group may have loose teeth. They are usually anxious and thus should be provided with proper psychological management including adequate reassurance and good rapport. Routine blood examination such as hemoglobin percentage, total and differential counts, bleeding time, clotting time, prothrombin time and hematocrit should be done. Urine analysis, particularly for specific gravity, albumin and microscopic examination is also needed. Blood should be grouped and cross-matched.

Premedication is usually with syrup trimeprazine 3 mg/kg or diazepam 0.4 mg/kg orally about 90 minutes before induction of anesthesia. Atropine sulfate 0.02 mg/kg should also be given for its vagolytic action to prevent bradycardia produced by halothane, mechanical stimulation and succinylcholine, if used for intubation. Older children may have usual premedication with pethidine and atropine or promethazine combination. Essential anesthesia requirements include the following:

a. Access of patent airway.
b. Sensitive airway reflexes are to be obtunded.
c. Good mandibular and pharyngeal muscular relaxation.
d. Blood transfusion may be needed. A functional IV line is essential.
e. Likelihood of vagal and sympathetic stimulation.
f. Monitoring of vital signs and ECG is essential.
g. Early return of reflexes.
h. A properly working sucker machine should always be ready at hand in operation theater and in recovery room.

Anesthesia

Induction of anesthesia may be either intravenous or by inhalation. Intravenously, thiopentone and suxamethonium in usual clinical doses may be given. By the inhalation route, nitrous oxide, oxygen and halothane sequence may be used. Nasotracheal intubation is helpful when only tonsillectomy is to be done, but in the case of adenoidectomy, orotracheal intubation is justified. In such cases, adequate care should be taken so that the tube or its connections are not compressed by the blade of the mouth gag. A sand bag should be placed below the shoulders to extend the head and neck.

Anesthesia is maintained with nitrous oxide, oxygen and halothane with spontaneous or assisted ventilation using Jackson Rees modification of Ayre's technique. Monitoring of pulse, respiration, blood pressure, ECG and body temperature should be done. Careful monitoring of the depth of anesthesia is also needed. At the end of surgery, the child should be well awake and responding with airway reflex intact to protect from any aspiration in the upper airway.

In adult patients, tonsillectomy can be done under local anesthesia and sedation, but, on the whole, general anesthesia is usually preferred. The insufflation method of anesthesia without endotracheal intubation or open drop anesthesia using either diethyl ether or chloroform was very popular at one time for guillotine tonsillectomy. But these anesthetic techniques are not recommended in modern anesthesia as these have inherent dangers of uneven anesthesia, respiratory obstruction and aspiration of blood.

Postoperative Care

Analgesics should be given at the end of anesthesia and the child should be in a pain-free state in early postoperative period. Careful observations should be made to detect any bleeding, airway obstruction and aspiration, any undue swallowing, pallor, restlessness, unexplained tachycardia, retracted respiration, vomiting, cyanosis and so on should be detected early and managed. The child should be placed in a lateral position, hips elevated by a pillow, head down turned to one side and extended and upper hand under the chin. This is the so-called posttonsillar position.

Postoperative Bleeding Tonsil

Tonsillar bleeding following tonsillectomy is not an uncommon complication and it may fatally, if not tackled immediately and tactfully. Usually, the child is awake, restless, anxious and pale, skin is moist, blood pressure is low, pulse is rapid and respiration hurried. Stomach may be full with swallowed blood, blood vomiting may also occur. On the whole, the child is hypovolemic, hypotensive, tachycardiac and hypoxic. Under such circumstances, it is necessary to anesthetize the child again, so that the bleeder may be ligated and the source of blood loss stopped. Meanwhile, blood should be cross-matched and a coagulation profile should be obtained to detect any defect.

Preparation of the patient

The vascular volume should be restored adequately. A large functional IV line is essential to administer crystalloid solutions and for blood transfusion. All clots should be removed from the mouth and pharynx with a large suction catheter. A nasogastric tube may be passed to suck out most of the gases and liquid from the stomach. But care should be taken not to cause further trauma to tonsillar fossa.

Anesthesia

With proper resuscitation, blood pressure should return towards normal and the heart rate should begin to slow down. No premedication, particularly sedation is usually necessary.

Awake intubation may be tried, but it is difficult in the case of an anxious patient. Rapid sequence induction with atropine sulfate (0.02 mg/kg), thiopentone sodium (2 mg/kg) and suxamethonium (2 mg/kg) IV is usually satisfactory. Full dose of thiopentone is avoided as severe hypotension and even cardiac arrest may occur in such critically ill patients. Orotracheal intubation is done with Seillick's maneuver. Some prefer a breathing induction with nitrous oxide, oxygen and halothane or isoflurane. But with this technique there is danger of regurgitation, vomiting and aspiration of blood into the tracheobronchial tree. In such cases, induction of anesthesia should be done with the child on his side and in a slightly, head-down position to avoid aspiration as far as practicable.

Careful monitoring of pulse, blood pressure, body temperature, ECG, CVP and depth of anesthesia is essential during and after anesthesia. Fluid therapy should be adequate. Blood loss should be replaced. Orogastric tube, if not inserted earlier should be given before extubation. The air and blood should be sucked out. Extubation should be done while the patient is well awake and in a lateral position.

Repeated intubation may cause laryngeal edema or subglottic edema, particularly in children in the postoperative period. There may be hoarse cry, difficulty in respiration, inspiratory stridor and cyanosis. This should be detected early and treated accordingly.

The hemoglobin level should be checked to confirm adequacy of blood replacement. Postoperative analgesia is often needed, but over-sedation should always be avoided, as it may cause respiratory depression. One should be alert, as there is a possibility of further bleeding.

Tonsillar Abscess

Acute infection of tonsil may result in peritonsillar abscess or quinsy. These patients may have respiratory difficulty and laryngoscopy and endotracheal intubation may be difficult. Such a child is usually pyrexic and toxic. However, the child should be made afebrile as far as practicable.

The child may be premedicated with only atropine sulfate 0.02 mg/kg IV or glycopyrrolate 0.004 mg/kg IV. Sedatives should not be given as these may cause respiratory depression. Anesthesia is induced by inhalation of nitrous oxide, oxygen and halothane. Muscle relaxants should not be given as these may cause airway obstruction. Endotracheal intubation should be done when child is deeply anesthetized. Anesthesia is maintained with nitrous oxide and halothane. Extubation should be done, when the child is fully awake.

Adenoidectomy

Adenoidectomy is usually combined with tonsillectomy. Preanesthetic assessment, preparation, premedication and anesthesia are mostly similar to those for tonsillectomy. However, oral endotracheal intubation is recommended and a throat pack is advisable. The adenoids are curetted and the postnasal space packed for hemostasis. After a few minutes, this postnasal pack is removed and after removal of throat pack, the child is turned to lateral side. Then the extubation should be done when the child is well awake.

Postoperative adenoidal bed hemorrhage may occur. It can be controlled safely with a cuffed nasal tube which can compress the raw area without obstructing respiration. This type of placement of nasal tube can be easily done without anesthesia. Postoperatively, vital signs should be adequately monitored.

Choanal Atresia

It is a congenital condition involving membranous or bony occlusion of the posterior nares. It causes respiratory distress in the newborn, particularly when the occlusion is complete. Neonates are obligatory nose breathers; so such nasal obstruction can be easily relieved by establishing a patent oropharyngeal airway. The airway must be maintained until nasopharyngeal airway is obtained. The immediate management should be done by transnasal puncture and dilatation. However, definitive repair can be performed later. Choanal atresia is diagnosed by passing soft rubber catheters through each nostrils.

The newborn presents with severe respiratory distress and needs immediate care and maintenance of the airway. Adequate ventilation should be given with the continued use of oropharyngeal airway.

Newborn may be premedicated with only atropine sulfate 0.02 mg/kg IM before induction or IV at the time of induction. Awake orotracheal intubation may be easily performed. Anesthesia may be induced and maintained with nitrous oxide, oxygen and halothane. The pharynx should be well-sucked very gently at the end of anesthesia. Extubation should be done when the baby is fully awake. Constant care should be taken; otherwise, pulmonary aspiration may occur after the operation.

Definite repair is usually done in later childhood and at that time no other special anesthetic problems are apprehended.

ANESTHESIA IN EAR SURGERY

Ear surgery includes both minor and major procedures, including delicate microsurgery. The risk of surgical procedures in these case itself is less in comparison to that in general surgery. The main risk is mostly related to the patient's age and medical condition and, hence, needs careful anesthetic management. Some special anesthetic management should also be borne in mind, as a good and skillful anesthetic management largely contributes to a successful surgical outcome.

Common ear surgery includes stapedectomy, tympanoplasty, mastoidectomy, ossicular reconstruction and so on. The basic principles of anesthesia are mostly conventional and similar to those in other branches of surgery. The choice of management of anesthetic methods is wide open and should not pose additional risk to the patient provided a basic pediatric circuit like Jackson Ree's modification of Ayre's T-piece is used.

Some specific anesthetic problems are as follows:
1. The child may need repeated surgical procedures and hence be very anxious and apprehensive.
2. Communication may be difficult due to impaired hearing.
3. Ear surgery may involve delicate procedures under microscopic vision. A little blood may obscure the very small surgical field. Some degree of controlled hypotension may be beneficial.
4. Absolute control of airway is essential.
5. Child may have serious systemic diseases and thus need preoperative evaluation and preparation before subjecting to anesthesia.
6. Vasoconstrictor drugs like adrenaline, if needed, should be used with caution, particularly during halothane anesthesia.
7. Some children may have history of taking drugs such as steroids. This should be taken into account and adequate preparation is made.
8. Nitrous oxide and middle ear pressure need special attention. Middle ear and paranasal air sinuses are normal body air cavities—open, nonventilated spaces. Middle ear is intermittently vented through Eustachian tubes. During nitrous oxide inhalation, nitrous oxide enters faster than nitrogen can leave.

    This causes an increase in pressure inside. Passive venting may occur by Eustachian tube at a pressure of about 200 to 300 mm water pressure. If the tube is blocked, the pressure may reach even 375 mm water pressure in adults within 30 minutes of nitrous oxide anesthesia.

    On the other hand, when nitrous oxide is discontinued at the end of anesthesia, nitrous oxide is rapidly absorbed and as a result a marked negative pressure may develop. It is said that with abnormal Eustachian tube -285 mm H_2O pressure may occur within 75 minutes after stoppage of nitrous oxide anesthesia. This may cause hemotympanum and even disarticulation of stapes.

    Nitrous oxide may transiently worsen middle ear function. Increased middle ear pressure may even cause rupture of tympanic membrane. Thus, the following recommendations are made. Halothane-oxygen sequence may be adopted avoiding nitrous oxide.

Nitrous oxide should be discontinued 15 minutes prior to final closure of middle ear. Middle ear should be flushed with air prior to closure.
9. A smooth induction and a smooth emergence are necessary. Extubation of trachea should be without cough, bucking and straining.
10. Emesis in early postoperative period should be prevented by suitable antiemetic given preoperatively or about 30 minutes before extubation. Oral prochlorperazine may be continued 2 to 3 days postoperatively,
11. Nasal airways may be compromised by bleeding, edema, change of position of head and even inadvertent kinking or extubation of endotracheal tube.
12. Hypotensive anesthesia in the field of ENT surgery, particularly in microsurgery is controversial. Controlled hypotension has got its own disadvantages and is not without its mortality and morbidity, particularly in children. Some advocate a modified controlled hypotension technique with the help of tubocurarine and halothane aided with a mild head up-tilt posture and controlled ventilation. Tachycardia may be prevented with the help of beta blockers. A systolic pressure of about 70 to 80 mmHg in older children may be sufficiently low to minimize bleeding rather than a bloodless operative fluid.
13. In selective cases the infiltration of adrenaline may be needed to achieve a more or less bloodless operative field. Topical application of adrenaline may also be needed. But it may cause arrhythmia during halothane anesthesia. In enflurane anesthesia adrenaline can be used more or less safely.
14. Short surgical procedures such as stapedectomy may be carried out by providing sedation, local anesthesia supplemented with adrenaline. Nausea and vomiting can be prevented with the help of antiemetics like prochlorperazine.
15. Some patients may have associated congenital deformities of the upper airway which predispose them to ear disease, as for example cleft plate and Pierre Robin syndrome. These should be checked properly.
16. For certain operative procedures like ossicular reconstruction, the surgeon may intend to assess hearing during operation. In such cases, neuroleptanalgesia may be helpful, particularly in older children.

Minor Operations like Myringotomy

Premedication: Sedation is usually necessary. Trimeprazine or diazepam with or without atropine may be given in the case of children.

Induction of anesthesia may be either intravenous or inhalational, particularly in children. Anesthesia is usually maintained with nitrous oxide, oxygen and halothane.

Anesthesia for Middle Ear Surgery

Smooth anesthesia is essential, coughing, bucking or straining may increase venous pressure and may lead to excessive oozing from the operative field. Premedication may be given with pethidine and atropine in usual clinical doses in the case of older children. Trimeprazine or diazepam is usually satisfactory in smaller children. Anesthesia is induced with thiopentone and suxamethonium, following orotracheal intubation; anesthesia is maintained with nitrous oxide, oxygen and intermittent doses of pethidine and a muscle relaxant.

The operation of myringoplasty and tympanoplasty are usually lengthy and provision of an ischemic filed may be beneficial. Some degree of hypotension may be achieved, using halothane or enflurane in combination with tubocurarine and IPPV and a slight head up-tilt. Blood pressure must be monitored and use of pulse monitor is always helpful. ECG and CVP monitoring may also be done. Nitrous oxide anesthesia may increase the middle ear pressure and may cause dislodgement of grafts. Some anesthetists suggest the use of oxygen-nitrogen mixture in place of oxygen-nitrous oxide mixture to obviate such problems. If labyrinthine function seems to be disturbed, an antiemetic may help to control postoperative vertigo and vomiting. Proper sedation and analgesia are needed.

ANESTHESIA FOR NASAL AND SINUS SURGERY

The common operations in children include nasal polypectomy, correction of deviated nasal septum, reduction of nasal fractures, reconstructive plastic procedures of the nose, surgical treatment of epistaxis and surgery of frontal, maxillary and ethmoidal sinuses.

These patients may have compromised airways before surgery because of bleeding, infection, tumor, polyp and abnormal anatomy of the upper airway. Nasotracheal intubation is absolutely contraindicated in such cases. Children with nasal polyps may present as a complication of cystic fibrosis.

In nasal surgery, the tracheobronchial tract must be protected against inhalation of blood both during and after operations in the nasal cavities. Use of posterior pharyngeal pack is absolutely essential in such cases to absorb blood.

The patients should recover in the semiprone position with the head and neck at a lower level than glottis (tonsillar position). Early return of reflex activities is most important. Nasal packs given during operation may cause uneasiness, restlessness and anxiety in early postoperative period.

Minor Surgery of the Nose

This may be done under local anesthesia. Nasal packing is done with either 2% lignocaine or 4% cocaine with adrenaline (1 in 100,000). This is often used for hemostasis even when general anesthesia is administered.

Cocaine should be used with sensible precautions for its toxicity and interaction with adrenaline. The maximum safe dose of cocaine is roughly 3 mg/kg. A drop of 4% cocaine is said to contain about 1 to 2 mg cocaine. The synergistic effect of cocaine on adrenaline may be dangerous, particularly in patients with hypertension. However, the addition of adrenaline may not help to increase the vasoconstriction caused by cocaine. Topical adrenaline does not retard the absorption, nor prolong the action of cocaine.

Major Surgery of the Nose

This should always be done under general anesthesia. The choice of anesthetic agents and techniques are mostly conventional. Volatile anesthetic agents may be used with spontaneous or assisted ventilation using Rees modification of Ayre's technique. Not much muscle relaxation is usually needed in such cases, but airway management by an endotracheal tube is essential. To minimize bleeding and to provide a reasonably dry workable surgical field during operation, modified controlled hypotension technique may be adopted in the case of older children, with adequate precautions.

Sinus surgery may be associated with large blood loss. Adequate replacement therapy and blood transfusion are needed. Hypertension during anesthesia should be avoided at all costs. Postoperative surgical complications, particularly intracranial problems such as brain abscess, meningitis and so on should be borne in mind. Extubation should always be done when the child is fully awake. Analgesics are needed in postoperative period. Humidified oxygen should also be administered.

Epistaxis

Common causes of epistaxis include trauma, hypertension, leukemia, bleeding dyscrasia, medications like coumarins, aspirin, etc. Surgical management usually include—(a) Packing the nose of postnasal space, (b) ligation of internal maxillary artery and anterior ethmoidal artery and, on some occasions external carotid artery.

Anesthesia in such cases may be problematic. The child may be hypertensive, anxious, hypovolemic and tachycardiac. Stomach may be full with swallowed blood and there are all possible risks of aspiration. Nasogastric tube is contraindicated in such cases. The case is more or less an emergency one.

General anesthesia should be given very carefully. The child should be sedated with adequate barbiturates or diazepam. Analgesics may also be given. A large functional intravenous line is absolutely essential. Blood transfusion is often needed. A rapid sequence of induction with thiopentone and suxamethonium with Sellick's maneuver is mostly satisfactory, but thiopentone should only be given after adequate resuscitation. Orotracheal intubation and a pharyngeal pack should be given. Maintenance of anesthesia may be done with nitrous oxide, oxygen and halothane. Hypoxia, hypercarbia and further hypotension should be avoided. All vital signs should be monitored. Orogastric tube should be introduced before extubation of endotracheal tube to suck out the gastric contents.

ENDOSCOPY

Endoscopy is a common procedure in infants and children. It is often indicated for diagnosis or therapy. The common procedures are direct laryngoscopy, bronchoscopy and esophagoscopy. Diagnostic indications include evaluation of stridor, dysphagia, etc. and therapeutic endoscopy includes removal of foreign body or polyp, cauterization of papillomatosis, etc.

Special problems related to endoscopy are as follows:
a. Child is already with airway problems.
b. Child may be with tracheostomy.
c. It may be difficult to maintain adequate ventilation during endoscopy, as the child is already with a very narrow airway.
d. Trauma and bleeding may occur.
e. Subglottic edema may occur in postoperative period.
f. All equipment such as laryngoscopes, endotracheal tubes, suction apparatus, etc. should be kept ready at hand.
g. Emergency tracheostomy may have to be done in critical situations. Thus, tracheostomy set should be kept ready and the endoscopist must be competent to tackle the situation.

Laryngoscopy

Laryngoscopy can be done without anesthesia in neonates, but infants and older children need general anesthesia. These patients should be adequately evaluated in the preoperative period. The child may have some degree of respiratory obstruction. Heavy sedation should be avoided in premedication. Diazepam may be given orally. Atropine sulfate 0.02 mg/kg IV should be given at the time of induction. Anesthesia may be induced with nitrous oxide, oxygen and halothane. Intravenous induction is contraindicated in such cases. At the time of laryngoscopy, anesthesia may be maintained with oxygen and halothane. Insufflated into the pharynx. Ventilation and pulse should always be monitored.

Endotracheal tube of a smaller size may be used, but it may get into the surgeon's field of vision. Jet injectors are not much helpful, particularly in infants and may cause problems. The child should be closely observed in the immediate postoperative period. There may be irritant cough and laryngospasm.

Laryngomalacia

Here the cartilages of the larynx are not fully matured and there is tendency for the epiglottis or one of the arytenoid cartilages to prolapse into the glottis on inspiration and thus cause inspiratory stridor. Though the condition is selflimiting and no special treatment is needed, laryngoscopy is indicated to diagnose and rule out the other causes of stridor. It should be noted that it can be well-diagnosed in lighter plane of anesthesia as the stridor usually disappears during deeper plane of anesthesia.

Laryngeal papilloma

It may cause severe respiratory tract obstruction. The condition may need repeated laryngoscopy and resection as recurrences are common until adolescence. Hoarseness and dyspnea are usual symptoms. A large papilloma may completely obstruct the glottis.

Anesthetic management may need special considerations. The laryngeal inlet may be difficult to visualize. At the time of induction, there may be complete acute airway obstruction. Intravenous induction is contraindicated in such cases. Endotracheal intubation should be avoided, as it may implant papilloma in lower airways. Laser treatment demands a clear view of the larynx and immobile vocal cords.

The child should be premedicated with atropine sulfate IV at the time of induction. Inhalation induction (N_2O, O_2 and halothane) followed by laryngoscopy and lignocaine spray to the larynx seems to be a safe technique in such cases. In cases of obstruction, endotracheal intubation may be needed. During laser treatment, special care is needed. Patient's eyes should be covered and all inside the operation theater should wear eyeglasses. Oxygen should be used in reduced concentration to limit the conflagration at the lesion. Care should be taken as it may ignite explosive anesthetics or endotracheal tubes.

Bronchoscopy

Bronchoscopy is indicated in children for removal of secretions and foreign bodies, diagnosis of respiratory diseases and treatment of atelectasis.

General anesthesia is usually satisfactory, but it should be combined with topical spray to larynx and trachea to prevent laryngospasm and undue straining during the light plane of anesthesia.

The child should be carefully assessed in preoperative period, particularly the respiratory status. Heavy sedation should be avoided in premedication. Atropine sulfate IV should be given at the time of induction. Inhalational induction is preferred with N_2O, O_2 and halothane. When the child is anesthetized, the mask is removed, laryngoscopy is done and the larynx, trachea and bronchi are sprayed with lignocaine (maximum safe dose 3 mg/kg). The anesthesia is continued with O_2 and halothane under face mask for about 5 minutes to get the optimum effect of lignocaine. Then the bronchoscope is inserted. Oxygen and halothane mixture is supplied through the side arm of the bronchoscope and the spontaneous ventilation is maintained. Ventilation is better assisted as the resistance to ventilation is high through a small bronchoscope.

During the procedure, heartbeat and ventilation should be monitored. In presence of respiratory failure, a venturi device may be helpful. Complications of bronchoscopy may include hemorrhage, pneumothorax, stridor and so on.

At the end of the procedure, there should be rapid return of reflexes. The child should be placed in the lateral position afterwards to allow drainage of blood, secretions, etc. Humidified oxygen should be given. The child should not be allowed any feed, for at least 2 hours after lignocaine spray.

Bronchography

Bronchoscopy is also done for bronchography. As usual, the child is anesthetized and bronchoscope is introduced. Then under direct vision, the contrast medium is passed through a narrow catheter into the lobe to be examined. The child should have quiet, shallow and spontaneous ventilation during radiography. Coughing, bucking, etc. may cause bad quality films.

General anesthesia is satisfactory in children. But with severe bronchiectasis, profuse sputum and diminished respiratory reserve may cause problems. Endotracheal anesthesia may also be employed. A skilled team of anesthesiologist, endoscopist, radiologist and nurses is necessary for such procedures. Suction apparatus must be readily available to clear the bronchial tree before the introduction of dye, at the end of the procedure and as an emergency at any time. At the end of bronchography, the patient should be well awake and turned on the side.

Esophagoscopy

Esophagoscopy in children is usually indicated to dilate a stricture or for removal of a foreign body. Some specific problems related to anesthesia may be present. In small children, esophagoscopy may press the trachea causing obstruction in ventilation even when the endotracheal tube is in place. The child should be adequately anesthetized during the procedure. Otherwise, coughing or straining may even cause esophageal trauma and perforation. In presence of stricture in the lower esophagus, there may be food and secretion in the upper dilated segment and thus there is a chance of aspiration during anesthesia.

The child should be adequately sedated and premedicated with atropine sulfate. Endotracheal anesthesia is mostly satisfactory. Intravenous induction (thiopentone and suxamethonium) can be done. Airway should be secured rapidly. Cricoid pressure should be used, as there is a risk of regurgitation and aspiration. Armored endotracheal tube is less likely to be compressed by the esophagoscope. Controlled ventilation may be employed by administering intermittent doses of muscle relaxants like vecuronium or atracurium. Ventilation should always be monitored during the procedure.

Esophagoscopy may cause trauma and bleeding after biopsy or in presence of esophageal varices. The child should be fully awake at the end of the procedure. Pharynx should be adequately cleared of blood, secretions, etc. and the child turned on the side.

LASER MICROSURGERY

The use of fiberoptic instruments, the operating microscope and the carbon dioxide laser has developed the microsurgery and brought it to a very successful stage. Laser light energy is being used as a surgical tool. The CO_2 laser light is absorbed by all biological tissues and it rapidly vaporizes intracellular water. The laser energy rapidly dissipates in tissues with a high water content. The adjoining tissue is unaffected. Laser therapy can be applied to cure patients having various leisons, such as nasal, oral or laryngeal papilloma, subglottic stenosis, subglottic hemangioma, nodules, tumors and so on. Laser therapy provides excellent hemostasis, minimal postoperative edema and rapid healing. Surgical excision is mostly accurate and precise.

The argon and ruby lasers are mostly used in the ophthalmic surgery. Argon laser is also being used in the plastic and dermatologic surgery. In neodymium-ytrium-aluminium garnet (Nd: YAG) laser, tissue penetration is less controllable.

To prevent thermal injury from the laser beam, the operation theater personnel must wear glasses and patient's eyes should also be protected. CO_2 laser does not penetrate cornea, but argon and Nd: YAG laser can penetrate. Surrounding healthy tissue should also be protected and covered with wet sponges. Constant vigilance and monitoring of vital signs are needed even in recovery rooms. Drapes should be minimum as paper and cloth drapes are combustible. Inhalation injury can occur in patients and operation theater personnel. Laser beam can be reflected by polished shiny surface. The laser should be properly used to minimize the energy emitted.

Latex, rubber, silicone and plastic endotracheal tubes can absorb CO_2 laser energy and even ignite. Wrapping the endotracheal tubes in aluminium foil tape may be helpful to protect the tube from thermal damage. Various metallic tapes are also being used. Laser-guard protective coating is also very much efficient. Foil wrapped tubes may kink, irritate the mucosa and even obstruct the airway. Insufflation with endotracheal tube or jet ventilation may also increase the hazard of fire.

In spite of all precautions, ignition of endotracheal tube can occur. In such cases, the flow of oxygen should be discontinued and immediate disconnection of endotracheal tube is needed. The flaming endotracheal tube should be removed. Chest radiography and bronchoscopy are needed to know the extent of thermal injury. Management should be according to the degree of injury and may include humidification of inspired gases, assisted ventilation and steroids. Tracheostomy may also be needed in some cases.

ANESTHESIA FOR TRACHEOSTOMY

Preservation of the airway by tracheostomy is a major procedure that requires careful evaluation, adequate planning and enough skill and experience. Many a time it is a life saving procedure and may have to be carried out as an emergency case. The main indications of tracheostomy are as follows:

1. To relieve obstruction in the upper respiratory tract, not relieved by other means.
2. To maintain long-term IPPV.
3. To prevent inhalation of foreign materials where there is failure of swallowing or absence of laryngeal reflexes.
4. For suction of the trachea and bronchial tree when there is inability to cough out the secretions.
5. Narrow subglottic stenosis, gross papillomatosis of larynx and severe epiglottitis.

Ordinarily tracheostomy should be done as an elective case, except in cases with acute upper airway obstruction, where the emergency tracheostomy is needed. Upper airway obstruction may be due to foreign bodies, exudate, burns, large tumors, trauma, etc. Elective tracheostomy should always be done on the operating table with adequate light, sterile conditions, proper patient position and experienced surgical and anesthetic care.

The Advantages of Tracheostomy

1. It overcomes upper airway obstruction
2. It reduces respiratory dead space significantly
3. It allows effective suction from the respiratory tract
4. It prevents aspiration
5. It facilitates long-term ventilation.

General anesthesia is usually preferred and endotracheal intubation should be done to maintain a clear patent airway. Endotracheal tube in situ also helps the surgical procedure. The passage of a bronchoscope may also help. However, general anesthesia without endotracheal tube may be provided if there is no airway problem. But a marginal airway may become completely obstructed in deeper planes of anesthesia.

The head is extended and a midline incision is made. The trachea is usually opened through the third and fourth cartilages. In children, a vertical slit is preferred in the trachea instead of flap; no cartilage should be excised in children. It helps to reduce the danger of subsequent stenosis or collapse. However, hemostasis should be secured and the tube inserted and adequately fixed.

Side effects of tracheostomy include loss of voice, loss of expulsive cough and loss of physiological filtering, humidifying and warming mechanisms.

Metal tracheostomy tubes consist of an outer tube with flanged ends carrying tapes and an inner tube. The inner tube can be removed for replacement and for cleaning. The outer tube is not usually disturbed for 7 days and this allows the formation of a good track. The inner tube can be changed frequently.

Polyvinylchloride (PVC) tracheostomy tubes can also be used satisfactorily as these are pliable, nonirritant and are single tubes gently curved with a lower angle. Some have curved wings which allow comfortable and secure fixation. Recommended sizes are as follows: 2 years: 16 to 18 FG; 2 to 5 years: 20 FG; 5 to 10 years: 22 to 24 FG, adult male: 36 FG; adult female: 32 FG.

In the immediate postoperative period, the child should have a chest X-ray to detect any emphysema and to check the position of tracheostomy tube. Extra humidity is needed in the atmosphere. Saline instillation into the trachea and repeated tracheobronchial toilet are often needed. In children with respiratory inadequacy appropriate concentration of oxygen should be added to respiratory gases to overcome the continuing danger of hypoxemia. Close and constant observation of the child is necessary.

Complications Common to Tracheostomy

1. *Pneumomediastinum or pneumothorax*: It may be due to opening of the cervical pleura or due to air tracking down the mediastinum through the incision or from a displaced tracheostomy tube. The incidence is high in low tracheostomy.
2. Hemorrhage and bleeding into the trachea from an operative wound.
3. Erosion of tracheal wall.
4. Insertion of tube in a false tract.
5. *Laryngeal stenosis*: It is mostly due to division of the cricoid or first tracheal cartilage.
6. *Retained tube*: It may be caused by excision or necrosis of cartilage causing tracheomalacia and subsequent collapse when the tube is removed.
7. Beside all these, infection, tube obstruction, accidental extubation and endobronchial intubation can also occur. Pulmonary complications like atelectasis are also common.

Discontinuation of Tracheostomy

When the need of tracheostomy is over, it can be removed. The wound will heal automatically within 7 days. No secondary closure of the wound is needed. During this period the patient can cough or talk by occluding the gap by his finger. Sometimes a speaking tube can be provided to allow speech and at the same time suction can be done at the time of need.

CHAPTER 14

Anesthesia for Ophthalmic Surgery

In recent times, the use of general anesthesia in ophthalmic surgery has increased, particularly in pediatric cases. General anesthesia has some positive advantages to offer. Endotracheal anesthesia can provide satisfactory conditions for most procedure. Careful skilled anesthesia can efficiently eliminate coughing, retching and vomiting during anesthesia and in postoperative period. A relatively bloodless operative field can also be achieved. Patient's cooperation is not needed and movements of the head can be avoided in general anesthesia.

SPECIFIC PROBLEMS

The specific problems related to ophthalmic procedure are as follows:
1. Children are usually anxious, fearful and noncooperative. They need tactful and sympathetic management, personal persuasion and reassurance. General anesthesia is needed in most children.
2. *Intraocular tension*: The pressure in the anterior chamber of the normal eye is approximately 10 to 22 mmHg. It can be measured by manometry or tonometry. Tonometry indicates a measure of impressibility of the cornea, which depends mainly on intraocular pressure (IOP). IOP is mainly determined by the balance between the production of aqueous humor by the ciliary body and its drainage into the canal of Schlemn.
    a. During tracheal intubation, coughing, bucking, retching and vomiting, venus pressure increases and there is increase in IOP.
    b. Temporary increase in blood pressure raises IOP.
    c. Hypoxia and hypercarbia raise IOP.
    d. Squeezing will cause increase in IOP.
    e. Atropine causes only a slight increase in IOP, but a considerable increase in cases with closed angle glaucoma. Its use in premedication is not usually contraindicated except in patients with closed angle glaucoma.
    f. Suxamethonium IV causes an increase in IOP. The increase occurs

within 30 seconds and lasts for about 6 minutes. Pretreatment with nondepolarizing muscle relaxants or diazepam or self-taming with suxamethonium may help to reduce the increase in IOP to some extent. However, suxamethonium is contraindicated in patients undergoing intraocular surgery, children with penetrating eye injury and in patients with glaucoma.

    g. Ketamine has generally little effect on IOP, but it may sometimes increase IOP.

    h. All potent inhalation anesthetic agents (except nitrous oxide) decrease IOP.

    i. Barbiturates and narcotic analgesics decrease IOP.

    j. Nondepolarizing muscle relaxants lower the IOP.

    k. Diuretics lower IOP and may inhibit the increase in IOP caused by suxamethonium.

    l. Arterial hypotension, hypocapnia and high blood PO_2 decrease IOP.

    m. Retrobulbar block and manual massage of globe also lower IOP.

3. *Oculocardiac reflex*: Traction of the extrinsic muscles of the eye may cause bradycardia and even cardiac arrest. This reflex effect is mediated on the afferent side by ciliary nerves and on the efferent side by the cardiac fibers of vagus. It is powerful in children. Prevention can be attempted with IV atropine and retrobulbar block. Heart rate and ECG must be monitored during manipulation of eyes and all possible resuscitative measures and drugs should be available in the crisis period.

4. Intraocular surgery and surgery of nasolacrimal duct and eyelids usually need a bloodless operative filed. Care should be taken not to increase the bleeding at least. Induced hypotension is not usually required. But smooth general anesthesia, a good patent airway, good positioning (slight head up tilt) and smooth maintenance of anesthesia with halothane, avoidance of coughing, straining or vomiting are mostly satisfactory to achieve a relatively acceptable bloodless operative field.

5. Some cases with glaucoma or strabismus may be under treatment with long-acting cholinesterase inhibitors. These drugs may cause toxic symptoms like nausea, vomiting and abdominal pain. Suxamethonium may cause prolonged apnea in such cases. Ecothiopate lowers plasma cholinesterase activity after about 1 month of therapy and its effect may last 4 to 6 weeks after discontinuing therapy.

6. Adrenaline and phenylephrine applied to conjunctiva during surgery may cause adverse systemic effects. It may cause arrhythmias and hypertension. It may be dangerous during halothane anesthesia.

7. Suxamethonium may cause contracture of the extraocular muscles. It may interfere with forced duction testing, if done within 15 minutes. Forced duction test is usually performed by the ophthalmologist during surgery to estimate the amount of restriction in the movement of the extraocular muscles. If succinylcholine is being used, communication with the surgeon is essential.
8. Anesthesia in ophthalmic surgery must be in deeper planes. Smooth induction, even maintenance and smooth extubation and recovery are also essential.
9. Postoperative analgesia should be given. But nausea and vomiting in the postoperative period must be prevented by all possible means. Prochlorperazine or perphenazine at the end of anesthesia may be helpful.
10. *Malignant hyperthermia*: It is a genetic disease of muscle often triggered by surgery and anesthesia causing a fulminant and life-threatening hypermetabolic state. Patients with ptosis or strabismus are said to be prone to suffer from malignant hyperthermia. Any other occult myopathies may also be present. They may have a positive family history of the disease.

The agents that can trigger the disease may include depolarizing muscle relaxants and all potent anesthetics including halothane and desflurane. Local anesthetic agents, barbiturates, nitrous oxide, narcotics and nondepolarizing muscle relaxants are mostly safe.

The disease may occur intraoperatively with a rapid steep rise of temperature, muscle rigidity, dysrhythmias, rhabdomyolysis, hypercarbia, acidosis, hyperkalemia and increased plasma catecholamines. Masseter muscle rigidity following succinylcholine may also occur in such sensitive patients. A muscle biopsy and contracture test are indicated in these patients. A creatine phosphokinase (CPK) level above 20000 IV strongly suggests malignant hyperthermia susceptibility. In the late stage myoglobinuria, disseminated intravascular coagulation and renal failure can occur.

Essential treatment of malignant hyperthermia should include discontinuation of succinylcholine, and potent inhaled anesthetics, 100% oxygenation, adequate ventilation, administration of bicarbonate and dantrolene 2.5 mg/kg IV. Patients should be cooled by ice water, lavage of gastric, rectal and peritoneal cavities with iced saline solution and IV administration of refrigerated fluids. Adequate monitoring of vital signs, early recognition of the syndrome and aggressive immediate management are vital.

ANESTHETIC MANAGEMENT

All these children who have to undergo ophthalmic surgery should be adequately assessed in the preanesthetic period, whatever minor procedure it might be. The child may be tense and nervous and should be dealt with proper sympathetic approach. The use of opiates in premedication is usually avoided as most of them may cause vomiting. Diazepam may be given orally about 90 minutes before anesthesia. Atropine sulfate 0.02 mg/kg should be given at the time of induction, particularly where oculocardiac reflex is a problem.

In minor case, nitrous oxide, oxygen and halothane sequence is the most satisfactory method of anesthesia. Halothane is nonirritant to respiratory tract and provides smooth anesthesia with a rapid and quiet awakening. Halothane lowers IOP and does not cause vomiting.

However, the induction can also be made with thiopentone and muscle relaxants followed by endotracheal intubation and maintenance with nitrous oxide, oxygen and halothane using Rees modification of Ayre's technique. Suxamethonium is contraindicated in the cases of intraocular surgery, in the cases with glaucoma or penetrating eye injury. Controlled ventilation using a muscle relaxant like pancuronium or vecuronium or atracurium is also frequently used, particularly in neonates and small children and also in very long procedures. The use of light anesthesia and muscle relaxants facilitates a speedy recovery. Endotracheal intubation and extubation should be smooth and coughing and vomiting should always be avoided. Hypoxia, hypercarbia and hypotension should not occur in the perioperative period.

Anesthesia for Surgical Correction of Strabismus

Surgical correction of strabismus is the common operation in children. It may have some anesthetic problems as,
1. Oculocardiac reflex.
2. *Oculogastric reflex*: Vomiting is common after eye muscle surgery.
3. *Malignant hyperpyrexia*: Children with strabismus are very prone to develop malignant hyperpyrexia. Thus, adequate investigations and preventive measures should be taken.
4. Postoperative pain may be severe.
5. Some patients may have been using ecothiopate iodide. Its interaction with suxamethonium should be borne in mind.

Anesthesia

Usually, the heavy sedation is avoided and administration of only atropine IV at the time in induction is necessary. Intravenous induction with thiopentone and suxamethonium, endotracheal intubation and maintenance of anesthesia with nitrous oxide and oxygen using Rees modification of Ayre's technique seems to be most satisfactory. Halothane may be used for spontaneous ventilation, otherwise, controlled ventilation using nondepolarizing muscle relaxants like vecuronium or atracurium is helpful. Monitoring of pulse, respiration, body temperature and ECG is essential. Prochlorperazine IV may be given during anesthesia to reduce postoperative vomiting. Extubation should be done when the patient is fully awake. Analgesics should be given to alleviate pain in the postoperative period.

Probing and Syringing of the Nasolacrimal Duct

It is a minor procedure. Inhalation anesthesia with nitrous oxide, oxygen and halothane under face mask is usually satisfactory. But it should be noted that after probing, saline is syringed through the duct and this may enter the nasal cavity and pharynx. Care should be taken; otherwise aspiration in the respiratory tract may occur. To avoid the problem, endotracheal anesthesia may be the choice.

Anesthesia for Intraocular Surgery

The surgical procedures include cataract surgery, treatment of detached retina and so on. Here also the problem of oculocardiac reflex should be borne in mind. IOP may be affected by anesthetic drugs and techniques, hypoxia, hypercarbia and blood pressure. Coughing and straining may increase the IOP. Induction of anesthesia and emergence should be as quiet and smooth as possible. Vomiting should be avoided as far as practicable.

Adequate sedation and atropine should be given in premedication. Inhalation or intravenous induction is satisfactory. Suxamethonium is better avoided. Endotracheal intubation should be smooth and anesthesia may be maintained with nitrous oxide, oxygen and halothane allowing spontaneous ventilation in minor procedures. Otherwise, controlled ventilation using nondepolarizing muscle relaxants should be employed. Extubation should also be smooth and no coughing or straining is allowed during recovery. In the postoperative period, adequate sedation, analgesics and antiemetics may be needed.

Anesthesia in Cases of Glaucoma

Acute closed angle glaucoma results in a severe risk to IOP and needs urgent treatment. IOP may be reduced with a combination of miotics, IM acetazolamide or IV osmotic diuretics. Peripheral iridectomy is done to relieve the increased IOP. The operation is preferably done under general anesthesia. Retrobulbar injections are contraindicated as there is a danger of retrobulbar hemorrhage and subsequent extrusion of eye contents. Atropine and suxamethonium are somewhat contraindicated in this condition.

Chronic simple glaucoma (open angle glaucoma) is mostly controlled by topical miotics and oral acetazolamide. Failure of such therapy necessitates surgical intervention. Some patients may use anticholinesterase drugs which may cause problems following use of suxamethonium and may produce prolonged apnea.

The anesthetic management is mostly rational with all sensible precautions.

Anesthesia for Penetrating Eye Injury

Penetrating eye trauma is a relatively common injury in children. It may be serious and may be associated with presence of intraocular foreign bodies. It is mostly the emergency procedure. Retrobular block is contraindicated as it may cause retrobulbar hemorrhage and there is danger of extrusion of eye contents. Any increase in IOP may result in loss of vitreous humor. Thus, suxamethonium should not be used in such cases. Inhalational anesthesia may be difficult as the positioning of face mask may not be satisfactory and there is risk of pressure over the injured eye. Patient may have a full stomach and thus preventive measures should be taken against acid aspiration syndrome.

Atropine may be given IV at the time of induction. Analgesic may be given in presence of pain. Induction of anesthesia should be done with thiopentone and muscle relaxants. Endotracheal intubation is mandatory. Anesthesia is maintained with nitrous oxide, oxygen and halothane. Ventilation may be controlled using nondepolarizing muscle relaxants. At the end of anesthesia, adequate decurarization should be done and the child should be extubated when he is fully awake.

Drug Interactions

Children with glaucoma might have been treated with some drugs and these may cause problems during anesthesia.

1. *Acetazolamide*: It is diuretic and thus may produce dehydration and some electrolyte imbalance.
2. Adrenaline used topically may have systemic absorption significantly. Precautions should be taken, particularly during halothane anesthesia.
3. Ecothiopate iodide is a potent anticholinesterase. Suxamethonium may cause prolonged apnea.
4. A topical beta-blocker, timolol maleate used topically, may have significant systemic absorption. Precautions should be taken as in cases of oral beta-blockers.

CHAPTER 15

Anesthesia for Dental Surgery

Special features and problems related to dental anesthesia in children are as follows:
1. Most operations are elective and rarely life saving. Patients are mostly ambulatory and operations are undertaken as day case surgery.
2. Preoperative assessment is usually quick and there is little or no time of laboratory investigations. Preoperative preparation is minimum. Delayed recovery is unwanted and the child is expected to return home on the day of operation.
3. Children require mostly general anesthesia for dental procedures. Local anesthesia has very limited scope in this context.
4. Airway is shared by the surgeons. Inhalation of blood, debris or vomitus may occur. Surgeon needs a wide unobstructed mouth and the anesthetist a clear unobstructed airway.
5. Anesthesia should be smooth and quick, spontaneous breathing is preferred. Jaw should be well-relaxed. No coughing, retching, nausea and vomiting are wanted. Recovery should also be quick.
6. Anesthesia apparatus should be ready well in time. Suction apparatus, a good operation table and life saving drugs should always be available.
7. Posture: When seated on a dental chair, general anesthesia may cause hypotension. Supine position is always preferred.
8. Children may be apprehensive and they should be tactfully managed.
9. Nasotracheal intubation may be helpful in most cases.
10. It should be ensured that no foreign bodies remain in the airway at the end of the procedure.

ANESTHETIC MANAGEMENT

Preoperative Assessment

All children should be adequately assessed in the preoperative period. Medical history is important. Enquiry should be made regarding certain preexisting or past diseases such as cardiac disease, lung disease, rheumatic fever, hypertension, kidney disease, diabetes, blood disease, epilepsy, any nervous trouble. It should be noted whether the child is allergic or not. The child may be on a medicine that may cause severe drug interaction during anesthesia.

Clinical examination should be proper and adequate. There may be trismus, retropharyngeal abscess, nasal obstruction, obesity, mouth sepsis, loose teeth and so on. These have definite anesthetic implications. Enquire about cough, sputum, cyanosis, edema, etc. A thorough examination of cardiovascular system and respiratory system is essential.

Investigations should include blood examination (Hb%, TC, DC, BT and CT), blood sugar estimation and urine examination.

Preparation of the Patient

Children are usually anxious and nervous. They should be tackled with sympathetic reassurance and a good rapport. More careful attention should be given to children who have undergone repeated surgery. No food or drink should be allowed for at least 4 hours before induction of anesthesia. In the case of children, bladder should be emptied before sending the patient to OT. Shoes should be taken off and no tight clothing allowed. Loose teeth should also be taken into account.

No premedication is usually necessary. Narcotics are avoided as these delay the recovery. Atropine sulfate 0.02 mg/kg IV at the time of induction is always helpful.

Induction of anesthesia may be either inhalational through nasal mask or intravenous. Inhalation induction with nitrous oxide, oxygen and halothane is usually satisfactory in children. Halothane is nonirritant and provides quick induction and quick recovery. Prolonged halothane anesthesia may cause hypotension. Inhalation anesthesia may cause hypoxia due to respiratory obstruction or hypotension. Fainting, postural hypotension, sore throat, nausea and vomiting, soft tissue trauma, aspiration, etc. may also occur. Masks may be disliked by some children. Oxygen should be given judiciously and never be less than 30%. Throat pack should be given very carefully and correctly taking care not to push the tongue against posterior pharyngeal wall. It should prevent only oral breathing. A tail should be kept outside. Pack should be removed after the end of the procedure. Complete recovery is essential before discharge.

Intravenous induction can also be employed. Ketamine 2 mg/kg IV may be used satisfactorily. Diazepam is also used IV for sedation. However, complications of intravenous induction include overdose, venous thrombosis, pain, extravascular injection, intraarterial injection and so on.

Endotracheal intubation is mandatory when protection and maintenance of airway is otherwise difficult, as in the following:
a. Difficult access to operation site as in impacted wisdom teeth
b. Prolonged operating time, extended surgery
c. Excessive bleeding
d. Anatomical causes: Short neck, small mouth and macroglossia
e. Major oral or maxillofacial surgery
f. Mentally handicapped child
g. Obstruction in nasal airway.

Endotracheal intubation may be done under either inhalational induction or IV induction with a short-acting muscle relaxant like suxamethonium. Intubation may be done either orally or nasally. Nasal route provides access to either side, but care should be taken as it may cause damage to adenoids. Oral tube should be moved on either side during the procedure. The pack should be placed more posteriorly, if intubation is done.

Standard anesthetic technique includes induction with thiopentone and suxamethonium, nasotracheal intubation and maintenance of anesthesia with nitrous oxide, oxygen and halothane allowing spontaneous ventilation. In controlled ventilation, muscle relaxants like vecuronium or atracurium may be used.

During the procedure, pulse, respiration, blood pressure, body temperature and ECG should be monitored. An intravenous infusion should always be established and maintenance fluids given. At the end of the procedure, adequate decurarization is needed and a clear patent airway must be ensured prior to extubation. Postoperative analgesics may be needed.

On rare occasions, the jaw may be accidentally dislocated during the procedure. In such cases, it should be promptly reduced by downward and forward traction of the mandible. Postoperatively, the child should be placed in lateral position with a slight head down tilt and proper suction should be done frequently.

FILLING AND RECONSTRUCTION OF TEETH

This is usually done under general anesthesia. Standard endotracheal anesthesia should be employed. During forceps extraction or drilling, nonexplosive agents should be used as sparks are created.

The use of air turbine dental drills, the air jet may cause surgical emphysema and mediastinal emphysema which can rapidly extend into the neck leading to airway obstruction and possible pneumothorax. The condition should be detected early. If it occurs, nitrous oxide should be discontinued. Ventilation may have to be supported in cases of pneumothorax.

Eyes should be protected from the drilling dust or debris by applying suitable ointments. At the end of the procedure, mouth and pharynx should be thoroughly cleared by suction to get a clear patent airway.

Adrenaline is sometimes used topically by dentists. Significant systemic absorption may occur and caution is needed in the use of volatile agents, particularly halothane. Hypercapnia should be avoided.

COMMON COMPLICATIONS FOLLOWING DENTAL PROCEDURES

a. Airway maintenance both with or without endotracheal tube may be difficult. Secretions, bleeding and foreign bodies may cause respiratory problems.
b. Cardiac dysrhythmias may occur in unpremedicated children, particularly following halothane anesthesia. This may be due to light anesthesia, elevated endogenous catecholamine secretion and trigeminal nerve stimulation. Deepening of anesthesia or local anesthetic block can reduce the incidences and severity of dysrhythmias.
c. Subcutaneous emphysema may occur over the face and neck by air driven ultrahigh speed dental instruments. It may extend to cause pneumothorax and even air embolism. Air may also cause swelling of tongue and oral tissues and airway obstruction. Adequate precautions and early detection are needed. Nitrous oxide should be discontinued; otherwise, expansion of gas volume may occur. A chest radiograph is always helpful.
d. Bacteremia can occur after dental extractions and nasotracheal intubations. Patients with poor dental hygiene or periodontal infections may suffer bacteremia even in the absence of dental procedures. Children at risk of developing bacterial endocarditis should maintain a good oral health. In such cases prophylactic antibiotic therapy is recommended for dental, oral or upper airway procedures.

CHAPTER 16

Anesthesia for Plastic Surgery

This particular discipline, 'plastic surgery', usually involves reconstruction of damaged or deformed tissues, the removal of surface tumors and cosmetic alteration of some body features. In children, major plastic surgery includes repair of cleft lip and palate, excision of cystic hygroma, reconstructive surgery for burns and burn contracture, craniofacial reconstructive procedures, repositioning of skin and pedical grafts, etc.

Some *specific problems* related to plastic surgery may be enumerated as follows:

1. Children may be grossly deformed due to previous trauma and serious disease, and they are prone to psychological upsets. This may be accentuated by repeated surgery and anesthesia, long confinement and rehabilitation. Thus, a very sympathetic, careful and considerate approach is essential to tackle the child psychologically.
2. Some patients may be having some drug treatment. This should be noted carefully to avoid adverse drug interactions during anesthesia.
3. Children should have no local or generalized infection. State of nutrition and hematocrit should be at acceptable levels as these largely dictate the outcome of the procedure.
4. Blood loss may be considerable in some cases. Blood transfusion is essential in such cases.
5. Many operations are time-consuming and have ill effects of prolonged anesthesia and surgery.
6. Smooth general anesthesia and quiet recovery are required; otherwise, grafts may be dislocated and delicate sutures damaged. Postoperative analgesia should be adequate.
7. One congenital anomaly may commonly be associated with others. This aspect needs careful examination, particularly for congenital heart lesions.
8. Patients with burn contracture of neck and face may lead to difficult intubation. It should be assessed carefully in the preoperative period.

They may have some respiratory problems for which adequate care should be taken during anesthesia.

ANESTHESIA FOR REPAIR OF CLEFT LIP AND PALATE

Cleft lip and cleft palate are common, being as many as 1 in 1000 live births. These congenital defects may be associated with other congenital lesions, like congenital heart disease, Pierre-Robin syndrome, Treacher Collins syndrome and subglottic stenosis. The condition may cause airway problems and lead to difficult intubation.

Cleft lip should be operated as early as possible, even in the neonatal period. But it may increase the incidence of neonatal mortality and morbidity. In the neonatal period, there may be deficiency of tissue to repair it adequately. Cleft lip is usually repaired at 2 to 3 months of age and palate at 18 months to 2 years of age.

Preanesthetic check up should be adequate. Proper examination of cardiovascular system and respiratory system should be made. There may be other congenital defects. Blood examination should include the Hb percentage, TC, DC, BT and CT. Hb should be 10 g% or higher, WBC count should be less than $10000/mm.^3$ Throat swab culture is needed to detect any infection. Examination of mouth may give an indication of potential intubation problems. Cleft lip should be operated usually adopting the rule of 10, that is, Hb 10 g% or higher, 10 weeks of age and 10 lb body weight.

Preanesthetic preparation is essential. No feed or drink is allowed for at least 4 to 6 hours prior to anesthesia. Before that, clear fluid may be given. No solid food is allowed after midnight. Atropine 0.02 mg/kg may be given in premedication 45 minutes before anesthesia. Older children may also receive pethidine 1 to 2 mg/kg IM or trimeprazine 3 mg/kg orally.

Induction of anesthesia may be done with inhalation method. Nitrous oxide, oxygen and halothane may be used, particularly in presence of doubt about the ease of endotracheal intubation. Alternatively, intravenous method with thiopentone and suxamethonium may be adopted.

Orotracheal intubation is essential. Selection of adequate size is most important. Throat pack is given only in case of cleft lip. Endotracheal connection should be more curved and longer. Worcestor connection is mostly helpful. This is to avoid pressure over the tube by the Boyle Davis gag.

Anesthesia is maintained with nitrous oxide, oxygen and halothane with Jackson Rees modification of Ayre's technique. Fresh gas volume should be 2.5 to 3 times the minute volume of the child. Anesthesia may also be maintained with nitrous oxide and a muscle relaxant and controlled ventilation. Anesthetic machine should be placed at the foot end of the child.

Several special features should be noted. There may be *subglottic stenosis* at the level of cricoid. This is the narrowest part of the larynx in children. Undue trauma at the site may cause glottic edema in the postoperative period. Laryngoscopy may be difficult in the left side cleft, where the blade of laryngoscope sinks, in projecting or anteriorly displaced maxillae, and in presence of micrognathia, retrognathia, etc. Bilateral clefts often have a freely mobile premaxilla which is very prone to be traumatized during laryngoscopy.

Endotracheal tube and its connection must be in midposition of lower lip to obviate distortion of the face. Eyes should be protected with some bland eye ointment. Head may be placed in a stable position in a ring and neck extended by pacing a sand bag below the shoulders. During extension the bevel of the tube may come against trachea and cause obstruction: In such cases, extension should be reduced and adjusted accordingly.

Monitoring of pulse, respiration, blood pressure, body temperature and ECG is essential. Precordial stethoscopy may be helpful in monitoring heart and breath sounds. Blood loss should also be estimated.

Fluid therapy should be adequate. Hartmann solution or 5% glucose saline solution may be given. Blood loss above 10% of the estimated blood volume must be replaced by blood. Blood loss in palatal surgery usually needs blood transfusion.

Recovery should be immediate after the end of operation. Laryngeal reflexes should be adequate and the child should be well awake before he is sent to ward. Pharyngeal airway tube should be avoided. Slow gentle suction may be allowed. Baby's arms are to be splinted to prevent interference with the wounds (elbow restraint). Following cleft lip surgery, a Logan bow is frequently used to take tension off the newly sutured lip. In posterior pharyngeal flap cases, some degree of nasal obstruction may occur. The child may have to breathe through the mouth. A small nasal tube is usually kept in situ following such operations. In check flap cases, blood loss is usually more and it should be replaced. Postoperative sedation and analgesia may be given with pethidine hydrochloride 1.5 to 2 mg/kg IM or codeine 1 to 1.5 mg/kg IM.

Anesthetic complications may include obstruction in the endotracheal airway, inadvertent extubation and even cardiac arrest. Postanesthetic complications like airway obstruction, bleeding, aspiration, glottic edema, bronchiolitis, hypothermia, etc. may also occur. Other complications include breakdown of sutured tissue, scarring and persistent palatal opening. Delayed wound healing, diarrhea and otitis media may also occur in postanesthetic period.

BURNS

Burns are classified in three degrees such as first degree erythema, second degree partial thickness skin loss and third degree full thickness skin loss. The rule of nines is used to express the extent of burn injury as a percentage of total surface area. Each upper extremity accounts for 9%, head 9%, each lower extremity 9%, front and back of the trunk each 18% and perineum 1%; total being 100%. In infants, this is somewhat modified to allow for relatively large head. Here each limb accounts for 10% each, head 20%, and 20% each for the front and back of the trunk.

Systemic effects of a severe burn are widespread. Stress response increases the circulating catecholamines, cortisol, antidiuretic hormone, renin, insulin and glycogen. The patient suffers from severe shock, impaired liver function and renal dysfunction.

Following thermal injury there is enormous fluid loss from the circulation and this necessitates massive intravenous infusion to match this in the initial period. Body weight and percentage of surface area affected should be estimated. If the burn is more than 15% in adults and 10% in children, transfusion is indicated. Hematocrit, Hb percentage, electrolytes and pulse and blood pressure should be measured. Fluid volume for replacement can be calculated as body weight in kg multiplied by area of burns as percentage, divided by 2 in ml for every 4 hours for the first 12 hours, then every 6 hours for next 12 hours and then finally over a third 12 hours period.

Another regime of crystalloid resuscitation for burn victims (children) in the first 24 hours is 3 to 4 ml/kg/% body surface area burned. Half the calculated volume is given over the first 8 hours and the rest is administered over the next 16 hours.

The ideal fluid for replacement is plasma. At least half the amount should be plasma and the rest may be the other plasma expanders. Clinical conditions may, of course, modify the regime. The IV therapy should be monitored with the clinical condition of the patient, central venous pressure measurement, hematocrit estimation and measurement of urine volume and specific gravity.

Besides fluid replacement, care should be taken in respect of both ventilation and perfusion. The clear patent airway should be secured and 100% oxygen should be given. The patient may even need endotracheal intubation and IPPV. Such cases also need humidification of inspired gas, physiotherapy and bronchial suction. Respiratory injury may be caused by heat or by inhalation of smoke or chemical fumes. Thermal injury may affect the upper airway resulting in ciliary damage, mucosal edema, surfactant depression and epithelial destruction. There may even be mucosal sloughing and alveolar edema. The use of X-ray, blood gas analysis and fiberoptic bronchoscopy may help to assess the extent of damage.

Basal metabolic rate may be increased enormously due to hypercatabolism. When oral intake is impossible parenteral nutrition is highly indicated.

Special Anesthetic Problems

1. The anesthetist may be involved with acute burns at an early stage when hypoxia is life-threatening. The child may be admitted in ICU under his care.
2. Burns dressings need anesthesia. In such cases repeated anesthesia makes the patient anxious and apprehensive. Severe emotional problems may also result from the accident and disfigurement.
3. In the early stage of burns to the head and neck, raw and painful tissue may cause difficulty in application of face mask.
4. In the late stage of burns, contracture of face and neck, difficulties may arise in intubation. Movements of the neck and temporomandibular joints may be grossly restricted making laryngoscopic intubation difficult.
5. Blood loss during operation is usually massive and thus blood transfusion is needed.
6. Hepatic dysfunction is common following major burns.
7. Pseudocholinesterase level becomes low after burns. It may take even 3 months to come to normal.
8. Suxamethonium is contraindicated in burns. It may cause cardiac arrest secondary to hyperkalemia. Potassium releasing action of suxamethonium begins about 5 to 15 days after thermal injury and persists for about 3 months. This abrupt release of potassium is mostly due to increased chemosensitivity of the muscle membrane as a result of development of receptor sites in the extrajunctional areas (Yao and Artusio, 1985).
9. Nondepolarizing muscle relaxants are needed in high doses to get the desired effect. It may be due to abnormally high volumes of distribution, an increased glomerular filtration rate resulting in high output, increasing drug elimination, excretion of drug in burn wound exudate and increased plasma protein binding (atkinson and Adams, 1985).
10. Recovery from anesthesia should be smooth. Postoperative analgesics are helpful. Patient should be quiet; otherwise, recent graft areas may be damaged.

Burns Dressings

Cleaning and debridement of the wound and redressing are most painful and thus adequate pain relief should be provided. Several analgesic techniques are employed in such cases.

a. *IV analgesics*: A combination of phenoperidine and droperidol may be useful. Nausea, vomiting and respiratory depression may occur. Close monitoring of vital signs is needed.
b. *Entonox*: It is 50% nitrous oxide in oxygen. It provides good analgesia.
c. Volatile anesthetics like methoxyflurane and trichlorethylene may also be used satisfactorily in air with a draw-over vaporizer.
d. *Ketamine*: This is a powerful analgesic and may be given IM or IV. Dysphoria and hallucinations are not common in children. Recovery is somewhat slower following ketamine anesthesia. Ketamine can also be used as slow IV infusion (0.1% solution in 5% dextrose) for pain relief.

NECK CONTRACTURE

Children with neck contracture may pose difficulty in laryngoscopy and intubation. Thus, proper preanesthetic assessment is essential.

If there is no airway problem, the anesthetic management is rather easy and similar to that in other surgical disciplines. The child may be premedicated with pethidine hydrochloride and atropine sulfate in the usual doses. Induction may be either through inhalation (N_2O, O_2 and halothane) or intravenous (thiopentone + relaxant). It is followed by endotracheal intubation, and anesthesia is maintained with nitrous oxide, oxygen and halothane. In controlled ventilation, relaxants are used. All the usual parameters should be monitored. Blood loss should be measured and replaced accordingly.

If there is anticipated difficult intubation, blind nasal intubation under inhalational anesthesia may be attempted. Many times it is very difficult to pass the tube as the scar tissue has distorted the anatomy of the airway. Alternatively, under ketamine anesthesia the scar tissue may be released and then laryngoscopy and direct vision intubation can be performed. Once the airway is established, the standard technique of anesthesia should be adopted.

Recovery from anesthesia should be quiet. Postoperative analgesia should be provided adequately.

ANESTHESIA FOR CRANIOFACIAL DYSOSTOSIS

This involves extensive reconstruction, and specific anesthetic problems related to it are as follows:

1. In the case of severe deformity, it may pose difficulty in intubation.
2. Extensive reconstruction is a major procedure. It is time-consuming.
3. Blood loss may be massive and blood transfusion is always needed.
4. Manipulation of the eye may initiate oculocardiac reflex and may result in cardiac arrest.
5. Deformity of the cranium may cause increase in intracranial pressure.
6. Smooth induction and smooth recovery are essential.

Anesthetic Management

Child should be thoroughly assessed preoperatively. Craniofacial deformity may be associated with other congenital anomalies. Routine investigations should be done. Premedication should include a sedative drug and atropine sulfate.

Induction of anesthesia may be either intravenous or through inhalation. In cases of anticipated difficult intubation, blind nasal intubation may be tried under inhalation anesthesia. If intubation is impossible, tracheostomy may have to be done. Once the airway is secured, anesthesia is maintained with N_2O, O_2 and a muscle relaxant and controlled ventilation using Rees modification of Ayre's technique. All vital signs, ECG and CVP should be monitored. Blood loss is measured and adequate replacement is provided. Following craniotomy, if the brain mass needs reduction, frusemide may be given IV. The child should be fully decurarized at the end of anesthesia and extubation done when the child is fully awake. Postoperative sedation and analgesia are also needed.

EXCISION OF CYSTIC HYGROMA

Cystic hygroma or lymphangioma may present at birth as a multiloculated cystic swelling in the neck. Rarely, it may occur in axilla. Usually, the tumor is large and may extend intraorally. Involvement of the base of the tongue and oropharynx is common and may cause airway obstruction. Intrathoracic extension can also occur.

The intraoral extension of cystic hygroma may pose difficult intubation. Intravenous induction is contraindicated as it may make ventilation impossible in the apneic patient. It is better to maintain spontaneous breathing under inhalation induction and then intubation can be performed. In worst cases, tracheostomy may be needed.

Complete surgical removal of the tumor may be impossible. Blood should be available for transfusion. The child should not be extubated until fully awake.

CRANIECTOMY

Strip craniectomy is usually done for premature fusion of sagittal sutures to decompress the brain and to allow normal brain growth. Operation is performed as early as possible after diagnosis. The major problems are that the procedure is time-consuming and exposed to massive bleeding from dural venous sinuses and exposed bone margins. An intravenous line must be well-established during operation. Blood loss should be measured and adequate blood replacement provided. Vasoconstrictors may be used by surgeons, but care must be taken to limit the total dose, particularly during halothane anesthesia.

MAJOR ORAL AND MAXILLOFACIAL SURGERY

Major oral and maxillofacial procedures are needed for congenital abnormalities, the removal of tumor and mostly for trauma. Fractures of maxilla and mandible may be associated with fracture of cervical spine, head injury and even chest and abdominal injury.

Bilateral fractured mandible may cause acute airway obstruction. If the patient is conscious, it may be relieved by placing him in prone position; otherwise, emergency intubation is indicated. The child may have full stomach. Swallowed blood and loose teeth may be there. Associated fracture of cervical spine may make the patient unstable and proper care is needed during laryngoscopy. Extensive tissue damage and distortion of facial contour may make mask anesthesia impossible. All these factors should be considered while choosing the anesthetic technique. In worst cases, a preliminary tracheostomy may be required. Surgical procedure may be either interdental wiring or open reduction and wiring. Thus, the mouth is wired closed after the procedure. In such cases, postanesthetic vomiting is mostly hazardous and may be fatal.

The child with fractured mandible should be assessed carefully. All precautions against full stomach should be taken. No heavy sedation is needed, but atropine should be given. 'Crash' induction is preferred with thiopentone, suxamethonium and Sellick's maneuver. Nasotracheal intubation is always helpful. Anesthesia should be maintained with N_2O, O_2 and a relaxant with controlled ventilation. Before fixation of jaws, the pack is removed and suction is used to remove the blood clots and debris from the mouth and pharynx. Adequate decurarization should be done. Nasotracheal tube may be kept in situ until the patient is fully awake, and preferably during transportation to the recovery room. Nausea and vomiting should be avoided as far as practicable and prochlorperazine may be given before the end of anesthesia. Close observation of the patient is needed. The wire cutters must be available at hand at all times.

Postoperative edema may compromise the airway and if it is anticipated, nasotracheal tube may be kept in situ for another 24 to 48 hours. Prophylactic antibiotics and dexamethasone should be given to reduce the edema. Analgesics should be used cautiously as overdose may cause respiratory depression.

Removal of Interdental Wiring

General anesthesia is usually needed for removal of interdental wiring in children. Jaw movement may be extremely restricted, mostly due to prolonged immobilization. It may cause difficult laryngoscopy and intubation. Anesthesia may be induced and maintained with nitrous oxide, oxygen and halothane. Great care should be taken to ensure that the patient's airway is clear and patent.

ANESTHESIA FOR CONDYLECTOMY

Various problems due to pathology of the temporomandibular joint and of the mandible itself present formidable challenges in airway management to the anesthesiologist. Ankylosis of temporomandibuliar joint, either bony or fibrous, occurs mainly due to trauma and also from infection of middle ear. Mandible becomes hypoplastic in these cases and the line of dental bite becomes oblique. Inability to open the mouth makes direct laryngoscopy impossible. In such cases, the insertion of nasotracheal tube by a blind technique is extremely essential to maintain satisfactory anesthesia for procedures like condylectomy. Blind nasal intubation avoids the need of tracheostomy which has its own hazards, morbidity and mortality.

Preanesthetic assessment is essential. Investigations should include standard hemogram, urine analysis and X-ray of temporomandibular joints. Adequate oral hygiene should be maintained with proper mouth wash. Premedication should include a sedative drug and atropine. Blind nasal intubation should be done following inhalation induction. Once the airway is ensured, anesthesia may be maintained with N_2O, O_2 and halothane or a muscle relaxant and controlled ventilation in the usual manner.

CHAPTER 17

Anesthesia for Day Case Surgery

Day case anesthesia comprises a large section of pediatric anesthesia in a big general hospital. The admission of a child, surgical treatment under anesthesia, recovery and discharge occur in the same day. The advantages of day stay surgery are numerous. It provides shorter waiting time for operation, recovery of the child in his own home, and avoids psychological trauma of prolonged separation from home and parents. It is mostly economical. It reduces the cost of care and there is less risk of hospital acquired infection.

Day case anesthesia seems to be more challenging than anesthesia for major surgery. Thus, the operating room must be well-equipped with anesthetic machine, suction apparatus, anesthetic drugs and equipment and life saving emergency drugs. There should be some beds for admission of some patients who are not fit for discharge on the same day. Adequate nursing care should also be available. Standard of surgery, anesthesia and nursing care should be the same as for indoor patients. Facilities of resuscitation must also be provided. Increased medicolegal risk in day case surgery and anesthesia should also be borne in mind.

Day case anesthesia has some specific requirements. Anesthesia should be at the particular depth, necessary for operation. There should be rapid, smooth and pleasant anesthesia and rapid awakening at the end of the surgical procedures. It should have minimum side effects and absence of anesthetic complications.

SELECTION OF PATIENTS

Selection of patient for day case surgery is initially done in the outpatient clinic in different surgical disciplines. Any minor surgical procedure expected to last less than 1 hour can be undertaken, provided there will be no massive tissue trauma, no undue hemorrhage and no severe postoperative pain. Various general surgical procedures like eversion of sac, circumcision, excision of superficial lipoma, cyst, rectal polyp, etc. hernia repair, cystoscopy, endoscopy, submucous diathermy and so on are suitable for day case surgery. Procedures of other disciplines may include antral washouts, laryngoscopy, removal of foreign bodies, particularly from upper airway or esophagus, extraction of tooth, examination under anesthesia, particularly eye, cryotherapy, physiotherapy, radiological investigations and so on. A large number of minor orthopedic procedures, such as reduction of fractures, manipulation and plastering of telepes, etc. are also included in day case surgery.

After initial selection, the child should be referred to outpatient anesthesia clinic to assess the physical status of the child and for final selection. The child should be of fitness rating equivalent to ASA grade 1 or grade 2. A thorough clinical examination should be done.

PREANESTHETIC ASSESSMENT

Every patient must be examined carefully. It will help in assessing the physical status and establishing a relationship with the child. Children are usually nervous and fearful. They should be tackled with sympathetic attitude and reassurance.

The clinical assessment should include the name, age, weight, length/hight of the child, relevant history of past and present illness, drug therapy, allergy, any history of cold and cough, any bleeding problem, any congenital abnormality and any anatomical deformity which may make venepuncture or laryngoscopy and intubation difficult. Details of any previous anesthesia should be noted. Past history of major illness like diabetes, asthma, cystic fibrosis, tuberculosis, rheumatic fever, heart disease, liver disease, kidney disease, anemia, jaundice, convulsions, glaucoma and so on should be checked. Clinical examination of respiratory system and cardiovascular system should be done. Pulse, respiration, blood pressure and body temperature should be noted. Minimum investigations should include standard hemogram and urine analysis. Recording of all these informations is essential.

The anesthetist must ensure that consent forms have been completed and the parents are informed of the surgery. Child should be admitted on the day of operation well in time for completing paper work, premedication and other preparations.

PREANESTHETIC PREPARATION

Children should have nothing to eat or drink after midnight on the day before operation. Infants and small children below 4 years, however, should be given liquid feed, even milk at least 6 hours before anesthesia.

On admission on the day of operation, the child should be treated as an inpatient.

Premedication is needed in children to allay anxiety, to prevent pain and to control the vagal reflex activities. Mild sedative may be beneficial, but the drug should not have hangover effect and prolong recovery time. Oral diazepam (0.05 mg/kg body weight) may be helpful when given at least 90 minutes before induction of anesthesia. Children over 5 years of age are usually cooperative and may not require sedation. The routine use of atropine in premedication is also controversial. Atropine sulfate is a good vagolytic and antisialogogue agent, but it may cause cardiac arrhythmia, flushing of face, dryness of mouth and rise of body temperature, particularly in children. It can be given in a dose of 0.02 mg/kg IM at least 45 minutes before anesthesia or IV at the time of induction of anesthesia.

The child should have identification wristlet before sending him/her to the operating room.

ANESTHETIC MANAGEMENT

Induction of anesthesia may be through either inhalation or intravenous technique. Both the techniques are satisfactory and the child may be allowed to choose the technique. However, when the veins are accessible, IV induction is mostly pleasant and preferable.

Of the different intravenous agents, thiopentone, methohexitone, etomidate and ketamine are mostly satisfactory. The awakening time is usually rapid with all these agents. With thiopentone, induction is smooth, but there is a hangover effect. Methohexitone has little hangover effect, but can cause pain on injection. Etomidate also produces pain on injection. Ketamine IV is most pleasant and produces total analgesia. It can cause hallucination and emergence reactions, but the incidence is rare in the case of children. Ketarnine can also be used by intramuscular route in a dose of 8 to 10 mg/kg when body veins are not accessible. Ketamine may prolong recovery time. Propofol infusion may also be used, often combined with a short-acting narcotic drug like alfentanil, and a short-acting muscle relaxant like atracurium depending upon the surgical procedure.

The inhalation method of induction is also popular. Some children may dislike injections and prefer inhalation. Nitrous oxide, oxygen and halothane sequence is being widely used with good results. Halothane causes rapid, smooth induction and recovery. Other volatile agents like enflurane or isoflurane can also be used. Ether and 50% cyclopropane in oxygen can also be used, but these are not used in modern anesthesia due to their various disadvantages. Stage of excitement of ether anesthesia is notorious and both ether and cyclopropane should be avoided during diathermy.

Endotracheal Intubation

In short surgical procedures, endotracheal intubation is not usually necessary. Unnecessary endotracheal intubation should be avoided as intubation has its own hazards. However, endotracheal intubation should always be done whenever indicated. In such cases, intravenous induction with thiopentone and a muscle relaxant like suxamethonium is always preferred. Laryngoscopy and intubation should always be atraumatic. With inhalation induction, intubation should be done at deeper planes of anesthesia. Suxamethonium should be used with caution; it can cause muscle pains, particularly in older children.

It is said that muscle relaxants should be avoided in day case anesthesia unless the indication is strong. Amongst nondepolarizing muscle relaxants, vecuronium and atracurium can be used satisfactorily. Both the drugs are intermediate acting muscle relaxants. Duration of clinical relaxation is approximately 15 minutes and these are mostly without any serious side effects. Moreover, atracurium is degraded in the body by Hofmann reaction. Gallamine and pancuronium are not much suitable in the case of children as they cause tachycardia. Whenever nondepolarizing muscle relaxants are used, adequate decurarization must be ensured at the end of anesthesia.

Maintenance of Anesthesia

Anesthesia can be maintained with nitrous oxide, oxygen and halothane with spontaneous ventilation using Rees modification of Ayre's technique in most cases. It can also be maintained with nitrous oxide, oxygen and a muscle relaxant with controlled ventilation. Sometimes, it can be supplemented with volatile agents and analgesics. Analgesics may prolong the awakening time. Of the volatile agents, halothane is most popular.

Local Analgesia

Local analgesia has a limited value in the case of children, though it is advantageous in the case of adults. Children are mostly noncooperative and they choose 'sleep' during the procedure. However, the caudal anesthesia with light inhalational analgesia may be used for circumcision. A penile dorsal nerve block is also a recognized technique for circumcision.

Monitoring during Anesthesia

All the usual vital signs should be monitored. Pulse, respiration, blood pressure, body temperature and ECG monitoring is essential. Anesthetic machine and its functioning should be regularly checked. Standard of monitoring in day case anesthesia should not deviate from that in inpatient anesthesia.

RECOVERY

The child should be well awake before leaving the operation theater. Restoration of all protective reflexes must be ensured. Then the child is kept in the ward until ready to return home and discharged. In the ward, nursing care should be available. Here also the standard resuscitation drugs and equipment must be available.

Postoperative Sedation and Analgesia

Postoperative analgesia may be needed in the case of some children. But subsequent sedation may delay discharge. However, oral analgesics like aspirin or codeine or paracetamol are often advised and may even be continued at home. Parenteral analgesics may be needed, if the pain is severe. Presence of parents in the postoperative period may lessen the restlessness of the child.

Complications and Sequelae

Postanesthetic complications and sequelae in day case anesthesia are mostly of minor type. Pain, nausea and vomiting, restlessness, drowsiness, sore throat, etc. are common. Of these, pain at the operation site is the commonest. This should be tackled with proper analgesics.

Sometimes, the child may need admission, particularly in the case of major anesthetic complications and unexpected surgical findings and complications.

DISCHARGE

Every child should be examined by the anesthetist before discharge. Child should be well awake, and pulse, respiration, blood pressure and body temperature should be within normal limits. Minor complications, if any, are already tackled. Necessary advice should be given to parents, particularly regarding medications. The child should always be accompanied by parents or responsible attendant. The child is usually very appreciative of early return to his relatives and home environment. Parents should be warned that their child must not ride bicycle or engage in serious activities for 24 hours. If any problem arises in the home, parents should be advised to take the followup service from the hospital.

Guidelines for safe discharge after day case surgery
1. Stable vital signs—Respiration, heart rate and blood pressure
2. Maintains airway unassisted
3. Conscious-May doze, but awakens easily
4. Body temperature normal–No fever, no hypothermia
5. No active vomiting, no vertigo
6. Able to tolerate oral fluids
7. Absence of surgical bleeding
8. No threat of dehydration, no hypovolemia
9. Pain adequately controlled
10. Responsible escort available

CHAPTER
18

Anesthesia for General Surgery

The domain of general surgery is widespread and it mainly involves abdominal surgery, repair of abdominal wall defects, herniotomies and minor procedures like tongue tie, circumcision, orchidopexy and so on. There are certain congenital defects that may need surgery during the neonatal period and they demand special care and considerations. Some emergency cases like diaphragmatic hernia, tracheoesophageal fistula, intestinal obstruction, actute abdomen, etc. may have to be tackled and the emergency cases have their own problems and dangers. These patients should be properly evaluated and managed accordingly. Some cases may involve patients with full stomach and necessary precautions should be taken against acid aspiration syndrome. Some procedures may be time-consuming and may be associated with considerable blood loss. Need for blood transfusion and its hazards should be borne in mind.

The basic principles of anesthesia, in this discipline are mostly similar to those in other branches of surgery. But the anesthetic technique and agents should be chosen according to the need of the individual child.

Monitoring should be adequate and all the usual parameters (pulse, respiration, blood pressure, body temperature, ECG, etc.) should be considered. Special care should be taken for preterm babies, newborn and neonates.

ANESTHESIA IN CONGENITAL DIAPHRAGMATIC HERNIA

Congenital diaphragmatic hernia is not an uncommon disorder, the incidence being 1 in 2260 of all births and it involves about 8% of all major anomalies. It may be of various types. Of these, left-sided Bochdalek (posterolateral) type is most common. It may be of eventration type where whole diaphragm is membranous. Hiatus hernia is situated at the esophageal opening, which is congenitally widened. It is usually associated with short esophagus.

Diagnosis

The baby is apparently normal after birth. Herniated bowel filled up with gas or food may lead to cardiorespiratory embarrassment, dyspnea and cyanosis. There may be diminished movement and breath sound on the affected side of the chest. Borborygmi may be heard over the chest. The mediastinum may be deviated to the contralateral side. Abdomen is usually empty and scaphoid. X-ray chest shows that the heart is pushed to right side and stomach and intestines may be inside the chest. There may be other congenital abnormalities like malrotation of gut, congenital heart disease and renal or neurologic abnormalities.

The case should have a differential diagnosis with certain diseases like congenital lung cyst, congenital heart disease with dextrocardia, esophageal atresia with or without tracheoesophageal fistula and pneumonia with pneumatocele.

Preanesthetic Preparation

The baby should have careful preanesthetic evaluation. Nasogastric tube should be applied and frequent suction should be done. Blood grouping and cross matching are essential. A cut down intravenous line is indicated and infusion with one-fourth or one-fifth glucose saline should be started. Vitamin K 1mg IM is given. The baby should be nursed on semiupright position, slightly rolled to the affected side. It is better to keep the baby in an atmosphere with high humidity and oxygen enrichment. It helps to relieve the gaseous intra-abdominal pressure. High humidity prevents drying of secretions and reduces insensible water loss. In presence of metabolic acidosis, sodium bicarbonate may have to be given. Arterial or capillary blood gas should be monitored.

In presence of severe cardiorespiratory distress, the resuscitation should be initially by endotracheal intubation and controlled ventilation. Positive pressure ventilation using bag and mask may be detrimental, as expansion of the viscera in the hernia further compresses the contralateral lung and heart. Pneumothorax is an ever present danger in such cases.

Anesthetic Management

If the baby is in poor condition, no premedication should be given; otherwise, atropine sulfate may be given about 45 minutes before the induction of anesthesia.

Conscious or awake intubation is mostly satisfactory in neonates. In some cases, induction may be needed with nitrous oxide, oxygen and halothane under face mask. Positive pressure should be avoided as it may further distend the bowel and increase distress. Nitrous oxide should be given cautiously or avoided as it may distend gas containing herniated viscera. Orotracheal intubation should be done and anesthesia maintained with oxygen and halothane using Jackson Rees modification of Ayre's technique. Muscle relaxants should be used to facilitate controlled ventilation. Endotracheal pressure should not be above 25 to 35 cm water pressure; otherwise, rupture of alveoli may occur. Internal bleeding from hypoplastic or collapsed lung may also occur. Monitoring of airway is always helpful.

Pulse, respiration, blood pressure, body temperature and ECG should be monitored. Precordial stethoscope should be placed. Blood loss should be estimated. Blood gas and acid-base status should be checked frequently and corrected as indicated.

The operation is a major and lengthy procedure. It involves thoracoabdominal approach and massive blood loss. All these factors may have some implication for the outcome of the surgical procedures.

Postoperative Care

The baby should be kept in oxygen-enriched high humid atmosphere. Estimated blood loss should be replaced. But over transfusion or over infusion is harmful. Fluid therapy should be adequate. Tube feeding may be started after the return of peristalsis. Intrapleural drain is to be removed after full expansion of lungs. Chest X-ray should be done daily to detect it. Frequent gastric suction and pharyngeal suction should be done. Antibiotics, sedatives and sodium bicarbonate to treat metabolic acidosis, are also needed. Postoperative respiratory assistance is mostly needed when the respiratory status is not satisfactory. If hypoxemia and acidosis persist even with controlled ventilation, a positive end expiratory pressure (PEEP), and the use of 100% oxygen and administration pulmonary vasodilator (tolazoline) may be helpful. Tolazoline can be given in a dose of 1 mg/kg body weight systematically or infused in pulmonary artery. Attempts should be made to keep arterial oxygen tension at 80 to 90 mmHg. As some of these babies revert to fetal circulation with right to left shunting through patent ductus arteriosus, pulmonary vasodilatation may be considered helpful and the baby may respond with improved oxygenation and lowered pulmonary artery pressure.

Prognosis of congenital diaphragmatic hernia largely depends on the degree of pulmonary hyperplasia. Pulmonary hyperplasia seems to have no effective treatment, but extracorporeal membrane oxygenation (ECMO) may be tried with the hope to rest the lung while providing adequate oxygenation for survival and repair of lung parenchyma and restructure of the pulmonary vascular bed. Here the lung should be ventilated with low pressures (20 cm with PEEP of 5 cm H_2O) and FiO_2 of 0.21 to 0.3. As lung function improves, ECMO should be weaned accordingly. The technique is expensive and risky and requires a vascular shunt and heparin.

Complications

These may include vomiting, aspiration, respiratory inadequacy, postoperative pain, abdominal distension, pulmonary infection, wound infection, nutritional deficiency and so on.

Successful outcome of the surgical procedure depends on early diagnosis, nasogastric suction, adequate fluid therapy, pre and postoperative respiratory assistance and adequate surgical, anesthetic and nursing care.

Mortality depends on several factors such as age, prematurity, situation, size and type of gap in diaphragm, degree of obstruction, if present, pulmonary infection, hypoplasia of lungs, delay in diagnosis, poor surgical care, poor anesthetic care and presence of additional congenital abnormalities.

ANESTHESIA IN TRACHEOESOPHAGEAL FISTULA

It is also a common congenital anomaly and requires immediate surgical management. Usual types of tracheoesophageal fistula are as follows:
1. Esophageal atresia with no tracheoesophageal fistula.
2. Esophageal atresia with tracheoesophageal fistula. The upper end ends in a blind pouch and the lower esophagus joins the trachea near its bifurcation. It is seen in nearly 80% cases.
3. Esophageal atresia, the upper segment communicates with trachea.
4. Esophageal atresia, both segments communicating with trachea. The H type fistula is the second most common form. Diagnosis is difficult and usually delayed.
5. Esophagus is continuous but there is fistulous communication with the trachea near its bifurcation.

Clinical Features

There is excessive frothy mucus from the mouth. There may be periodic cyanotic attacks and respiratory difficulty. There is persistent vomiting, particularly after each feed. Nasogastric tube is usually arrested at some part of the esophagus. There are associated pneumonitis and atelectasis. Abdominal X-ray shows excessive air in the stomach. X-ray following introduction of opaque dye through Ryles tube shows blind pouch. If there is fistulous communication, the dye may enter into the lungs.

If the condition persists for a prolonged period of time, there may be aspiration pneumonitis, atelectasis and bacterial pneumonitis leading to sepsis, shunting, hypoxia, hypercarbia and acidosis. Blood examination and blood gas analysis are always helpful. A complete physical examination is essential.

Preoperative Preparation

Suction through a soft nasogastric tube and tracheobronchial toilet should be done. A broad spectrum antibiotic is used to control the infection. Vitamin K 1mg IM should be given. All feeds should be withheld. Baby should be kept in oxygen-enriched high humid atmosphere. Blood should be cross-matched and a cut down intravenous line must be kept. Infusion with one-fifth glucose saline is given. If the dehydration is not apparent, fluid replacement may be approximately 4 ml/kg/hour making allowance for suction.

Anesthetic Management

Usually, no premedication is needed. But often atropine is indicated to reduce the secretions and to prevent the bradycardia associated with halothane anesthesia. Awake or conscious intubation is mostly satisfactory. Anesthesia is maintained with nitrous oxide, oxygen and halothane with spontaneous ventilation using Rees modification of Ayre's technique. If the ventilation is inadequate, controlled ventilation should be done very cautiously; otherwise, excessive positive pressure will distend the stomach. It is preferable to maintain spontaneous ventilation till chest is opened and fistula clamped. Then controlled ventilation may be instituted. Nondepolarizing muscle relaxants like vecuronium or atracurium may be given intermittently, if needed.

Monitoring of vital signs like pulse, respiration, body temperature and ECG is essential. Blood loss should also be monitored and estimated blood lost must be replaced.

Special problems of tracheoesophageal fistula related to anesthesia may include pulmonary complications secondary to aspiration, possibility of intubating the fistula and inflation of stomach by anesthetic gases through the fistula. Surgical procedure involves right thoractomy, closure of fistula and anstomosis of upper and lower esophagus. Gastrostomy may be needed in some cases.

Postoperative Care

The baby should be kept in oxygen-enriched incubator. Chest X-ray should be done daily to detect atelectasis, and hemopneumothorax. In presence of pulmonary complication or respiratory inadequacy, respiratory assistance is indicated in postoperative period.

Fluid therapy should be adequate. Body temperature should be kept normal as far as possible. Antibiotics are needed to control and prevent infection. Sedation may be given judiciously, whenever needed.

Postoperative Complications

Some complications may exist prior to surgery such as continuing pneumonia and problems related to other congenital anomalies. Other complications include wound infection, pulmonary infection, aspiration pneumonitis, mediastinitis, pneumothorax, anastomotic leaks, esophageal stricture, recurrent fistula and so on.

Mortality depends on age, prematurity, associated congenital anomalies, preexisting lung complications, delay in surgery, poor surgical and anesthetic care, type of esophageal atresia and gap between upper and lower esophagus and presence of fistulous communication.

Success of surgical procedure depends on early diagnosis and early operation, absence of other congenital abnormalities, satisfactory body weight, good team work including skilled surgical, anesthetic and nursing care.

ANESTHESIA IN CONGENITAL PYLORIC STENOSIS

Congenital hypertrophic pyloric stenosis usually occurs in babies of 3 to 8 weeks of age. It is a common surgical problem in neonates. The essential pathology is the hypertrophy of the muscle of the pyloric sphincter with subsequent obstruction leading to persistent vomiting, dehydration, electrolyte imbalance and acid-base imbalance.

The operation pyloromyotomy is indicated in neonatal period or in early childhood. Before operation, the condition is to be finally diagnosed with the pathognomonic features such as absence of bile staining of the vomitus, presence of visible peristalis and a palpable pyloric mass. Differential diagnosis with other congenital conditions such as hiatus hernia, duodenal atresia, malrotation of gut, Meckle's diverticulum, etc. should also be done.

Associated metabolic problems in such patients occur secondary to protracted vomiting and the baby is usually alkalotic, hypokalemic, with hypochloremic alkalosis and sometimes hyponatremic. Severe dehydration may cause circulatory shock, lack of adequate perfusion and impaired hepatorenal functions. To assess the severity of fluid and electrolyte imbalance and to monitor therapy, several investigations such as blood count, urine analysis, serum electrolytes, blood urea nitrogen, blood gas analysis and ECG should be carried out. Medical management of the baby with pyloric stenosis is urgent and essential. Circulatory support should be provided with adequate fluid replacement and electrolyte with the necessary ions to correct the deficit. Ringer lactate may be given initially and then one-half strength 5% glucose saline. Potassium should also be added to correct hypokalemia and this may help in the correction of alkalosis. However, potassium should only be given when renal function is established.

Preanesthetic Preparation

Hypertrophic pyloric stenosis should be medically treated to stabilize the infant and the surgical intervention should be made as an elective case.

The fluid and electrolyte therapy should be started to prepare the child and it may take 24 to 72 hours depending upon the severity of the case. Nasogastric suction must be carried out through a nasogastric tube frequently before induction of anesthesia. Premedication is usually atropine sulfate 0.02 mg/kg given 60 minutes before anesthesia. No sedation is usually needed.

Anesthetic Management

Induction of anesthesia is made by the inhalational method with nitrous oxide, oxygen and halothane under a face mask. Halothane provides a safe, smooth and rapid induction. In older children, intravenous technique may be used. This is followed by orotracheal intubation. Anesthesia is maintained with nitrous oxide, oxygen and halothane using Jackson Rees modification of Ayre's technique. At the end of operation, decurarization with atropine and neostigmine should be done, if a nondepolarizing muscle relaxant is used. Monitoring should include blood pressure, ECG, rectal temperature and precordial stethoscope. Blood loss is usually not much. An intravenous line should always be there and adequate fluid therapy is always indicated. Hyperventilation should be avoided as it may worsen the preexisting alkalosis. This may lead to slow return of respiration at the end of anesthesia. Nasogastric tube should be aspirated well prior to endotracheal extubation.

Postoperative sedation is not usually required, particularly in neonates, but older children may need it. Early oral feeds should be allowed as far as practicable. The feed may be started with clear fluids 6 to 12 hours postoperatively.

The baby should be carefully observed in the postoperative period for signs of respiratory inadequacy. This may be due to general anesthesia, preexisting metabolic alkalosis and decreased body temperature. Hypoventilation may predispose to atelectasis. All these should be borne in mind.

Postanesthetic complications may also include gastroenteritis, dehydration, wound infection, aspiration and so on. Hypoglycemia may occur, if intravenous fluids containing glucose are discontinued before oral intake is adequate.

ANESTHESIA IN SURGERY OF ABDOMINAL WALL DEFECTS

From time to time, children, particularly neonates are presented for anesthesia for repair of abdominal wall defects. These defects are mostly congenital. A simplified working classification of abdominal wall defects can be outlined in the following order.
1. *Congenital defects*:
    a. Diastasis recti: Upper midline protrusion of the abdominal wall between the right and left rectus abdominis muscles.
    b. Exomphalos (omphalocele): Defect in the closure of umbilical ring through which viscera covered within a sac herniates. It may be major or minor.
    c. Gastroschisis: Failure of closure of abdominal wall on either side through which protrusion of viscera occurs.
    d. Omphalomesenteric duct remnants: (i) Umbilical polyp, (ii) umbilical sinus, (iii) persistent vitelline duct, (iv) cystic remnant of vitelline duct and (v) Meckel's diverticulum.
    e. Urachal defects: (i) Urinary fistula, (ii) urachal sinus and (iii) urachal cyst.
    f. Complete exstrophy of urinary bladder due to failure of closure of the infraumbilical anterior abdominal wall.
    g. Prune belly syndrome: Absence of abdominal musculature, poor respiratory effort and renal anomalies.
    h. Hernias in the anterior abdominal wall.
2. *Infections of abdominal wall*:
    a. Dermatoses
    b. Subcutaneous infections
    c. Nectrotizing fasciitis
    d. Omphalitis.
3. *Abdominal wall tumors*:
    a. Lipoma
    b. Hemangioma
    c. Neurofibroma.
4. *Miscellaneous*:
    a. Incisional hernias
    b. Burst abdomen.

These abdominal wall defects very often need surgical intervention and thus may pose various problems in anesthetic management, though the basic principles of anesthesia are similar to those for other pediatric surgical procedures.

Gastroschisis

It is a rare congenital full thickness defect in the anterior abdominal wall through which evisceration occurs. The term "gastroschisis" is derived from the Greek word meaning separator or splitting of the belly. The extraumbilical location of the defect, normal appearance and insertion of the umbilical cord and absence of a sac or its ruptured remnants are its main diagnostic features. It is common in males, in prematures and is on the right side of the umbilical cord. The size of the defect may vary from 2.5 to 15 cm and may extend from xiphoid process to pubis. The whole of the gut may be matted due to adhesions and reduced in a mass. The adhesions usually resolve within a week or two. It may be of 2 types—Antenatal and perinatal type. In the antenatal type, the peritoneal cavity is abnormally small due to long standing evisceration in intrauterine life. In the perinatal type the cavity is usually normal, most probably due to evisceration in late pregnancy just before or during active labor. Replacement of the contents and closure of the abdominal cavity are obviously difficult in the antenatal type. An intermediate type may also occur.

There may be associated conditions like prematurity, other gastrointestinal malformations, congenital heart disease and so on. There may be heat loss from exposed viscera, and severe fluid and electrolyte imbalance from the transudation of fluid into bowel. Hypoglycemia is common in such cases. Postoperative ventilatory inadequacy may occur following primary closure due to high intra-abdominal pressure.

Anesthetic management

The baby should be nursed in a semiupright position in a pediatric incubator. Nasogastric suction will help to decompress the bowel. The exposed viscera should be wrapped in a wet towel to minimize heat and fluid loss. An intravenous line should be established and fluid therapy started to correct hypovolemia. Blood should be cross-matched.

Usually, no premedication is necessary. Induction of anesthesia may be with nitrous oxide, oxygen and halothane under a face mask. Following orotracheal intubation, anesthesia is maintained with oxygen and halothane using Rees modification of Ayre's technique. Intermittent doses of nondepolarizing muscle relaxants are needed for controlled ventilation. Nitrous oxide may cause further bowel distension.

The baby should be decurarized and well awake prior to extubation. In the postoperative period nasogastric suction should be continued. If there is impaired ventilation, respiratory assistance is indicated. Fluid and electrolyte balance should be meticulously maintained as severe disturbances may occur from transudation of fluid and heat loss from large exposed abdominal contents. Prolonged intravenous feeding may be helpful in such cases. Electrolyte and acid-base status should be checked regularly.

Exomphalos (Omphalocele)

In omphalocele there is a herniation into the umbilical cord and thus the umbilical cord is continuous with the apex of the sac. The exomphalos sac may be intact or may sometimes rupture before, during or after birth with prolapsed abdominal contents coming through it. The incidence may vary, from 1 in 5000 to 1 in 10000 live births. It may be a part of Beckwith-Wiedemann syndrome, which consists of high birth weight, exomphalos and persistent hypoglycemia. So, preoperative blood sugar estimation is essential in such cases.

Surgical treatment is usually done by excision of sac, if present, and repair of abdominal wall. Ventilation may be impaired during closure of abdomen due to restriction of diaphragmatic movement. In the massive type, use of a sialastic pouch may be helpful, in augmenting the abdominal wall temporarily. Complete repair is undertaken later as the abdominal cavity grows.

The condition may need operation on an emergency basis. Delay invites infection and bowel distension. Omphalocele may be associated with other congenital anomalies. Heat loss may occur from exposed viscera. Fluid and electrolyte imbalance and hypovolemia may occur from transudation of fluid into bowel.

Anesthetic problems and their management are mostly similar to those for gastroschisis. Peritonitis and prolonged ileus are common complications. Continuous nasogastric suction, intravenous alimentation, adequate maintenance of fluid and electrolyte balance, postoperative ventilatory support and meticulous care of the baby are needed for the better outcome of the surgical procedure though the overall mortality is fairly high.

Prune Belly Syndrome

The syndrome involves agenesis of the anterior abdominal musculature causing the skin over the abdomen to wrinkle like a prune. The degree of muscular defect may vary and involve one or both sides of the abdomen.

The costal margin is usually flared and the sternum becomes prominent. Abdomen is bulky. The upper parts of the recti and oblique muscles are usually present. The syndrome is seen only in male babies.

Associated urinary tract abnormalities are common and their severity varies with the deficiency of abdominal muscles. The urinary bladder is usually large and the urachus may be patent as far as umbilicus. There may be dilatation of ureter and pelves of the kidneys depending on the back pressure effect of urine. Testes are always undescended. Anomalies of gut may induce volvulus or intestinal obstruction.

The babies with prune belly syndrome may have renal dysfunction, acidosis, dehydration, urinary tract infection and even septicemia in the preoperative period. The poor musculature of abdominal wall restricts the normal pulmonary function, interferes with the ability to cough and clear the secretions and thus predisposes to various chest complications following anesthesia and may necessitate short-term respiratory support.

Surgical intervention may be needed to restore normal function of urinary tract and to preserve or improve the renal function.

Degree and severity of renal dysfunction should be carefully assessed in the preoperative period. Nephrotoxic drugs should be avoided. Drugs which are primarily excreted in urine should be used very cautiously in reduced doses. Antibiotic cover may be needed to prevent or treat chest and/or urinary tract infection. Extreme care should be taken as the abdomen is abnormally very lax. But if needed, atracurium seems to be the best as its excretion is independent of kidney and liver function. Pancuronium and vecuronium may be used cautiously in reduced doses. Gallamine should be avoided as it is entirely excreted in urine. Ventilation should always be controlled. Extubation should be done when the baby is well awake and very active.

In the postoperative period respiratory parameters must be carefully monitored. Ventilatory support is often helpful. Hypoventilation and a reduced effort of cough may cause retention of sputum and respiratory failure.

Bladder Exstrophy (Ectopia vesicae)

It is a rare congenital malformation and affects nearly 1 in 2000 babies. It is 3 times more common in males than in females. There is a failure of growth of the skin of anterior abdominal wall in the midline below the umbilicus and the urinary bladder and the ureteric orifices are visible. The size of exstrophy may vary and it may even be the same as that of a normal bladder. There is complete epispadius. The recti muscles may be present but widely separated and the intra-abdominal pressure forces the bladder forward to come to the surface. The testes are retained within the abdomen. The pubic bones do not meet in the midline and the pelvis becomes malformed. Exposed bladder mucosa become hyperemic, friable and infected. Hydroureteronephrosis may develop due to edema and fibrosis of ureteric orifices causing urinary outflow obstruction. Definitive surgical intervention is needed even in neonatal period before infection and ureteric problems arise.

The anesthetic management of such a case is usually problematic. It is a time-consuming major surgery. The surgical procedure involves closure of the detrusor muscle and abdominal wall and reconstruction of the bladder neck and posterior urethra and reimplantation of the ureters. If bladder closure is not possible, urinary diversion may have to be made.

General anesthesia with a potent inhalational agent or narcotic and a muscle relaxant is mostly acceptable. Endotracheal intubation should always be done. Controlled ventilation is instituted using Rees modification of Ayre's technique. Initially, the baby is positioned prone for bilateral osteotomies of the iliac bones and thereafter made supine for normal mobilization and closure of the bladder. Adequate care is needed during change of posture. Blood loss should be monitored as severe blood loss is expected. So, adequate blood should be available for transfusion. Two reliable intravenous lines should always be established. While the baby is prone, adequate padding under the pelvis and chest is essential; otherwise, pressure on the inferior vena cava will decrease the cardiac output and increase the bleeding. Prolonged anesthesia and surgery may induce hypothermia, particularly in an air-conditioned theater, so preventive measures should be adopted to conserve the body heat. Monitoring of vital signs is essential. Sometimes serial hematocrits estimation of electrolytes and glucose and blood gas analysis may be helpful.

Incisional Hernia

It is mostly due to misplaced incision, insecure suturing, hematoma formation and sepsis. It may also be iatrogenic when the surgeon intentionally closes the abdomen only by suturing the skin and leaving the cut peritoneum unsutured. Increase in intra-abdominal pressure by cough or intestinal distension may disrupt the peritoneal sutures leading to incisional hernia.

Preoperative assessment is important in such cases. Repair of hernia may cause restriction of diaphragmatic movement, thereby leading to dyspnea and hypoxia. The use of abdominal binder in the preoperative period and respiratory physiotherapy are often helpful in tackling the postoperative respiratory difficulties.

General anesthesia together with a muscle relaxant is usually the method of choice for anesthesia. Ventilation should always be controlled. However, spinal or epidural analgesia may be helpful in older children in selective cases.

Extubation should be smooth and no coughing or bucking should be allowed; otherwise, undue strain on suture lines may disrupt the operative wound.

Blood loss should be measured and lost blood should be replaced adequately. Postoperative analgesia may be needed. Acid-base status should be monitored to detect any hypoxia or hypercarbia. Care should be taken to protect the lungs from aspiration of stomach contents during induction of anesthesia and from infection and atelectasis after operation.

ANESTHESIA IN BILIARY ATRESIA

Biliary atresia may be either congenital or due to postnatal inflammation. Atresia of bile ducts may be extrahepatic, but more commonly it is intrahepatic. The incidence of biliary atresia is said to be 1 in 25000 live births. It may be associated with other congenital anomalies like malrotation of gut, congenital heart disease and so on.

Surgical exploration of bile ducts and intraoperative cholangiography are usually needed to confirm the diagnosis. Surgical procedure is mostly hepatic portoenterostomy (Kasai operation). The operation should be done as early as possible, preferably before 12 weeks of age.

Anesthetic problems in such cases of biliary atresia are numerous. The problems related to neonatal anesthesia are always there. Surgical procedure is time-consuming and blood loss may be severe. Hepatic function is mostly impaired. The babies may have coagulation abnormalities due to hypoprothrombinemia. Intraoperative radiographs are often needed. Good muscular relaxation is needed during dissection of bile ducts. If the jaundice is severe (bilirubin level is more than 17 mg/100 ml), there is a risk of brain damage (kernicterus).

Anesthetic Management

The baby should be properly evaluated in preoperative period. Standard hemogram and coagulogram are needed. Serum bilirubin level should be determined. Vitamin K_1 1mg should be given two or three times preoperatively. Blood should be cross-matched and adequate blood transfusion may be necessary.

Premedication should be given with atropine sulfate 0.02 mg/kg IV at the time of induction. No sedative is needed. Conscious or awake intubation is mostly satisfactory. In some cases, thiopentone and suxamethonium may be used IV in small doses. Following orotracheal intubation, anesthesia may be maintained with nitrous oxide, oxygen and nondepolarizing muscle relaxants like vecuronium or atracurium in incremental doses. Controlled ventilation should be maintained using Jackson Rees modification of Ayre's technique.

The usual parameters of vital signs should be monitored. Fluid therapy should be adequate. Blood loss should be estimated and lost blood replaced. Body temperature should be kept normal as far as practicable. Postoperatively, intravenous alimentation may be useful in such cases as it is difficult to provide a satisfactory carbohydrate intake orally. In severe case of jaundice, exchange transfusion should be considered to avoid brain damage.

ANESTHESIA IN BOWEL OBSTRUCTION

Bowel obstruction may be due to an atresia anywhere from duodenum to anal canal. Malrotation of gut, volvulus, intussusception, meconium ileus, reduplication of gut may also cause intestinal obstruction. Intestinal obstruction is one of the common surgical emergencies in pediatrics.

The major anesthetic problems may be of various types. Fluid and electrolyte imbalance may be there, and its severity increases with delay in diagnosis and operation. Abdominal distension may cause cardiorespiratory embarrassment. Aspiration pneumonitis is a common complication. Adequate precaution should be taken against regurgitation and aspiration during induction of anesthesia. Dehydration, shock and acidosis usually complicate the condition. There are always risks of intestinal perforation and septicemia in such cases. Associated conditions such as prematurity, congenital heart disease and other congenital anomalies may also be there.

Anesthetic Management

The baby should be carefully evaluated in the preoperative period. Adequate fluid replacement and correction of acid-base imbalance and electrolyte imbalance are essential. Several investigations like hemogram, serum electrolytes, blood gas analysis and urine analysis should be done. X-ray abdomen may also be helpful. A nasogastric tube should always be in place as frequent suction is needed for decompression. Vitamin K 1mg IM is indicated in neonates and infants.

Atropine sulfate 0.02 mg/kg should be given at the time of induction. Awake intubation is usually done in neonates and in children in extremis. The possibility of regurgitation and aspiration should be borne in mind. Induction of anesthesia can also be made with nitrous oxide, oxygen and halothane by the inhalation method or crash induction using suxamethonium. Maintenance of anesthesia is usually done with nitrous oxide, oxygen and halothane. Relaxants may also be used and controlled ventilation instituted using Rees modification of Ayre's technique. Nitrous oxide may cause further distension of the gut and so it is better to be avoided. Extubation should be done at the end of anesthesia, when the baby is fully awake and adequate decurarization has been done. Monitoring of vital signs should be adequate. Fluid therapy and blood replacement should be meticulous. Prolonged intravenous feeding in the postoperative period may be required.

Duodenal Atresia

Duodenal obstruction may be due to complete atresia, stenosis, intraluminal diaphragm or annular pancreas. Stomach and proximal duodenum are dilated. There is vomiting and it may be bile stained, if the obstruction is below the ampulla of Vater. Weight loss, hypochloremic alkalosis and dehydration are common. There may be associated anomalies like malrotation of gut, esophageal atresia, imperforate anus, Meckel's diverticulum and congenital diseases.

Anesthetic management should be meticulous in such neonates. Pneumonitis and atelectasis may occur from pulmonary aspiration. Gastric distension may cause cardiorespiratory embarrassment and thus needs frequent nasogastric suction. Fluid, electrolyte and acid-base imbalance should be corrected. Hypothermia and shock should be prevented.

Jejunal/Ileal Atresia

These atresias are also not uncommon. The proximal intestine may dilate enormously and the bowel wall may show congestion and necrosis. Bile stained vomiting is common. Meconium peritonitis may occur. It may be associated with other congenital abnormalities.

The main anesthetic problems include gross distension, cardiorespiratory embarrassment, aspiration, fluid, electrolyte and acid-base imbalance, bowel infarction, bacterial or meconium peritonitis and so on.

Malrotation and Volvulus

The gut may take various abnormal positions and there may be strangulation due to volvulus. Abdominal distension and bleeding per rectum are usual findings. The condition may be associated with other anomalies like exomphalos and duodenal atresia.

The anesthetic problems include huge abdominal distension, fluid and electrolyte losses secondary to vomiting, pyrexia, bowel infarction and septicemia. Fluid therapy and blood loss replacement are essential during surgery.

Meconium Ileus

Some patients with cystic fibrosis may present with meconium ileus. Here the distal ileum is obstructed by inspissated meconium. The condition may be complicated with different atresias, volvulus, perforation, gangrene and meconium peritonitis. In some selected uncomplicated cases, enema may help to relieve obstruction; otherwise, laparotomy is indicated. Surgical procedure may need resection of nonviable segment of intestine and ileostomy. The degree of obstruction and presence of complications make the anesthetic management problematic. Atropine given in such cases may cause the respiratory secretions viscid. As the babies mostly have respiratory problems due to cystic fibrosis (mucoviscidosis), care should be taken to humidify the respiratory gases, particularly in the postoperative period.

Hirschsprung's Disease

The disease is common, the incidence being 1 in 5000 live births. It involves a functional obstruction due to the absence of ganglia in the distal colon and rectum. Clinical features include vomiting, reluctance to feed and abdominal distension within a few days of birth. In the newborn, there may be failure to pass meconium. Erect X-ray of abdomen may show multiple fluid levels as in typical low intestinal obstruction. Rectal biopsy is needed to confirm the diagnosis. Usually, colostomy is done in the neonatal period for temporary relief of obstruction and a later 'pull through' operation like Duhamel's operation is undertaken at about 6 to 9 months of age. In the neonate, the anesthetic management may be problematic mostly due to huge abdominal distension, general ill health, fluid and electrolyte imbalance and presence of other anomalies. The "pull through" operation is usually time-consuming and blood loss may be extensive.

Anorectal Anomalies

These are mostly due to embryological failure of differentiation of the cloaca and urogenital sinus. High anomalies include rectal agenesis where the rectum ends above the levator ani muscle and low anomalies like covered anus where the rectum passes to end close to the perineum. High anomalies may be associated with rectourethral or rectovaginal fistula. Other associated congenital anomalies like congenital heart disease, esophageal atresia, Hirschsprung's disease, vertebral and skeletal anomalies should also be borne in mind.

Surgical procedure for the covered anus such as anal 'cut back' is usually simple and performed in lithotomy position. High anomalies are temporarily managed with colostomy and later at about 6 to 9 months of age 'pull through' operation (posterior sagittal anorectoplasty) is done. Anesthetic management is mostly similar to that in other procedures of pediatric surgery.

ANESTHESIA IN 'ACUTE ABDOMEN'

In pediatric practice acute conditions of the abdomen may often need emergency surgery. The conditions usually include acute appendicitis, perforated Meckel's diverticulum, intussusception and so on.

These patients need special care in anesthetic management. The child may be toxic and pyrexic. There may be fluid and electrolyte imbalance, mostly due to vomiting. As the case is emergency one, there is always risk of full stomach and hence of regurgitation and aspiration of gastric contents in the tracheobronchial tree. In case of intussusception, there may be a massive loss of blood and fluid and occasionally extensive gangrene, and all these make the condition worse. Persistent postoperative ileus and venous thrombosis and infection may be serious for the outcome of the procedure. In children, 'silent' bowel leakage may produce sudden shock and collapse from toxemia.

The child should be carefully assessed in the preoperative period. Fluid, electrolyte and acid-base imbalance should be corrected as far as practicable. If the patient is pyrexic, body temperature should be reduced towards normal by cooling, ice sponging, ice bags, etc. Atropine should not be used in such cases. As the child is more or less with full stomach, a nasogastric tube should be passed for suction of the gastric contents. In presence of 'acute abdomen' the gastric emptying is usually delayed. All precautions against regurgitation and aspiration should be taken. A reliable intravenous line should be guaranteed.

Investigations should include hemogram, serum electrolytes, blood gas analysis and urine analysis. X-ray of the abdomen is often needed for diagnosis. Premedication with only atropine 0.02 mg/kg is usually satisfactory.

Crash induction may be advantageous in such emergency cases. After preoxygenation for 4 minutes, thiopentone 4 mg/kg and suxamethonium 2 mg/kg should be given IV. Cricoid pressure is applied to prevent aspiration. Endotracheal tube should be passed quickly. Once the endotracheal airway is secured, anesthesia may be maintained with nitrous oxide, oxygen and halothane with some nondepolarizing muscle relaxants like vecuronium and atracurium. Controlled ventilation may be instituted using Rees modification of Ayre's technique.

Monitoring of vital signs like pulse, respiration, blood pressure and body temperature is essential. Fluid therapy should be cautious and blood transfusion may be necessary. At the end of surgery, extubation should be done after reversing the effects of the muscle relaxants and when the child is fully awake. Postoperative analgesics should be given as required.

ANESTHESIA FOR SPLENECTOMY

Splenectomy in children may have to be undertaken in cases of idiopathic thrombocytopenic purpura (ITP) or thalassemia major or trauma. In ITP, there is excessive destruction of platelets by the spleen due to presence of an antiplatelet factor. The condition may sometimes be complicated with severe intracranial bleeding or gastrointestinal hemorrhage. Splenectomy in such cases causes a definite improvement. In thalassemia the primary defect is a slow rate of hemoglobin synthesis and there is always low level of hemoglobin. Here splenectomy is usually done empirically with the hope of lessening the destruction of red blood cells in spleen. In case of trauma or intra-abdominal injury, splenectomy may have to be done, if there is splenic rupture.

Special anesthetic problems may include severe anemia. Anemia may be severe with Hb 5 to 7 g% in thalassemia cases. Repeated blood transfusion may cause hemosiderosis and impair myocardial and liver function. In ITP, platelet count is low and this cannot be improved satisfactorily even with transfusions. Thus, there is always a risk of bleeding even with minor trauma. Some patients may have a steroid therapy and these patients need adequate steroid cover in the perioperative period. In cases of trauma, the child may be in shock and may need emergency laparotomy. In these cases adequate resuscitation should be done beforehand. Blood is needed to replace blood loss. There is always a risk of regurgitation and aspiration of gastric contents in the tracheobronchial tree and, therefore, all possible precautions should be taken.

The patient should be well-prepared in elective cases. Anemia should be corrected as far as practicable. Blood should be kept ready for transfusion. Platelet concentrate may be needed after the removal of spleen.

Induction of anesthesia is usually intravenous with thiopentone and suxamethonium in usual clinical doses. The level of pseudocholinesterase may be low in anemic patients. Following endotracheal intubation, anesthesia should be maintained with nitrous oxide, oxygen and a muscle relaxant (nondepolarizing) with controlled ventilation using Rees modification of Ayre's technique. During endotracheal intubation, trauma should be avoided as it may cause bleeding, particularly in cases of ITP. Hypoxia, hypercarbia and hypotension should always be avoided. At the end of anesthesia extubation should be done after adequate reversal of muscle relaxant and when the child is fully awake. Fluid replacement should be meticulous. Postoperative sedation and analgesia are always advised.

ANESTHESIA IN PHEOCHROMOCYTOMA

Pheochromocytoma is a relatively rare condition in children. It usually occurs in the adrenal medulla and may be bilateral. In some cases, it may occur in any sympathetic ganglion. Adrenaline and noradrenaline are the principal hormonal secretions when the tumor occurs in adrenal medulla. But when it occurs in sympathetic ganglion, it produces mostly noradrenaline. The principal symptoms include sustained or episodic hypertension, palpitations, headache, blurred vision, fits, sweating, etc. Clinical signs essentially include hypertension, increased basal metabolic rate and oxygen requirements, hemoconcentration, increased blood levels of glucose, lactic acid, and free fatty acids. There may be retinopathy and renal pathology. Diagnosis may be confirmed by estimation of plasma catecholamines level or of their metabolite 3-methoxy-4-hydroxy-mandelic acid. The tumor may be localized by selective arteriography, aortography or pyelography following an adrenergic blockade or by CAT scan. Surgical removal of all tumor tissue should be the treatment.

Anesthetic management of such cases is usually problematic. Adequate control of blood pressure may sometimes be difficult. There may be cardiac arrhythmias. Extensive blood loss may occur during surgery. Severe hypertension may occur during manipulation of the tumor and severe hypotension may occur after its removal. There is arteriolar constriction with increased systemic arterial pressure and venous constriction with a reduced blood volume.

Hypoxia and hypercarbia may increase the secretion of catecholamines and thus should be avoided during anesthesia and surgery. Some anesthetic drugs and muscle relaxants such as ether, cyclopropane, ketamine, suxamethonium, etc. may increase the release of catecholamines. Halothane should also be avoided as it may sensitize the heart to catecholamines. Curare and alcuronium may release histamine and aggravate catecholamine secretion.

Preparation for anesthesia and surgery should be started well in advance to control the hypertension and to produce a good adrenergic receptor blockade preoperatively. Phentolamine or phenoxybenzamine can be used as these (alpha-adrenergic blockers produce vasodilatation causing hypotension and reducing the ratio of blood volume to capacitance. Adequate blood volume should be maintained by infusion of fluid, preferably under CVP monitoring. In presence of tachycardia, a beta-adrenergic blocker is also indicated.

A good premedication may help to reduce catecholamine release. Atropine is usually avoided as it increases metabolic rate and heart rate. Premedication should provide adequate sedation.

As in such cases sudden changes of blood pressure can occur, monitoring should be started before induction of anesthesia. Central venous pressure measurement, electrocardiography and direct arterial pressure measurement should always be done. Urinary output should also be measured. At least two good venous accesses must be established for rapid infusion, blood transfusion and administration of drugs. Certain drugs should be readily available to tackle the emergency situation. These drugs include phentolamine to lower blood pressure, propranolol to treat arrhythmias, isoprenaline to increase the heart rate, noradrenaline to raise the blood pressure and sodium nitroprusside to produce hypotension. Adequate supplies of blood for transfusion should also be ensured.

Anesthesia should be induced with thiopentone 4 mg/kg and vecuronium 0.1 mg/kg or atracurium 0.5 mg/kg IV. Pancuronium, gallamine, tubocurarine or suxamethonium are not recommended as these may cause either tachycardia or hypertension. Anesthesia is maintained with nitrous oxide, oxygen and muscle relaxants with controlled ventilation using Jackson Rees modification of Ayre's technique. Analgesics may also be given IV. Normocapnia should be maintained. Blood gas analysis at frequent intervals may also be helpful.

During operative manipulation, a short-acting hypotensive drug like nitroprusside should be used to avoid hypertensive crisis. The abrupt release of catecholamines can be minimized by early clamping of the venous drainage. Arrhythmias can be well-treated with beta-blockers. Hypotension occurring after the removal of tumor should be better treated with fluid replacement rather than catecholamine (nonadrealine) infusion.

At the end of surgery, the child should be decurarized and extubation done when the child is well awake. Postoperative sedation and analgesia may be needed. Fluid therapy should be adequate. Blood glucose level should be checked at frequent intervals as hypoglycemia may sometimes occur following the fall in catecholamine level.

ANESTHESIA FOR MINOR SURGERY IN CHILDREN

Inguinal Herniotomy/Orchidopexy

These operations are common in early childhood. These are usually done as elective procedure. However, obstructed incarcerated hernia is rare in children and if it occurs, it should be treated as an emergency case.

Inguinal herniotomy and orchidopexy are usually minor procedures. The child should be assessed carefully in the preoperative period. The minimum investigations should include hemogram and urine analysis. The child should be premedicated with only atropine sulfate 0.02 mg/kg IV at the time of induction. Older children may need oral trimeprazine 3 mg/kg or diazepam 0.4 mg/kg at least 90 minutes before induction of anesthesia.

Induction of anesthesia is usually done by inhalation method with nitrous oxide, oxygen and halothane. Endotracheal intubation is usually done and anesthesia may be maintained with nitrous oxide, oxygen and halothane. In older children, of course, induction may be done with thiopentone and a muscle relaxant given IV. Anesthesia may be maintained with nitrous oxide, oxygen and a muscle relaxant with controlled ventilation. This is particularly helpful when a more extensive intra-abdominal exploration becomes necessary.

The child should be extubated when he is fully awake and after reversal of nondepolarizing muscle relaxants. Postoperative analgesics are needed. During anesthesia adequate depth must be maintained to protect against reflex disturbances such as laryngospasm during testicular manipulation and spermatic cord traction.

Circumcision/Urethral Meatotomy

It is the most common operation in children done in the pediatric outpatients department. The child should be assessed preoperatively and prepared adequately. Usually, only atropine sulfate is given in premedication about 60 minutes before induction of anesthesia. The anesthesia may be induced and maintained with nitrous oxide, oxygen and halothane under a face mask with spontaneous ventilation. Usually, no endotracheal intubation is needed.

In these cases, management of postoperative pain is essential. Analgesics should be given. Pethidine hydrochloride 1.5 mg/kg may be given IM. Caudal block or block of dorsal nerve of penis may be useful to provide analgesia in postoperative period.

Urethral meatotomy is a brief procedure lasting only a few minutes. It may be done under intravenous anesthesia with ketamine 2 mg/kg or propofol 2mg/kg.

Rectal Polyp

Excision of rectal polyp is also a minor procedure, but it needs adequate muscular relaxation. Rectum should be kept empty as far as practicable during operation. Usually, enema is given preoperatively. Here also only atropine sulfate 0.02 mg/kg IV should be given at the time of induction. Anesthesia may be induced and maintained with nitrous oxide, oxygen, and halothane under a face mask. Operation should be allowed when the child is under a deep plane of anesthesia.

Operation for Tongue-tie

This is also a very minor procedure done in the pediatric outpatients department. The problem lies in the fact that the operation is inside the oral cavity. There is a risk of aspiration of blood, etc. into the respiratory tract.

In this case also, only atropine is given at the time of induction. Induction may be done with nitrous oxide, oxygen and halothane. Endotracheal intubation is done in most cases and anesthesia maintained with nitrous oxide, oxygen and halothane. If bleeding occurs, frequent pharyngeal suctions should be done to remove blood. The child should be fully awake at the end of surgery. Analgesics are not usually needed in the postoperative period.

Cystoscopy

It is a common urological procedure in children. It usually requires general anesthesia via a face mask or an endotracheal tube with nitrous oxide, oxygen and halothane. Anesthesia should be adequate and deep prior to urethral instrumentation in order to prevent laryngospasm (Brener-Luckhardt reflex). Any body movement during instrumentation may cause urethral or even bladder injury. Postoperative analgesic may be needed in some cases.

CHAPTER

19

Anesthesia for Urological Surgery

Anesthesia for urological surgery in children involves a wide variety of clinical conditions ranging from short minor surgical procedures like circumcision, urethral meatotomy, cystoscopy, hypospadius to major procedures like bladder exstrophy, resection of Wilms tumor, Anderson Hynes operation and so on. Some patients may have good renal function, but some may have poor renal function. These patients may be suffering from anemia, uremia, etc. The surgical procedures may also be associated with extensive blood loss, fluid shifts, heat loss and other organ derangements. Thus, it is better to be familiar with some common urological conditions of children for better outcome of surgical and anesthetic procedures.

Some of the urological conditions such as circumcision, cystoscopy, orchidopexy and bladder exstrophy, etc. have been already discussed in the previous chapters. The rest will be discussed in the present chapter.

VOIDING CYSTOURETHROGRAMS

It is usually a minor procedure. In most children, it can be performed in waking condition without anesthesia. But in an uncooperative child, it may need general anesthesia with nitrous oxide, oxygen and halothane under a face mask. A deeper plane of anesthesia is needed before the urethral instrumentation. But all volatile anesthetics, barbiturates and atropine relax bladder muscle and the sphincter tone. So, anesthesia should always be lightened just after the instrumentation.

HYPOSPADIUS

Repair of hypospadius is most commonly performed in children. The cases are usually taken up as elective ones. No special anesthetic problems are usually faced, unless it is associated with other congenital anomalies and other systemic disorders. Endotracheal anesthesia with nitrous oxide, oxygen and halothane or muscle relaxants is mostly satisfactory.

Regional techniques such as caudal block using 0.25% bupivacaine with adrenaline may also be helpful, particularly in older children.

PYELOPLASTY/URETERAL REIMPLANTATION

These two are common urological surgical procedures in children. Pyeloplasty is done for ureteropelvic obstruction and ureteral reimplantation for vesicoureteral reflux.

These children should be carefully assessed in the preoperative period as they might have renal dysfunction. A thorough medical history and physical examination should be done. The assessment of renal function is essential and some investigations such as urine analysis, serum electrolytes, blood urea nitrogen, creatinine clearance, renal ultrasound and intravenous pyelogram should be done. In presence of renal parenchymal damage, either due to obstruction or due to chronic reflux, there may be hypertension. These patients may be under treatment with antihypertensive drugs and thus it is always recommended to continue the drugs throughout the perioperative period. Associated anemia, if present, should be adequately treated in preoperative period.

Routine preparation should be done. Adequate intravenous access is needed. All vital signs such as pulse, respiration, blood pressure, body temperature, CVP and urine output should be monitored. Blood loss may be profuse; hence, blood transfusion may be needed. Prolonged anesthesia and surgery in an air-conditioned theater may cause significant heat loss; thus, adequate preventive measures should be taken. The operation is usually in a lateral decubitus. This needs adequate padding of all pressure points and avoidance of extreme positions.

Induction of anesthesia with thiopentone and suxamethonium IV in usual clinical doses is satisfactory. Inhalation technique may be used in small infants. Endotracheal intubation should be done and anesthesia should be maintained with nitrous oxide, oxygen and nondepolarizing muscle relaxant (vecuronium or atracurium) with controlled ventilation. Adequate reversal is needed at the end of surgery. Postoperative analgesia is needed. Systemic narcotics may be given. Continuous caudal block may also be useful.

WILMS TUMOR

Wilms tumor is a relatively common neoplasm in children. It is also known as nephroblastoma and presents as an abdominal (retroperitoneal) mass. Abdominal pain and fever are the usual symptoms. The condition may be associated with other congenital anomalies. Hypertension may occur, most probably due to renal ischemia and release of renin from the tumor cells.

Hypertension may cause varying degrees of congestive cardiac failure. Local invasion by the tumor into the interior vena cava with subsequent embolization during operation may occur. Metastatic spread to lungs is also common. Chemotherapy may be helpful in some cases and it may consist of various drugs such as actinomycin, doxorubicin, cisplatin, etoposide and so on. All these drugs are mostly myelosuppressive in nature causing anemia, coagulation defects, debility, gastrointestinal disturbances and susceptibility to infection, etc. Moreover, doxorubicin is cardiotoxic and etoposide may cause hepatic and renal dysfunction. Thus, children being treated with these drugs may cause anesthetic problems.

Large abdominal mass may cause intestinal obstruction and increased intragastric pressure; thus, there is always risk of regurgitation and aspiration during anesthesia. It may necessitate a rapid sequence induction. Cardiorespiratory embarrassment may also occur with large intra-abdominal tumors. Blood loss may be massive and, therefore, enough blood should be available. An intravenous line should always be in place prior to induction. Preoperative evaluation should be made carefully and basic investigations should include hemogram, serum electrolytes, blood urea nitrogen, creatinine, coagulation profile, chest radiograph and intravenous pyelograms.

The usual technique of anesthesia may be employed with nitrous oxide, oxygen and halothane or muscle relaxants with controlled ventilation using Rees modification of Ayre's technique. Monitoring of usual vital signs including arterial blood pressure and central venous pressure is essential. Fluid therapy should be adequate and blood replacement is also required. Analgesics may be required in postoperative period. Hypertension may continue in postoperative period and requires antihypertensive therapy.

ANESTHESIA IN CHILDREN WITH CHRONIC RENAL DISEASES

Many children may have poor renal function due to some chronic renal diseases. These children always present some special anesthetic problems. These are as follows:

1. *Anemia*: Children with chronic renal diseases are usually underweight, thin and anemic. The anemia is mostly due to decreased erythropoietin formation, increased hemolysis, bone marrow depression, iron and folic acid deficiency and increased bleeding tendency. Anemia is mostly refractory to conventional drug therapy. Often, blood transfusion is needed. It is better to use fresh packed cells; otherwise, circulatory overloading and severe hyperkalemia may occur.

2. *Fluid balance*: Fluid overload may occur in both acute and chronic renal failure. It may lead to congestive cardiac failure and hypertension and this should be treated before anesthesia. Diuretics may be tried, and in resistant cases dialysis is indicated.
3. *Serum electrolyte changes*: Children with polycystic kidney or severe pyleonephritis may lose sodium, while with glomerulonephritis there are problems of sodium retention, hypertension and edema. Hyperkalemia is also common in chronic renal failure. It is often associated with metabolic acidosis. These should be corrected prior to anesthesia. Suxamethonium is contraindicated in presence of hyperkalemia. Hypokalemia may also occur in the cases of prolonged diuretic therapy. Potassium replacement may be needed before anesthesia.
4. *Acid-base imbalance*: Metabolic acidosis is common in such cases. The plasma bicarbonate level falls significantly.
5. *Coagulation defect*: This is most probably due to thrombocytopenia, decreased adhesiveness of platelets and increased capillary fragility. Renal disease may be associated with disseminated intravascular coagulation.
6. *Cardiovascular effects*: Hypertension may occur in advanced renal failure. It may be due to increased secretion of renin, angiotensin and aldosterone. Fluid retention may also be a factor. Heart failure may occur in chronic uremia; it is usually left-sided with consequent pulmonary congestion and edema. These children may be under treatment with antihypertensive drugs which may cause problems during anesthesia. Digitalis and diuretic therapy may also be problematic.
7. *Pulmonary and/or peripheral edema*: These are usually due to overloading of circulation, hypertensive cardiac disease or hypoproteinemia. Uremia may cause pericardial effusion. Large pleural or pericardial effusion may require paracentesis before operation to reduce the risk of cardiorespiratory embarrassment.
8. *Uremia*: Uremia causes drowsiness and coma. Electrolyte and fluid imbalance may aggravate the condition. Sedative drugs should be used very cautiously. Severely uremic patients should be treated with several measures such as elimination of infection, restriction of dietary protein intake and removal of extrarenal causes of renal dysfunction. In resistant cases hemodialysis is indicated preoperatively.
9. *Hemodialysis*: Immediate preoperative hemodialysis may cause some problems such as circulatory overload, enhanced digitalis toxicity and increased bleeding tendency. In case of over-correction of acidosis, serum calcium level may be reduced and tetany may precipitate. Children undergoing chronic hemodialysis may be carriers of hepatitis B

antigen and, thus, proper precaution should be taken by all concerned. These children with hemodialysis have a shunt or fistula in place and special care is needed to keep the device functioning at all times.
10. *Reduced immunity*: These children usually have low resistance to infection due to reduced immunity.
11. *Gastrointestinal disturbances*: Nausea and vomiting are common and may aggravate the fluid, electrolyte and acid-base imbalance.
12. *Concurrent drug therapy*:
    a. Diuretics may cause hypokalemia, alter acid-base balance and potentiate the antihypertensive drugs. Hypokalemia may precipitate digitalis toxicity and potentiate the action of nondepolarizing muscle relaxants.
    b. Antihypertensive drugs potentiate the hypotensive action of anesthetic drugs like halothane. Withdrawal of these drugs is not recommended, as it may raise blood pressure and take it out of control.
    c. Digitalis and other glycosides increase myocardial irritability and may cause cardiac dysrhythmias during anesthesia.
    d. *Beta-adrenergic blockers*: Larger doses of propranolol may potentiate the neuromuscular blocking effects of tubocurarine. Propranolol may cause bronchospasm. Practolol is cardioselective.
    e. Antibiotics may prolong the effect of nondepolarizing muscle relaxants.
    f. Many children are on long-term steroid therapy. They should continue steroid therapy pre-, per- and postoperatively.
    G. Some antimetabolites are highly protein-bound and thereby they may increase the bioavailability of other protein-bound agents by displacing them on the protein molecule. Drugs used in chemotherapy may have some ill effects and they can adversely affect the course of anesthesia.

Preanesthetic Assessment and Preparation

1. History of preexisting renal disease should be taken into account.
2. The type of operation and its approximate duration should also be taken into account.
3. Careful physical examination of the patient must be done. Anemia, hypertension, fluid imbalance, electrolyte imbalance, acid-base imbalance, dysfunction of liver and cardiorespiratory system may be present.
4. Body weight should be noted and due allowance made for any edema.
5. Investigations should include blood examination, blood biochemistry, urine examination, blood gas analysis, serum electrolytes, etc.

6. Circulatory overload, if any, should be treated adequately with judicious administration of diuretics.
7. If serum potassium is above 6 mEq/lit or in cases with severe acid-base derangement, hemodialysis may have to be considered preoperatively.
8. In presence of infection, adequate precautions and antibiotic cover are needed.
9. Blood should be cross-matched and be available during surgery.
10. Nephrotoxic drugs must be withheld. Current drug therapy should also be borne in mind.
11. The limb with a shunt or fistula needs special care. It should not be used for pressure readings or intra-arterial or intravenous lines.
12. Antihypertensive drugs must not be discontinued.

Anesthetic Management

A light premedication with benzodiazepines like diazepam is satisfactory. The drugs should be used in smaller doses than normally needed. Anesthetic management should aim to prevent and avoid further renal damage and to detect and treat the complications. Drugs which are primarily excreted in the urine should be avoided and, whenever used, the dose should be kept minimum. Atropine in premedication may be avoided as it causes extreme tachycardia, particularly in anemic children. In uremic patients, tolerance of sedatives, narcotic analgesics, anesthetic drugs and blood loss, etc. are reduced. The dose of barbiturates used for induction should also be kept minimum.

Anesthesia is induced with IV thiopentone 2–3 mg/kg and atracurium 0.5 mg/kg or vecuronium 0.1 mg/kg. Suxamethonium is contraindicated in hyperkalemic children. Inhalation technique with nitrous oxide, oxygen and halothane may also be adopted. Endotracheal intubation should be done and anesthesia maintained with nitrous oxide, oxygen and muscle relaxants with controlled ventilation using Jackson Rees modification of Ayre's technique. Halothane may be used but methoxyflurane is contraindicated due to its nephrotoxicity.

Monitoring of usual parameters of vital signs such as precordial stethoscopy, ECG, blood pressure, body temperature and CVP should be done. In selected cases blood gas study may be needed. Fluid replacement should be made with sensible precautions. Blood lost should be replaced as far as practicable. Urine output should also be monitored. Overtransfusion and potassium containing fluid infusion should be avoided. Muscle relaxants need adequate reversal at the end of surgery. Hypoxia, hypercarbia and hypotension should be avoided at all times.

Postoperative Care

The child should have a good ventilation and oxygenation in the immediate postoperative period. The electrolyte, fluid and acid-base status of the patient should be assessed and adequate therapy provided, whenever necessary. In cases of poor renal function, a short period of postoperative dialysis may be beneficial.

For postoperative pain, analgesics may be given in reduced doses. The effect should be monitored and supplements may have to be given, if necessary. Pulmonary infection is common. Antibiotics, if needed, should be based on culture and sensitivity tests. Nephrotoxic antibiotics should be avoided. Doses should be adjusted to avoid toxicity. Deep breathing exercises and general physiotherapy are helpful in the postoperative period.

CHAPTER 20

Anesthesia for Neurosurgery

Anesthesia for neurosurgery in pediatric cases may involve some special problems. These are as follows:
1. Raised intracranial pressure (ICP)
2. Surgical procedures are mostly lengthy. Severe blood loss may occur. Blood transfusion is always needed.
3. Surgical trauma may produce cerebral ischemia.
4. Maintenance of airway may be problematic in some cases.
5. Head-up or prone or lateral posture may be needed in some procedures which may adversely affect the physiology of the child.
6. Use of diathermy may necessitate the use of nonexplosive anesthetics and techniques.
7. Some children may have poor general health.

Anesthesia for neurosurgery requires conditions which will maintain adequate perfusion of brain with blood. This essentially depends on cerebral perfusion pressure. Cerebral perfusion pressure equals mean arterial pressure minus intracranial pressure. The cerebral perfusion rate is highest in children and decreases slowly with age. Anesthesia should also provide optimal surgical conditions by reducing brain volume and minimizing hemorrhage. General anesthesia is mostly satisfactory for neurosurgical operations in children. But care should be taken that the anesthetic drugs and techniques do not adversely affect the cerebral blood flow and intracranial pressure. Most of the inhalational anesthetics increase the ICP and most of the intravenous agents, with the exception of ketamine, decrease the ICP. Hypoxia and hypercarbia may increase the cerebral blood flow, while hypocarbia may decrease the cerebral blood flow. The anesthesia should have smooth induction and rapid and complete recovery. Postoperative analgesia, whenever required, should be given with extreme caution as these may cause respiratory depression.

CEREBRAL BLOOD FLOW (CBF)

Autoregulation of cerebral blood flow (CBF) ensures maintenance of constant blood flow within a widerange of systemic blood pressures between 90 and 180 mmHg, and even as low as 45 to 50 mmHg, when the child is in supine position. CBF is also related to venous pressure which may be influenced by gravity, intrathoracic and intra-abdominal pressure, blood volume, circulatory efficiency and venous tone. CBF varies directly with blood carbon dioxide tension when it is between 20 and 80 mmHg. Increase in blood oxygen tension reduces the CBF and the decreased oxygen tension increases the CBF. CBF is also regulated by cerebrovascular resistance depending upon the caliber of cerebral vessels and the viscosity of blood. Vasodilation of normal reactive cerebral vessels reduces blood flow in low resistance vessels and in areas which may have lost autoregulation due to cerebral infection or trauma (intracerebral steal). Vasoconstriction of normal reactive cerebral vessels may have the opposite effect. Pyrexia causes cerebral vasodilation, while hypothermia has the reverse effect.

Cerebral vasodilation may be produced by halothane, ether and chloroform. Inhalational agents mostly increase CBF and intravenous agents, with the exception of ketamine, either have no effect on CBF or decrease it. Muscle relaxants usually have no direct effect on CBF. Sodium nitroprusside inhibits cerebral autoregulation and thus may increase the intracranial pressure. But deliberate hypotension, on the whole, results in fall of CBF. Diazepam may cause reduction in CBF.

INTRACRANIAL PRESSURE (ICP)

Normally, intracranial pressure (ICP) ranges from 100 to 150 mm of H_2O above the atmospheric pressure. The source of this pressure is the secretory pressure of choroid plexuses. CSF pressure should be measured in the horizontal position with the spine and external occipital protuberance in the same line.

The ICP may be decreased in various conditions, such as in dehydration, in shock following blood loss, with elevation of head and following removal of a space occupying lesion. Normally, the ICP oscillates with the arterial pulse and also varies with respiration. Pressure usually falls in inspiration and rises in expiration.

The ICP may be increased during coughing, sneezing, straining and during defecation, etc. Raised intracranial tension may be found in craniostenosis, hydrocephalus, cerebral edema and with the head-down position. It may also occur with venous obstruction or with arterial dilatation or in presence of space-occupying lesion, like neoplasm, abscess or hematoma. Raised ICP may be worsened during general anesthesia, if associated with hypoxia, hypercapnia, coughing or straining.

Signs of Raised ICP

Clinical features arising from a raised ICP of slower onset usually include a history of headache, vomiting and papilledema. In presence of a space occupying lesion above the tentorium cerebelli, there are drowsiness and clouding of consciousness. Pupil on the side of the lesion dilates and reacts less to light and subsequently the pupil on the other side also dilates and both become unresponsive to light. Respiratory failure is common at this stage. When the lesion is in the posterior fossa, there are bradycardia, bradypnea, hypertension, drowsiness, clouding of consciousness and respiratory failure. When the cerebellar tonsils are pushed through the foramen magnum, the child holds his head very stiff, slightly retracted and turned to one side. In this position, the foramen magnum provides maximum diameter to accommodate the medulla and tonsils pushed through it. A hydrocephalic cry may also be noted. Loss of upward movement of the eyes also occurs in posterior fossa compression.

Reduction of intracranial tension may sometimes be needed. The usual methods are as follows: (a) ventricular tap, (b) spinal drainage, (c) use of hypertonic solutions IV, mannitol, urea, 50% sucrose, etc. (d) increasing head-up tilt, (e) lowering blood pressure, (f) hypothermia, (g) hyperventilation, (h) use of muscle relaxants to reduce intra-abdominal pressure and venous pressure, (i) use of steroids (Dexamethasone 0.015 mg/kg IV upto 10 mg decreases cerebral edema in response to surgical brain trauma) and (j) oral glycerol.

CEREBROSPINAL FLUID (CSF)

Cerebrospinal fluid (CSF) is formed from choroid arterial plexuses of the third, fourth and lateral ventricles by secretion or microfiltration. Meningeal and ependymal vessels and blood vessels of brain and spinal cord may also produce a little amount of CSF. It occupies the cerebral ventricles and the subarachnoid spaces surrounding the brain and spinal cord.

CSF passes from the lateral ventricles into the third ventricle through the foramen of Munro and then along the aqueduct of Sylvius into the fourth ventricle. CSF then passes through the lateral foramina of Luschka, Key and Retzius and the midline foramen of Magendie into the cisterna magna and throughout the subarachnoid spaces.

CSF is removed into the venous sinus of the brain through the arachnoid villi and into the lymphatic stream through the pacchionian bodies.

CSF acts as a fluid cushion to protect the brain and spinal cord from injury. It may also regulate the volume of cranial contents. It may have a slight function in the metabolic exchanges of nervous tissue.

CSF is clear and colorless with slight opalescence due to globulin with less than 5 lymphocytes/mm^3. Its specific gravity is 1003 to 1009. It is alkaline, pH being 7.6, with protein 20 to 40 mg/l 00 ml; sugar 40 to 80 mg%, sodium chloride 750 mg%, urea 10 to 30 mg/100 ml, bicarbonate 24 mEq/lit.

CSF is produced roughly 0.5 ml/minute in adults. The total volume is approximately 120 ml. Production of CSF should match removal or absorption to prevent an increase in intracranial pressure. If there is obstruction to the flow of cerebrospinal fluid, the intracranial pressure will increase and the ventricles upstream from the obstruction will dilate.

ANESTHETIC MANAGEMENT

The child should be preoperatively assessed carefully. ICP should be judged and the adverse effects of anesthesia on ICP should be taken into consideration. The presence of impaired consciousness, papilledema or neurological deficit should also be assessed. There may be dehydration and electrolyte imbalance due to excessive vomiting. These also need adequate attention. Some children may be under some medication like steroid, antihypertensive or anticonvulsant drugs and these may have some implications on anesthetic management.

The child with grossly elevated ICP may need some reduction in ICP by drug treatment or even ventricular drainage before operation. In presence of cerebral edema, steroid therapy should be started. Children receiving steroids should have adequate steroid cover during and after operation. Neurosurgical operations usually cause significant blood loss and thus blood should be cross-matched and available during operation.

Preoperative visit is essential. Child is usually anxious and fearful. Adequate reassurance and sympathetic explanation should be provided to the child.

Narcotic analgesics and heavy sedation are usually contraindicated. But diazepam may be helpful as it is anxiolytic, anticonvulsant and does not cause respiratory depression or any adverse effect on ICP in usual clinical doses. Atropine sulfate 0.02 mg/kg should be given at the time of induction for its antisialogogue and vagolytic effects. A nasogastric tube is always helpful to suck out the gastric contents.

Induction of anesthesia should always be smooth. No straining, coughing or bucking should be allowed. Hypoxia and hypercarbia should be avoided.

Drugs that increase ICP should not be used. Intravenous induction with IV thiopentone and suxamethonium is mostly satisfactory. Intubation should be smooth. A beta-adrenergic receptor blocker or lignocaine 1 to 1.5 mg/kg IV prior to intubation may minimize the rise of ICP associated with laryngoscopy and endotracheal intubation. Larynx and upper trachea may also be sprayed with 4% lignocaine. A nonkinkable endotracheal tube is preferred, particularly for surgery in prone position. The endotracheal tube should be fixed to the face with meticulous care after checking its position for correct placement.

Anesthesia may be maintained with nitrous oxide, oxygen and a nondepolarizing muscle relaxant (pancuronium, vecuronium or atracurium) with controlled ventilation using Jackson Rees modification of Ayre's technique. Analgesics may be given IV, whenever needed. Volatile anesthetic agents mostly increase CBF and, therefore, if used, should be in the lowest concentrations, compatible with adequate anesthesia. Controlled hyperventilation is often needed to reduce the brain volume and decrease the ICP during intracranial surgery and to improve the quality of cerebral arteriogram during neuroradiology. Adequate depth of anesthesia should always be provided.

An intravenous infusion should be started from the beginning of anesthesia. A second, separate infusion line may also be kept ready. The eyes should be well-protected with some bland eye ointment. There should be no stretching of peripheral nerves and vulnerable pressure points should be protected.

Posture during neurosurgery is important in order to provide a good operative access and to allow adequate venous drainage from the operative site by elevation of head above the level of heart. But excessive flexion or rotation of the neck may cause venous obstruction. The supine, lateral and prone positions are common. Sitting posture is usually discouraged. In prone position, meticulous care should be taken to support the body on the iliac crests and the chest, and to get free uncompressed abdomen and vena cava.

Monitoring during anesthesia is vital and it should include esophageal stethoscopy, direct intra-arterial pressure, CVP, thermometry, ECG, end-tidal carbon dioxide and serial blood gas analysis. Urinary output should also be measured.

Intravenous fluid therapy needs utmost care and precautions, whenever diuretics (mannitol or furosemide) are used. The schedule of fluid therapy may have to be modified according to the urine output. Blood transfusion is often needed. Blood loss is difficult to measure in cranitomies. Clinical assessment and hematocrit value will help in assessing the adequacy of blood replacement.

The children should be fully awake at the time of extubation. Reversal of nondepolarizing muscle relaxants should also be adequate. Hypoxia, hypercarbia and hypotension should be avoided; otherwise, brain edema may occur. In cases with anticipated brain edema or respiratory inadequacy, ventilatory assistance may be continued in the postoperative period. Betamethasone or dexamethasone should be started in anticipated brain edema. Some children may develop convulsions in the postoperative period and they should be treated with IV phenytoin. Postoperative sedation is often needed, but narcotic analgesics should be avoided.

Hypotensive Anesthesia

Induced hypotension may sometimes be needed in major craniotomies in children. But it should be done in well-selected cases and by expert anesthetist. The child must not have contraindications like diseases of heart, lungs, liver, and kidney, and metabolic disorders. Induction of anesthesia should be smooth, a perfect patent airway should be established and anesthetic depth should be adequate. Hypoxia, hypercarbia and tachycardia should be avoided.

A safe range of systolic blood pressure in the supine position ranges from 50 to 60 mmHg upto the age of 10 years and 70 to 75 mmHg in children above 10 years. Various drugs are used for induced hypotension, Halothane may be used in cases where short periods of hypotension are needed. Controlled ventilation and slight head-up tilt during halothane anesthesia are also helpful. Pentolinium or sodium nitroprusside can also be used to produce intentional hypotension. Pentolinium may cause dilatation of pupils which may remain dilated postoperatively. Sodium nitroprusside may interfere in cerebral autoregulation and increase ICP. It should be used after the skull is opened. Care should be taken to avoid cyanide poisoning with sodium nitroprusside, maximum dose being 3 mg/kg body weight.

Monitoring of pulse and blood pressure by direct artery catheterization is mandatory. Body temperature, CVP, urine volume, ECG and blood gas analysis should also be monitored. Fluid therapy should be adequate and blood loss should be fully replaced. Postoperatively, a careful check on vital signs should be kept.

ANESTHESIA FOR NEURORADIOLOGY

Anesthesia is often needed for neuroradiological investigations in children. It is mostly indicated in small children, noncooperative children, when the procedure is long and unpleasant, and when the child must be kept immobile. Some anesthetic problems may arise in such cases. The investigatory procedure is carried out in X-ray department, which usually lacks the facilities obtained in a well-equipped operation theater. Anesthesia may have to be given in difficult environment. The child may have increase in ICP and this has implications for the choice of anesthetic drugs and techniques. The use of a contrast medium carries some intrinsic risk. Anaphylactic and other hypersensitivity reactions may occur and thus resuscitative drugs and equipment should always be available. Anesthesia should be smooth and recovery should be rapid at the end of the procedure.

The child should be assessed preoperatively and a thorough clinical examination should be made. Usually, no sedatives and narcotics are needed. Atropine may be given IV at the time of induction. Intravenous induction of anesthesia with IV thiopentone and muscle relaxants, endotracheal anesthesia with controlled ventilation using Rees modification of Ayre's technique is mostly satisfactory.

In children with raised ICP, adequate measures should be adopted to attenuate the hypertensive response to laryngoscopy and endotracheal intubation.

Computerized Axial Tomography (CAT)

It is very commonly used investigation nowadays. The procedure is not uncomfortable, but requires complete immobility of the child. Older cooperative children may not need any anesthesia, but smaller children, noncooperative children need general anesthesia. Usual standard technique of general anesthesia may be adopted. Inhalational anesthesia with spontaneous ventilation or continuous IV sedation may also be used. Only plastic materials should be used in the breathing circuit as metal interferes with X-ray imaging.

Arteriography

Arteriography of the cranial vessels in children is usually performed under general anesthesia. The technique should include endotracheal intubation, muscle relaxation and hyperventilation. Hyperventilation improves the quality of radiographs, provided arterial carbon dioxide tension is maintained at about 30 mm Hg. Contrast medium is usually very hypertonic and, therefore, the dose should be kept minimum. Complications like bradycardia, hypotension, etc. may occur.

Air Encephalography and Ventriculography

In these procedures, air, oxygen or nitrous oxide is injected into the lumbar subarachnoid space, or directly into the cerebral ventricle. The passage of gas is governed by patient position and radiographs are taken in different postures of the child. Nitrous oxide anesthesia may increase the volume and pressure in the ventricular system, when air is used as the contrast medium. The use of nitrous oxide as contrast medium may obviate such problems. Usually, general anesthesia is needed for children, but hypoxia, hypercarbia and hypotension should be avoided. In older cooperative children, local anesthesia and sedation may be used.

Myelography

These studies can be performed under local analgesia and sedation in cooperative older children; otherwise, general anesthesia is needed. Anesthesia may be maintained with nitrous oxide, oxygen and halothane. Monitoring of pulse, respiration and blood pressure is essential.

HYDROCEPHALUS

Hydrocephalus is mostly due to obstruction in the outflow of the CSF. The obstruction may be within the CSF pathway, within the brain itself or it may be due to failure of absorption of the CSF by the pacchionian granulations. It is usually the result of brain tumor pressing the CSF pathways. Hydrocephalus may occur in aqueduct stenosis due to a congenital anomaly. It may be associated with Arnold-Chiari malformation where the cerebellum and medulla lie partly within the cervical spinal canal and in extreme causes the lower end of pons may be at the level of the foramen magnum. The other causes of hydrocephalus are meningeal inflammation leading to obstruction in subarachnoid space or the pacchionian granulations and interruption of the normal absorption of CSF. Hydrocephalus may result from the closure of a myelomeningocele.

Hydrocephalus may give rise to lack of activity, drowsiness, vomiting and convulsions. There is progressive enlargement of skull and a typical facial appearance develops. There are features of increased ICP, dulling of the mental faculties, low grade papilledema and squint.

Treatment of hydrocephalus by surgical means usually involves creation of CSF shunts. The common shunts are ventriculoperitoneal shunt (lateral ventricle to peritoneum) and ventriculoatrial shunt (lateral ventricle to right atrium). Here a tube is inserted into the lateral ventricle either to the peritoneal cavity or the right atrium and a oneway valve is incorporated.

Preoperative assessment should be carefully done. In presence of severely increased ICP, immediate ventricular tap is required to reduce the ICP. The child may often be apneic due to high rise of ICP. In such a case, the child should be intubated, properly ventilated and immediate ventricular tap should be done. Usually, no sedation is required, only atropine sulfate 0.02 mg/kg may be given IV at the time of induction.

Intravenous induction of anesthesia with thiopentone and suxamethonium in usual clinical doses may be done. Lignocaine 4% spray in the pharynx and larynx may help to attenuate the hypertensive response of laryngoscopy and intubation. Endotracheal intubation should be done, but difficulty is often faced due to large sized head. Anesthesia is maintained with nitrous oxide, oxygen and muscle relaxants (vecuronium or atracurium) with controlled ventilation using Rees modification of Ayre's technique. Hypoxia, hypercarbia and hypertension should always be avoided. Ketamine and volatile anesthetics should not be used. Hypertension due to increased ICP usually disappears when ICP is reduced. Blood loss is not much significant during the shunt surgery.

Some anesthetists advocate spontaneous ventilation during anesthesia using nitrous oxide, oxygen and halothane. Spontaneous ventilation helps to detect the rise of ICP as the patient becomes apneic on high rise of ICP.

Monitoring during anesthesia is vital and it should include monitoring of pulse, respiration, blood pressure, ECG and body temperature. Changes in blood pressure are common in shunt operation. Hypertension may also occur due to rise of ICP. Hypotension may occur following the ventricular tap.

In ventriculoatrial shunts, there is a risk of air embolism, while the vein is opened for insertion of the tubing. The tubing should be filled with either CSF or hypertonic saline before insertion into the vein; otherwise, the air inside the tubing may enter the vein. Controlled positive pressure ventilation may be useful in preventing air embolism. ECG monitoring is essential to detect the exact placement of the shunt tube in the right atrium. Insertion of the tubing inside the heart may pose some risk of cardiac arrest. Excessive drainage of CSF into the atrium may overload the circulation.

At the end of the procedure, extubation should be done after adequate reversal of nondepolarizing muscle relaxants and when the child is fully awake. Narcotic analgesics should be avoided.

MYELOMENINGOCELE/ENCEPHALOCELE

These defects result from the failure of the neural tube to close in the fetus. The incidence of encephalocele is less than that of myelomeningocele. Meningocele is the congenital herniation of the meninges protruding through an opening of the skull or spinal column. Myelomeningocele involves spina bifida with portions of cord and memebranes protruding. Encephalocele is the protrusion of brain through a cranial fissure.

When the defect is large, there are problems of fluid and heat loss during surgery. Often, there is rupture of membranes with consequent infection. Neurological deficit may also be there. The surgical procedure involves excision of sac and repair of the defect. Operation is usually done in the prone position. Blood loss may be significant, and, therefore, blood transfusion is needed during operation.

The baby is usually neonate and thus needs adequate care during anesthesia and surgery. The baby should be assessed preoperatively. There may be other associated congenital anomalies. The baby should be premedicated with only atropine sulfate 0.02 mg/kg IV at the time of induction.

Awake intubation is usually satisfactory in such cases. Otherwise, inhalation induction with nitrous oxide, oxygen and halothane is used. Endotracheal intubation may be a problem, particularly in babies with large occipital meningocele. Anesthesia may be maintained with nitrous oxide, oxygen and halothane. Controlled ventilation should be done as the baby is operated in the prone position. Muscle relaxant can be used intermittently. Rees modification of Ayre's technique is the standard circuit used in the case of these babies. The baby should be monitored with precordial stethoscope and ECG. Blood loss should be replaced as indicated. At the end of operation, the baby should be extubated when he is fully awake. Narcotic analgesics should be avoided. In cases of encephalocele, there may be some rise of ICP in the postoperative period. Thus, close observation and care are needed. The baby should be kept in an incubator and nursed prone on a frame.

CRANIOSYNOSTOSIS

It is the premature fusion or ossification of cranial sutures. It leads to a typical deformity and causes mental retardation. Surgical treatment involves craniectomy, that is, the division of skull along suture lines. The operation is time-consuming and massive blood loss from injured cerebral venous sinuses may occur. Adequate blood should be available during operation. In some extreme cases, raised ICP may be seen.

The child should be premedicated with atropine sulfate IV at the time of induction. Intravenous induction with thiopentone and suxamethonium may be satisfactory. Endotracheal intubation is essential and the tube should be well-secured in place. Anesthesia is maintained with nitrous oxide, oxygen and muscle relaxants with controlled ventilation using Rees modification of Ayre's technique.

Monitoring during anesthesia should be adequate. Fluid therapy and replacement of blood loss need special attention. The child should be wide awake at the time of extubation.

CEREBRAL TUMOR

Cerebral tumors may occur in childhood. Posterior fossa tumor is relatively more common than anterior and middle fossa tumors. The surgical procedure involves craniotomy and excision of the tumor.

These patients may have raised ICP and thus need special anesthetic care to provide satisfactory intracranial conditions for operation. There may be some associated metabolic, cardiac or respiratory disorders. These should be evaluated and treated preoperatively. The procedure is usually a major one and blood loss may be significant. Thus, adequate blood should be available during operation. Anesthesia should be smooth and hypoxia, hypercarbia and hypotension must be avoided. Drugs which increase ICP should not be used. Recovery should be rapid to allow accurate neurologic assessment postoperatively.

These patients should be carefully assessed and every attempt should be made to allay their preoperative fear, anxiety and tension. Usually, no sedation is required; only atropine should be given IV at the time of induction. Intravenous induction with thiopentone and suxamethonium is mostly satisfactory, but care should be taken that no straining or coughing occurs. Lignocaine 4% spray into the pharynx, larynx and upper trachea prior to intubation may attenuate the hypertensive response to laryngoscopy and endotracheal intubation. Anesthesia should be maintained with nitrous oxide, oxygen and a nondepolarizing muscle relaxant with controlled ventilation using Rees modification of Ayre's technique. Vecuronium or atracurium may be used satisfactorily. Controlled ventilation should provide arterial carbon dioxide tension of about 30 to 35 mmHg. Blood gas analysis should be done in these cases. A slight head-up tilt may be helpful in cases of anterior or middle fossa tumors. In posterior fossa tumor, the child should be kept in prone position with a slight head-up tilt and with thorax and abdomen kept free. Here nasotracheal intubation and fIrm fixation of the tube are essential.

Monitoring in these cases is most vital. Pulse, blood pressure, ECG, body temperature, CVP and urine output should be monitored. Fluid therapy should be adequate and replacement of blood loss is mandatory. Reduction of brain volume may be needed in some cases during operation.

The child should be fully recovered at the end of surgery. Narcotic analgesics are better avoided. Adequate watch and nursing care are required in the postoperative period.

HEAD INJURIES

Head injuries in children are not uncommon. These are mostly due to road accidents, but may occur as birth injury also. Subdural hematoma and subarachnoid hemorrhage may also occur. Anesthesia in cases of head injuries may be related to extracranial surgery in children with mild head injuries or intracranial surgery in severe head injuries. An anesthetist may also be involved in resuscitation and medical care of comatose children admitted in ICU.

Anesthesia for Head Injuries

Children with head injury should be properly assessed, particularly with regard to the cardiovascular, respiratory and neurological status. In emergency cases, the child may have a full stomach and, therefore, adequate precautions are needed to prevent aspiration. A nasogastric tube should be passed to make stomach empty by suction. The child may have other injuries on the body, particularly in thorax, abdomen or spine. The child may be comatose or unconscious. There may be respiratory inadequacy, for which immediate intubation and assisted ventilation with 100% oxygen are necessary. All children with head injury usually have some cerebral edema due to damaged cerebral blood vessels. Thus, there may be some degree of loss of autoregulation. There may be some rise of ICP and during anesthesia there is always a risk of further increase of ICP, particularly when volatile anesthetics are used. Hypoxia and hypercarbia also increase ICP and deteriorate the neurological status of the child. Hyperthermia may occur, particularly in cases with pontine hemorrhage and, therefore, adequate measures should be taken to bring down the temperature towards normal. In presence of hypovolemic shock, the etiology should be found out and adequate treatment should be provided.

Anesthetic management of such cases is mostly of the same standard as in neurosurgery. Endotracheal intubation is mandatory in such cases. Extreme care should be taken in the case of the child with associated cervical spine injury during laryngoscopy and endotracheal intubation. Reduction of cerebral edema may have to be done with IV mannitol or frusemide during anesthesia and surgery. In the case of unconscious children, the anesthetic requirements are minimal, but endotracheal intubation and adequate ventilation should always be maintained during anesthesia.

Management of Head Injuries

The child may be unconscious and there may be an airway obstruction. The child should be placed in the semiprone position and the airway should be cleared of any blood, vomit or secretions. In presence of respiratory inadequacy and impaired cough and swallowing reflexes, endotracheal intubation and ventilation should be done with 100% oxygen. Controlled ventilation may be helpful in producing mild hypocapnia. A nasogastric tube is always helpful in sucking out the gastric contents. Tracheostomy may be needed in some cases.

The cardiovascular status should be checked. Hypotension, whenever present, is mostly due to associated injuries. Bleeding from any site may occur and should be checked. Infusion should be started and blood transfusion may be carried out, whenever necessary.

Clinical assessment of neurological status and degree of coma should be carefully judged. Investigations like blood biochemistry, X-ray, scans and arterial blood gas analysis should be done.

Routine care of the eyes, mouth, joints, etc. is essential. An indwelling urinary catheter is also needed. Body cooling is often needed to reduce hyperthermia and cerebral metabolism.

Sedation is often necessary. Intramuscular phenobarbitone or pentobarbitone may be used for treating restlessness, but narcotics should always be avoided. Normal fluid requirements and appropriate electrolytes should always be administered. Parenteral feeding is also required.

Reduction of cerebral edema may be tried with intravenous hypertonic glucose, mannitol, frusemide or cortisone. Mannitol reduces the volume of intracranial water by extracting water from normal brain, but does not reduce cerebral edema *per se*. Frusemide may reduce CSF formation in addition to reducing intracerebral water.

The child with rapid decline in conscious level or sudden development of unilateral neurological signs, bradycardia with wide pulse pressure, with progressively spastic or flaccid musculature and also deep respiration, probably needs immediate surgical intervention.

Head Injury Associated with Spinal Cord Injury

Head injury associated with spinal cord injury/compression poses extra problems during anesthesia.
1. Suxamethonium should be avoided in such cases. There may be enormous release of potassium from the denervated muscles in response to suxamethonium. Serum potassium must be checked preoperatively.
2. Moving and positioning of these patients, particularly to the prone position need extreme care. Excessive movement may complete a partial transection of the spinal cord or markedly worsen existing damage.
3. Laryngoscopy and endotracheal intubation may be difficult and hazardous in such cases. Neck movement may be extremely limited or absent. The patient may be in rigid cervical collar or minerva plaster. Laryngoscopy and intubation should be better tried with the patient breathing spontaneously. All intubation aids including fiber optic bronchoscope should be available.
4. Mild degrees of hypoxia and hypercarbia may be lethal in such head injury cases.

CHAPTER 21

Anesthesia for Cardiothoracic Surgery

Thoracic surgery, particularly lung surgery is not much common in pediatric age group. However, lung surgery may be indicated for lung abscess, bronchiectasis, lung cysts, bronchogenic cysts and pulmonary neoplasms. Pulmonary arteriovenous malformation may also need lung surgery. Diagnostic biopsy may also be needed in some cases.

General assessment of children with these problems should be done carefully including their physical examination. Careful examination of the respiratory system is essential in these children presenting for thoracic surgery. Cyanosis may be present, either central or peripheral. There may be asymmetrical movement of chest, deviation of trachea or stridor. Auscultation may reveal crepitations or rhonchi.

Preoperative investigations should always be done. Full blood count, urine analysis, blood biochemistry, particularly blood glucose estimations should always be a routine procedure. Radiological examinations such as posterolateral and lateral X-rays of the chest are always helpful. Bronchography is needed in the child with bronchiectasis.

Pulmonary function should be evaluated as far as practicable, but it is difficult to obtain reliable data in the case of small and uncooperative children. Blood gas study is essential in such cases presenting for thoracic surgery, as it may dictate the appropriate inspired oxygen concentration during and after surgery.

SPECIAL PROBLEMS RELATED TO LUNG SURGERY

1. It is usually a major surgery and massive blood loss may occur. A reliable intravenous line must be established and adequate blood should be available for transfusion.
2. The child may be preoperatively ill-ventilated and when the thorax is opened, there may be major inequality of ventilation and perfusion.

Inspired oxygen concentration should be adjusted according to arterial blood gas studies.
3. Fluid therapy needs careful attention and even a mild fluid overload may be dangerous in children with already impaired pulmonary function.
4. In children with lung abscess or bronchiectasis, there is a chance of contamination of the normal lung during surgery and the lung segment may need to be isolated. Double lumen tubes and bronchial blockers are not available in appropriate sizes for small children. Selective intubation of either right or left bronchus may be helpful in some selected cases.
5. Preoperative physiotherapy is helpful to clear bronchial secretions, particularly in older children.
6. Preoperative bronchoscopy is sometimes used to remove the secretions.
7. Pulmonary arteriovenous malformation may cause large right to left shunt causing low arterial oxygen tension. In such cases, hypoxemia cannot be corrected by increased inspired oxygen concentration.
8. Postoperative analgesics are always needed as pain may limit coughing and deep breathing and cause atelectasis.
9. Postoperative respiratory care is essential.

ANESTHETIC MANAGEMENT

The child should be properly assessed preoperatively. Antibiotics may be needed, if infected sputum is present. Bronchodilator drugs and even corticosteriods may be used to reduce bronchospam. Adequate hydration, electrolyte correction and intravenous fluid therapy are often required preoperatively. The choice of premedication remains wide, but use of an anticholinergic drug is always advisable.

The child should be adequately preoxygenated with 100% oxygen using a face mask. Anesthesia is induced with IV thiopentone followed by suxamethonium. Orotracheal intubation is done and anesthesia is maintained with nitrous oxide, oxygen with intermittent narcotic analgesics and nondepolarizing muscle relaxants. Ventilation is controlled adequately. Inspired oxygen concentration should be such as to maintain arterial oxygen tension at about 100 mmHg and carbon dioxide level in between 35 and 45 mmHg.

A wide bore intravenous line must be established. Blood should be kept ready for necessary transfusion. The usual monitors should also be applied. Monitoring of blood gas is most important in such cases. Esophageal stethoscope and thermistor probe should also be there. After proper positioning of the child for thoracotomy, ventilation should be checked in all areas of lungs. Endotracheal tube may have to be sucked when there is excessive secretion. Ventilation should be well controlled and adequate.

Special precautions should be taken if one-lung anesthesia is given. The inspired oxygen should be increased and monitoring of blood gas studies is essential.

Following the operative procedure, adequate reversal of nondepolarizing muscle relaxants should be done. Lungs should be periodically inflated at the time of closure of chest. The chest drain should be checked regarding connection to under water seal. The child should have adequate spontaneous ventilation before extubation; otherwise, respiratory assistance must be continued in the postoperative period.

Postoperative Care

Postoperative analgesia is essential. Narcotic analgesics may be advised. Intercostal nerve blocks may be helpful. Monitoring of vital signs should be continued in the recovery room. Blood gas studies are essential to detect ventilatory adequacy. A chest radiograph should be done to detect pneumothorax or atelectasis, if any. Fluid therapy should be judicious and blood transfusion may be needed. Hemoglobin and hematocrit estimations are helpful.

CONGENITAL LOBAR EMPHYSEMA

A congenital emphysematous lobe may be large enough to compress the remaining normal lung. In such cases, there are subsequent mediastinal displacement, respiratory embarrassment and cyanosis. In extreme condition, it needs immediate surgical intervention and even lobectomy in early neonatal period. Obstruction of the bronchus supplying the distended lobe may also be due to abnormal blood vessels or bronchomalacia. Chest X-ray should always be done for proper diagnosis. Associated congenital heart disease, if any, should also be borne in mind.

Specific Anesthetic Problems

1. The patient is neonate and neonatal anesthesia requires specialized skill, experience and care.
2. There may be severe respiratory failure preoperatively.
3. Nitrous oxide anesthesia may further increase the volume and distend the lobe of the lung.
4. Positive pressure ventilation may also further distend the lobe due to ball-valve effect and cause respiratory distress.

Anesthetic Management

The baby should be properly assessed preoperatively. As the baby is with respiratory embarrassment, oxygenation is needed, but positive pressure ventilation should be avoided. A Ryles tube should be passed to empty the stomach. Vitamin K should be given IM. No premedication is usually necessary, but atropine sulfate 0.02 mg/kg can be given IV at the time of induction. Blood should be available for transfusion.

Usually, the bronchoscopy is needed before thoracotomy to exclude intraluminal obstruction, if any. In such cases awake intubation may be done gently and anesthesia maintained with oxygen and halothane. After bronchoscopy, endotracheal intubation with a proper-sized tube should be done and anesthesia maintained with spontaneous ventilation till the thorax is opened. At that time, ventilation should always be controlled with the aid of nondepolarizing muscle relaxants. Nitrous oxide can also be used at that time. High-inspired oxygen concentration is also advised. Following lobectomy, the remaining part of the lung is expected to expand gradually.

Usual monitoring of vital signs should be done. Adequate fluid therapy is needed. Blood loss should be replaced. Extubation should be done after using the reversal drug and when the baby is well awake.

The child should better be nursed in a pediatric incubator. Oxygen should be given to prevent hypoxemia. The chest drain with under water seal should be checked. Chest X-ray should be done in the postoperative period.

MEDIASTINAL TUMORS

Common mediastinal tumors in children may induce lymphoma, dermoid cysts and so on. Large tumors may cause acute airway obstruction and dyspnea. Difficult intubation may be anticipated in such cases. Endotracheal intubation may not relieve obstruction in some cases, where endobronchial intubation may help. This is mostly due to massive enlargement of hilar glands secondary to lymphoma.

The surgical procedure is usually a major one and massive blood loss may occur during surgery. Adequate blood replacement is needed.

The child should be carefully assessed and all necessary investigations should be done. Chest X-ray is essential. Some patients may be already treated with steroid hormones and cytotoxic drugs to reduce the hilar node enlargement. Therefore, interaction with anesthetic drugs should also be borne in mind.

No premedication is usually needed and only atropine sulfate may be given IV at the time of induction.

In cases of anticipated difficult intubation, all possible precautions and care should be adopted. Induction of anesthesia should be done by inhalation method. Following endotracheal intubation, anesthesia should be maintained with nitrous oxide, oxygen, muscle relaxants and controlled ventilation.

All usual monitors should be applied. ECG monitoring is essential. At the end of surgery, adequate reversal of muscle relaxants should be done and adequacy of ventilation should be checked. Fluid therapy should be carefully judged and blood transfusion may be needed.

Postoperative analgesia is usually needed. Chest X-ray should be done to detect any pneumothorax, if present.

ANESTHESIA FOR CARDIAC CATHETERIZATION

Cardiac catheterization involves passing a narrow catheter from the forearm vein into the right heart and pulmonary artery under radiographic control. The pressures at different chambers of the heart and pulmonary artery can be measured and blood samples can be taken for blood gas analysis. This cardiological procedure should be followed very cautiously as there is often risk of ventricular extrasystole and even ventricular fibrillation.

In older children, it can be performed under local anesthesia, but in small children it is better done in general anesthesia. In some cases, only heavy sedation may be needed. Several factors should be borne in mind. The child must be made immobile during the procedure. There should not be any interference with blood gas parameters. The hemodynamics of the child should be maintained as far as practicable. The procedure is done in dark X-ray room and no explosive agents should be used in that room. Pulse, blood pressure and ECG monitoring is essential. Oxygen enriched gas mixture should be avoided, as it may interfere with the results of blood gas analysis.

Halothane-air mixture can be used satisfactorily for induction of anesthesia by inhalation method. Intravenous ketamine can also be used. Blood pressure may rise, but usually returns to normal value before measurements are made.

Angiocardiography may be performed at the same time during catheterization. A large amount of radiopaque dye is passed through the heart and great vessels, and this is followed by high-speed serial radiography. Adverse reactions due to dye injection may occur. So, adequate precaution should be taken and steroid should be kept ready at hand. Other complications include blood loss due to repeated blood sampling, dysrhythmias, hypothermia, etc.

Cardioversion is mostly an emergency procedure. It is used to correct severe arrhythmia. Routine general anesthesia is needed and good oxygenation should be provided before the counter shock is applied.

ANESTHESIA FOR CARDIAC SURGERY IN CHILDREN

Cardiac surgery possess various problems for the anesthetist. These are as follows:

1. The affected children are mostly with diminished cardiac reserve. Therefore, anesthetic drugs should be used with adequate care. Oxygenation should also be adequate.
2. Various shunts may be present. In a child with right to left shunt, there may be low arterial oxygen tension, delayed uptake of inhaled anesthetic agents, risk of systemic emboli from venous air embolism, diminished arm-brain circulation time and thus chance of overdose of IV drugs. A child with left to right shunt may suffer from pulmonary hypertension and congestive cardiac failure.
3. An obstructive pathology may be associated with fixed cardiac output, myocardial hypertrophy and congestive cardiac failure.
4. Electrolyte disturbances may occur due to prolonged diuretic therapy.
5. Neonates may have low calcium and glucose levels.
6. The child may be with digitalis or beta-adrenergic blockers.
7. Polycythemia may be present. It increases the viscosity of blood and thereby increases the cardiac work. It increases the risk of thrombosis and may predispose patient to cerebral abscess.
8. There may be significant amount of blood loss during the procedure. Adequate replacement is essential. Overloading the circulation should, however, be avoided.
9. Surgical manipulation of the heart may initiate cardiac arrhythmias. So, adequate care and monitoring should always be provided.
10. In some cases, open heart surgery may be needed. If the heart is isolated from the circulation, adequate measures like hypothermia or use of cardiopulmonary bypass should be provided to prevent irreversible brain damage.
11. Associated congenital malformations, if any, should receive additional attention.
12. Cardiac anesthesia needs expert care and all requisite facilities must be available.

Routine Anesthetic Management

The child should be preoperatively assessed and a thorough physical examination, particularly of the cardiovascular and respiratory system should be done. All cardiological investigations should be done and ECG report and cardiac catheterization data should be judged. Other investigations, such as hemoglobin content, coagulation studies, estimation of electrolytes, urea and creatinine should also be done. Liver function tests and arterial blood gas analysis may also be helpful. Respiratory infection, if any, should always be treated adequately in the preoperative period.

The child may take some medications in the preoperative period. The common drugs are digitalis, beta-blocking agents, calcium antagonists, diuretics and even anticoagulants, and these may cause drug interaction and adversely affect the child.

There may be significant blood loss during surgery, so enough blood should be available at the time of need. Fresh frozen plasma and platelets may also be required.

Extensive and accurate monitoring is manadatory during and after anesthesia and surgery. It should include ECG, systemic arterial pressure, central and left atrial pressure, temperature and blood gas analysis. Electrolyte estimation and hematological analysis should also be carried out.

Most children may be sedated preoperatively with diazepam; otherwise, children may show increase in heart rate and arterial pressure prior to anesthesia and surgery. Opioid premedication may cause diminished cardiovascular and respiratory reserve. Atropine is best avoided in cardiac children because of its potent chronotropic effects.

All drugs including sodium bicarbonate, atropine, calcium gluconate, adrenaline, isoprenaline, etc. and equipment should be checked and kept ready.

Usual monitors such as precordial stethoscope, blood pressure cuff and ECG should be applied.

Induction of anesthesia should be rapid and smooth with no crying and struggling. Adequate preoxygenation should always be done. Induction of anesthesia may be undertaken with the standard agents like thiopentone in small doses and suxamethonium. If suxamethonium is not preferred, nondepolarizing muscle relaxants like vecuronium or atracurium can be used satisfactorily. Pancuronium may cause tachycardia and hypertension. Following endotracheal intubation, a suitable mixture of nitrous oxide and oxygen should be provided with controlled ventilation. Adequate doses of analgesics and muscle relaxants should be given. Hypertension, hypercarbia, hypocarbia and tachycardia should always be avoided and normocarbia should be maintained. Hypocarbia reduces the cardiac output, shifts oxygen dissociation curve to left, decreases myocardial and cerebral blood flow and decreases serum potassium level. Myocardial depressant drugs should be avoided and fluid balance should be adjusted accurately. High intrathoracic pressure should be avoided during IPPV in presence of cardiac shunts. Adequate oxygenation should be guaranteed; usually, 50% oxygen is enough for most cases. In presence of right to left shunt, increased inspired oxygen concentration may have little effect on the arterial oxygen tension. Intravenous drugs should be given in small doses, slowly in such cases as they act very rapidly.

A slow IV drip should be started with 5% dextrose solution before surgery. Blood should be kept ready for immediate transfusion. Blood pressure, pulse rate and ECG should be monitored. During manipulations of the heart, adequate care is needed as it may induce ectopic beats, arrhythmias, cardiac asystole or even ventricular fibrillation. Full oxygenation is mandatory during the surigical procedure.

Care should be taken that the lungs are fully expanded before chest is closed at the end of operation. The effects of muscle relaxants should be well reversed with atropine and neostigmine. The extubation should be done when the child is awake, and full tracheobronchial toilet should be done. Artificial ventilation may have to be considered in presence of hypoxemia, low cardiac output, pulmonary hypertension, hypothermia, etc.

The child should be kept in intensive care unit in the postoperative period as meticulous attention to respiratory care and constant expert nursing care are required. Controlled ventilation may be needed for a prolonged period. Monitoring of vital signs and blood gas analysis is essential. Narcotic analgesics and sedatives like morphine, diazepam, etc. are always needed. Fluid balance should be maintained and blood replacement should be adequate. Body temperature should be maintained at about 37°C. Special care is needed to ensure adequate nutrition.

PATENT DUCTUS ARTERIOSUS

Ductus arteriosus is a wide channel between the distal part of aortic arch and the pulmonary artery in fetal life. It conveys blood from the right side of the heart directly to the aorta and thus completely bypasses the functionless lungs. As the lungs expand after birth, the ductus gradually closes in about 4 weeks and it is then replaced by the ligamentum arteriosum.

If this closure does not occur, there will be persistence of ductus arteriosus resulting in blood flow from the high pressure aorta to the low pressure pulmonary artery, which is the reversal of blood flow seen in intrauterine life. This is common in preterm infants, prematurity, respiratory distress syndrome, neonatal asphyxia, hypoxia and acidosis. Patent ductus arteriosus causing a large left to fight shunt results in increased pulmonary pressure and right ventricular hypertrophy. As a small amount of blood passes through aorta, there will be low diastolic blood pressure and high pulse pressure. Ultimately, there will be hypertrophy of left ventricle.

Patent ductus arteriosus as the sole lesion in children may have clinical features like tachypnea, hepatomegaly, bounding pulse, loud, typical systolic and diastolic murmur. Cyanosis may not be marked unless other congenital abnormalities exist. Chest X-ray may show evidence of increased vascularity and echocardiogram findings of a large left atrium to aorta ratio. Diagnosis is confirmed by echocardiography. Initially the management should include fluid restriction, diuresis, mechanical ventilation and drugs like indomethacin.

Infants with certain types of congenital heart disease, such as tricuspid or pulmonary atresia may depend on the patency of the ductus to provide pulmonary blood flow. Ligation of patent ductus arteriosus in certain patients maintaining a right to left shunt across the ductus is usually not indicated and this may cause sudden right heart failure.

Optimum time for operation is 5 to 12 years of age. If the large shunt is not ligated, expectation of life is reduced.

Indomethacin, a prostaglandin inhibitor, may help in closure of the patent arteriosus. The drug is given 0.1 to 0.2 mg/kg, for several days. But the drug may cause renal damage and suppress bone marrow and, therefore, it should not be given to children with kidney failure and in presence of coagulopathy. Surgical treatment of the condition is the ligation of patent ductus arteriosus.

In most cases routine anesthetic management for thoracotomy is most suitable. Operative blood loss is usually not much and may not need replacement. But if any major vessel is damaged, blood loss may be severe. So, a good intravenous line should always be kept before anesthesia and operation and blood should be available at the time of need.

The child should be assessed carefully and monitoring of vital signs is essential during operation. During dissection near the vagus nerve, sudden bradycardia may occur. After ligation of ductus, reflex tachycardia may occur, the murmur may change and diastolic pressure may rise. In the postoperative period ventilatory assistance is mostly needed and the child should be kept in a pediatric intensive care unit.

COARCTATION OF AORTA

Coarctation of aorta may be of two types, preductal or postductal, according to its site in relation to the ductus arteriosus. The preductal or infantile type may occur in association with other anomalies like ventricular septal defect. Cardiac failure is the most common presenting feature in children below 6 months of age. The postductal or adult type may exhibit no symptoms in early childhood and may be diagnosed during investigation of hypertension in the upper limbs.

Resection of preductal (infantile) type of coarctation of aorta may be needed in certain cases. The affected children may have severe heart failure. They may be already under treatment with digoxin and diuretics which may have anesthetic implications. Assisted ventilation is mostly needed in these cases. Blood loss is usually much during resection and adequate blood should be kept ready during operation. The more complete the coarctation, the more the child will bleed from the chest wall and the less the change of blood pressure on clamping and releasing the aorta.

The child should be carefully assessed and all possible investigations should be done. Blood gas analysis is essential and abnormalities, if any, should be corrected. All drugs, including adrenaline, dopamine and steroids, and all monitoring equipment should be available during operation. Body temperature should be monitored and normothermia should be maintained. The method of general anesthesia may present a few problems and the generally adopted technique is based on the use of thiopentone, relaxant, endotracheal intubation and controlled ventilation with nitrous oxide and oxygen.

During operation when the aorta is clamped the blood pressure may rise, but the systolic pressure should not be allowed to rise above 80 mmHg. Sometimes, a hypotensive drug may be needed; low concentrations of isoflurane may be given to tackle the situation. After the removal of the aortic clamp, the circulation should be supported with IV infusion and vasopressor or drugs. The child should be treated in a pediatric intensive care unit in the postoperative period.

In postductal or adult type of coarctation of aorta also, there are several problems. Induced hypotension seems to have a useful place in anesthetic management of such cases. It should reduce blood loss during operation and make the dissection and resection easier. Clamping of aorta may compromise the blood supply to spinal cord. Induced hypothermia such as surface cooling may be helpful in such cases. Severe proximal hypertension following clamping of aorta may have to be treated with ganglion blockers. Here also adequate blood should be available at the time of need.

Routine anesthetic management is mostly satisfactory. All arrangements for surface cooling should be made. To induce hypotension, sodium nitroprusside infusion should also be available. Careful monitoring of vital signs is absolutely essential in such cases. At the end of operation, the child should be well awake and also able to move his limbs.

The child should be kept in an intensive care unit in the postoperative period. Continuous monitoring is needed, particularly of pulse, respiration, blood pressure, body temperature and blood loss. Reflex postoperative hypertension, mostly due to spasm in previously hypotensive vessels, may endanger blood supply of the bowel and there may be intestinal ileus due to mesenteric arteritis. Hypertension may persist for some days in the postoperative period and in some cases reserpine therapy may be needed to tackle the situation.

ANESTHESIA FOR NONCARDIAC SURGERY IN CHILDREN WITH CONGENITAL HEART DISEASE

Children with congenital heart diseases may often require anesthesia for noncardiac surgical procedures. They may pose potential problems and thus need a careful evaluation and extra care in anesthetic management. In elective procedures the child may be referred to cardiologists to bring the patient in optimal condition. These children carry extra risk and thus anesthesia must be carefully planned for a better outcome of the surgical procedures.

The child should be preoperatively evaluated regarding the type of cardiovascular anomaly and its present status. Other systems, particularly the respiratory system, should be thoroughly examined. Respiratory infection, if any, should be adequately treated. Suitable antibiotic prophylaxis must be ensured and it should be a routine in dental procedures, oropharyngeal surgery, gastrointestinal or genitourinary procedures and even in instrumentation of the respiratory tract.

All routine investigations should be carried out. If the hematocrit is above 45%, fluids should be given IV to avoid hemoconcentration and thus the risk of cerebral thrombosis. Adequate sedation should be given preoperatively to allay fear, anxiety and tension. Atropine sulfate is usually given IM in premedication. Coagulation studies should be done, particularly in children with cyanotic heart disease.

Anesthetic Management

All essential drugs and equipment, particularly for cardiopulmonary resuscitation should be readily available in the operation theater. Monitoring of vital signs including ECG is essential. A reliable intravenous line should be secured. Anesthesia may be induced with low doses of thiopentone IV given slowly. Endotracheal intubation may be facilitated with IV suxamethonium. Anesthesia should better be maintained with nitrous oxide, narcotic analgesic and a muscle relaxant with controlled ventilation. Vecuronium or atracurium can be used satisfactorily as they maintain cardiovascular stability. High concentration of oxygen should always be maintained and the ventilation should be monitored carefully. Proper monitoring of blood pressure and cardiac output is essential throughout the operative procedure by the Doppler device. In major cases, intra-arterial catheterization is desirable.

Extubation should be done when the child is adequately decurarized and fully awake. Edrophonium may be the drug of choice for the reversal as it has quick onset of action, long duration and minimum cardiovascular effect. Following extubation, the child should have stable circulation, good perfusion, no hypoxia and controlled normal body temperature.

The child should be monitored in the immediate postoperative period and adequate oxygenation must be ensured. Excessive narcotic sedation should be avoided. Fluid therapy should be adequate, but fluid overload must be avoided.

CHAPTER
22

Anesthesia for Pediatric Trauma

Trauma is common in pediatric age group and the mortality and morbidity due to trauma are also significant. Most children experience blunt trauma which may be due to falls, accidents, motor vehicle collisions, etc. Penetrating trauma can also occur. Injuries are often multiple and in different anatomical sites. Major trauma needs immediate evaluation of the condition and emergency care and resuscitation.

History is most important. Children, family members and/or bystanders can give relevant information regarding trauma or injury. Parents can provide past medical history and related injury. The type of injury should be determined and other possible hidden injuries should be also borne in mind.

Physical examination should be prompt particularly for airway patency, breathing and circulation. Vital signs should be checked frequently as these can change at any time. Central nervous system, cardiovascular system and pulmonary system need adequate monitoring to detect any derangements. Hidden bleeding can occur in chest, abdomen, pelvis and thighs, and these may need immediate care and even surgical intervention.

Laboratory investigations are extremely needed for exact diagnosis and these should be arranged without wasting time. Common investigations are:
1. Blood examination: TC, DC, Hb concentration, hematocrit, platelet count, prothrombin time, activated partial thromboplastin time, etc.
2. Blood biochemistry: Electrolytes, glucose, BUN and creatinine.
3. Urine examination.
4. Radiographic studies.
5. Electrocardiogram.

Monitoring the patient's vital signs is essential and it should include precordial stethoscope, noninvasive blood pressure cuff, electrocardiogram and pulse oximeter. Arterial catheters are inserted for frequent blood sampling. Central venous pressure and pulmonary artery catheters may be needed in selected cases.

Transesophageal echocardiography is often helpful in some cases.

BASIC RESUSCITATION

The basic principles of trauma resuscitation in children are mostly the same as those in adults. Primary survey is most important and it should be done rapidly but completely and systematically.

Airway

Airway should be checked carefully for patency or any obstruction including foreign bodies, facial fractures, and/or bleeding.

Child's ability to speak, cry and breathe spontaneously can indicate a patent airway. Look for any stridor which may suggest airway obstruction. Wheezing indicates bronchospasm. Flaring of nose and sternal retraction suggests airway obstruction. Airway injury can cause hoarseness and/or change of voice quality.

Management

1. Oropharyngeal secretion should be sucked out. Mouth and pharynx should be swept. Head extension with jaw thrust technique is helpful in cases with oropharyngeal obstruction.
2. Tongue obstruction is common in unconscious children. It can be managed with jaw thrust maneuver or by placing the chin in sniffing position. Cervical spine stabilization is most important in cases with suspected spinal injury. Neck should be kept in neutral position to get the maximum airway diameter.
3. Oral or nasal airways can be tried.
4. Endotracheal intubation and ventilation provide adequate oxygenation and ventilation particularly when conservative measures fail.
5. Traumatized children are mostly with full stomach. Endotracheal intubation with rapid sequence induction and cricoid pressure is advised to prevent aspiration. Awake intubation can also be tried.
6. Other options include surgical cricothyroidotomy or translaryngeal jet (needle) ventilation or lastly tracheostomy in extreme cases.

[Note: Adequate oxygenation is needed but hyperventilation should be avoided.
- Nasotracheal intubation is not much preferred due to the sharp angle between the nasopharynx and oropharynx and the small diameter of endotracheal tube that can be inserted through the child's nares.
- Position of the endotracheal tube should be confirmed with any change of posture or during transfer.]

Breathing

Ventilation should always be adequate. Controlled ventilation may be needed. Adequacy of ventilation is confirmed by capnography or blood gas analysis. Hypoxia and hypoventilation can cause cardiorespiratory arrest.

Vigorous assisted ventilation with high tidal volume should be avoided as it can cause barotrauma, bronchial injury, pneumothorax, etc.

A gastric tube should be passed to decompress the stomach. In cases with suspected basal skull fracture, the nasal route should be avoided.

Circulation

Pulse and blood pressure should be assessed carefully. Children tolerate shock badly and thus early detection and prompt fluid resuscitation are needed. Tachycardia may be the early indication of hypovolemic shock in traumatized children. Decreased capillary refilling, altered mental status and low-urinary output may indicate poor end-organ perfusion. Systolic blood pressure seems to be a good guide to volume status particularly in infants as it lies parallel with the intravascular volume. Blood volume in children is estimated as 80 ml/kg.

Pallor, mottling, sweating and coolness of the skin particularly in extremities are signs of hypovolemia. Metabolic acidosis is common in cases with hypovolemia due to impaired perfusion. It is mostly corrected by proper volume replacement. Sodium bicarbonate is better avoided except for severe acidosis.

INTRAVENOUS ACCESS

Large bore intravenous lines are to be placed preferable one on each side of the child in upper or lower extremities. A cut-down technique is mostly satisfactory. Long saphenous vein anterior to medial malleolus at the ankle, and veins of the antecubital fossa are the usual venous cut-down sites.

An intraosseous line may be helpful initially for immediate fluid resuscitation. It should be avoided in cases with fracture in the same leg, pelvic fractures or a conscious child. Intraosseous line is usually placed about 1cm inferior and medial to the tibial tuberosity. Prolonged intraosseous line should be avoided to decrease the risk of osteomyelitis.

FLUID RESUSCITATION

Fluid or volume resuscitation should be started with crystalloid to fill the vascular space. Ringer's lactate 20 ml/kg is given initially and it can be repeated twice. If no improvement occurs compatible blood transfusion is indicated. Basic fluid requirement is 100 ml/kg/day for 10 kg, plus 50 ml/kg/day for next 5 kg and plus 20 ml/kg/day for each kg above 16 kg.

Alternatively it can be calculated as	
For the first 10 kg	4 ml/kg/hour
For 10 kg to 20 kg	40 ml/hour plus 2 ml/kg/hour for every kg above 10 kg
Above 20 kg	60 ml/hour plus 1 ml/kg/hour for every kg above 20 kg

[Note:
- Glucose containing fluids are not indicated during resuscitation. These children are usually hyperglycemic due to high catecholamine response due to metabolic response of stress/injury.
- Careful monitoring of vital signs is essential during resuscitation.
- Monitoring of blood glucose is needed as the infants have limited glycogen reserve and can become hypoglycemic easily.
- Vasopressors may be indicated temporarily to promote central perfusing pressure.
- Hypoxia, hypercarbia and hypotension should always be avoided for best possible outcome.

BLOOD TRANSFUSION

Children tolerate blood loss badly. Traumatized children can loose sufficient amount of blood and these are mostly not measured. Large volume of blood may remain in hematoma or in body cavities. Thus it is very difficult to assess the actual blood loss. However the initial volume replacement should be tried with Ringer's solution or normal saline and then blood should be replaced in volumes sufficient to maintain the hematocrit at least at 30% or more. Crossmatched type specific whole blood should be given as early as possible. For more immediate needs for blood demand, transfusion of noncrossmatched 'O' negative blood can be given. 'O' negative packed red blood cells can also be used. Care should be taken to detect any source of ongoing bleeding and attempt should to made to stop it.

An extensive loss of blood in trauma usually require large amount of blood transfusion within a short period. Thus massive blood transfusion is possible in certain cases. In such circumstances some serious problems can arise.
  i. Metabolic acidosis: Sodium bicarbonate may be needed to correct it.
  ii. Citrate intoxication: It is mostly due to transfusion of citrated blood. Fresh frozen plasma or platelet suspension contain more citrate

than whole blood per unit volume. To treat the condition 10% calcium chloride 100 mg/kg should be given slowly preferably under electrocardiography control.
iii. Hyperkalemia can occur. It is usually treated with is calcium gluconate 100 mg/kg, sodium bicarbonate 1 to 2 mmol/kg and hyperventilation.
iv. Fluid overload. Diuretics may be needed to treat it.
v. Coagulation problems can occur due to low-platelet count and impaired function, deficiency of coagulation factors. These should be detected early and treat accordingly.
vi. Disseminated intravascular coagulation (DIC). This needs adequate attention and treatment. Replacement of coagulation factors and heparinization may be helpful.
vii. Hypothermia: All fluids and blood should be warmed at about 35°C before administration.
viii. Adequate precautions should be taken against mismatched blood transfusion. Blood transfusion should be given only, when it is indicated. Monitoring of vital signs is needed for early detection and immediate treatment and care.

SECONDARY SURVEY

The child should be thoroughly examined quickly. All the systems of the body need proper evaluation and some related investigations may be required to get a correct diagnosis and management accordingly.

- Neurologic evaluation and assessment of Glasgow coma scale score may be helpful.

Glasgow coma scale scoring in children	
A. Opening of eyes	
Spontaneous	: 4
To commands	: 3
To pain	: 2
No response	: 1
B. Verbal response	
Oriented	: 5
Confused	: 4
Inappropriate words	: 3
Incomprehensible	: 2
No response	: 1

Contd...

Contd...

Glasgow coma scale scoring in children
C. Motor response

Spontaneous : 6
    Withdrawal from touch : 5
    Withdrawal from pain : 4
    Flexion : 3
    Extension : 2
    No response : 1

Total Glasgow Coma Score 3 to 15

It is the most widely used scoring system to evaluate the severity of head injury. This scoring should be calculated in the early period as it helps much in patient care. This Glasgow Coma Score may be modified to same extent in case of babies and infants.

Secondary brain damage should always be prevented by maximizing the cerebral perfusion pressure with the aid of basic respiratory and cardiovascular resuscitation. Hypoxemia, hypercapnia and hypotension should always be avoided at all costs.

HEAD INJURY

i. Head injury is common in pediatric patients. Seizures and vomiting are common manifestations. Intracranial hypertension occurs due to diffuse hyperemia and edema. Early treatment to control intracranial tension is most important in such cases. Management should include to ensure a perfectly clear airway, adequate oxygenation and controlled ventilation. Computed tomography and magnetic resource imaging are needed to locate the traumatic lesion. ICP monitoring is essential. Increased intracranial tension should be treated with optimal positioning. Slight head up lift, controlled hyperventilation, diuretics like mannitol, frusemide, etc. Barbiturates can also help. Seizures should be treated with short-acting benzodiazepines, barbiturates. Electroencephalographic monitoring may be needed. Other measures should include general supportive care, maintenance of cerebral perfusion pressure, hemoglobin content, and arterial oxygenation.

ii. Intracranial lesions:

    Diffuse lesions are common in children and there may be concession or diffuse axonal injury.

    Localized lesions may be various types such as epidural hematoma, intracranial hematoma. Surgical intervention may be needed in certain cases.

    Skull fractures can also occur. It may be linear, complex or depressed. The fontanelles and sutures are open in children. Blood loss may be massive in some cases and blood transfusion may be indicated. Some cases may need surgical manipulation.

NECK INJURY

Neck injury is not uncommon in children. Children usually have shorter neck with a relatively large heavy head. Ligaments are lax and muscle power is less. The vertebral bodies show anterior wedging and the facet joints of C_1 to C_4 are horizontally placed.

Sublaxations of cervical spine are common alone or along with associated fracture. Atlantooccipital dislocation can occur and it is the separation of cranium from the cervical spinal column. It can cause proximal spinal cord injury. The condition is mostly fatal.

Cervical Spine Damage

Cervical spine fracture in children usually occurs between C_1 and C_3 whereas in adults in between C_4 and C_7. This is mostly due to motor vehicle accidents. Common manifestations include airway obstruction, subcutaneous emphysema, dyspnea, dysphagia, hypoxemia, esophageal tears and vascular disruption, hemorrhage, air embolism and so on. High cervical spinal cord damage can cause apnea and cardiac arrest. Pneumothorax and major vascular injury in the upper thoracic cavity may be associated with penetrating neck wounds.

Early relief of airway obstruction and controlled ventilation are most important in such cases. Careful orotracheal intubation is necessary without causing cord damage. Unnecessary head and neck movement must be avoided. Adequate precautions are needed to prevent aspiration.

Cervical spinal cord injury can occur without radiological findings. Thus many injuries may be overlooked. However, magnetic resonance imaging (MRI) evaluation of spine can help to demonstrate a cord contusion.

CHEST INJURIES

i. *Penetrating wounds*:
   - These are not uncommon in children.
   - These are similarly managed as in adults.
ii. *Hemothorax*: It may need initial drainage particularly when it is more than 20% of blood volume or when it is continuing bleeding. It needs thoracotomy.
iii. *Cardiac tamponade*: It can cause mechanical obstruction to cardiac action from direct compression over the heart or obstruction of venous return, ultimately leading to profound shock. It needs prompt resuscitation and immediate thoracotomy and drainage.
iv. *Tracheobronchial injuries*: It can occur in children. Most laryngeal injuries usually occur at or above the fourth tracheal ring. These children need early airway management and surgical intervention and repair.

v. *Tension pneumothorax*: It is the presence of air in the pleural space from an injury of chest wall (penetrating chest injury), fracture of ribs, lung laceration, etc. Air trapped in pleural cavity can shift the mobile mediastinum in children to opposite side of the chest and obstruct the venous return of the heart. Manifestations include dyspnea, tachypnea, cyanosis, hypoxemia, tachycardia, shock, muffled heart sounds, etc. Chest X-ray and CT scan can confirm the diagnosis. Needle decompression using 18 or 20 gauge needle is needed. Midaxillary line should be chosen as the site of need insertion and midclavicular second intercostal space should be avoided as it can injure pulmonary artery.
vi. *Pneumothorax*: Simple pneumothorax also needs urgent chest tube decompression. Adequate care should be taken to avoid lung damage.
vii. Rib fractures can also occur mostly due to blunt trauma with profound transmission of force/energy.
viii. *Lung contusion*: Simple lung contusion usually responds well in conservative management. Pulmonary physiotherapy and adequate oxygenation and general supportive care are required.
ix. *Ruptured diaphragm*: It can occur from blunt abdominal trauma. It is more common in children than adults. The condition needs thoracoabdominal repair.

ABDOMINAL INJURIES

Intra-abdominal injuries (blunt or penetrating) are common in children due to weak musculature and immature thoracic cage. Upper abdominal organs are more prone to trauma. These may be associated with other injuries of the body.

These children should be evaluated properly for exact diagnosis. Radiographic studies such as plain X-ray, CT with IV or central contrast, and ultasonography may be needed. Laboratory tests such blood examination (hemoglobin, hematocrit, prothrombin time, partial thromboplastin time, blood crossmatch, etc.) estimation of amylase or lipase, SGOT, SGPT, etc. and urine analysis may be required to come to a proper diagnosis and confirmation.

These children may pose different problems. Major hemorrhage may require massive blood transfusion. They may have full stomach and thus risk of aspiration is always there. Gastric distension from swallowing or from the act of crying can easily occur and interfere with respiratory effort. These children need nasogastric decompression. The extent of hypovolemic shock should be carefully assessed and adequate resuscitation is needed. Blood transfusion may be indicated.

Spleen Injury

Spleen injury is most common in intra-abdominal organ injury in children. They may have associated other abdominal injuries. Abdominal or shoulder pain with shortness of breath is common. Contrast CT scan can help its diagnosis. Most cases responds well with conservative treatment and do not require surgical intervention. In cases of hemodynamic instability, clinical deterioration or concomitant other intra-abdominal injury indicate operative intervention. These patients need appropriate blood transfusion. Postsplenectomy infection should always be prevented.

Liver Injury

Liver injury is also common in children and most injuries occur in right lobe. Patient needs proper assessment and exact diagnosis. Most patients need blood transfusion. Hemodynamically instability and clinical deterioration dictates early operation. Major liver resection may be needed.

Pancreas Injury

It can result from blunt abdominal injury. Duct transaction and contusion can occur patient usually complains epigastric pain and tenderness. Pancreatic contusion is usually treated conservatively, but major ductal injuries need early surgical intervention. Distal pancreatectomy with splenic preservation may be needed in certain cases.

Serum amylase and lipase estimations are helpful for diagnosis. CT with IV contrast medium is usually confirmatory.

Intestinal Injuries

These can result from blunt abdominal trauma. Injury is common points for fixation with jejunum terminal ileum, descending colon and pelvic colon. Careful clinical examinations, radiographic studies and CT scan are required for diagnosis. Laparoscopic exploration or even laparotomy is needed in selected cases.

GENITOURINARY TRACT INJURY

It is not uncommon in pediatric trauma patients. It is mostly due to blunt trauma but penetrating abdominal or back injuries also risk urinary tract injuries. Children usually present abdominal pain and hematuria. However the degree of hematuria may not always correlate with the severity of genitourinary tract trauma. Urine examination may reveal microscopic or frank hematuria. Kidney, ureter and bladder X-ray and intravenous pyelogram are mostly indicated. CT of the abdomen with intravenous contrast can confirm the diagnosis.

Renal Injury

Kidneys are relatively large in children and usually located in a lower abdominal region. Renal injury cases should be carefully assessed. Operative intervention may be needed in certain cases. Hypertension can occur afterwords postoperatively after injury to renovascular pedicle. These cases need blood pressure check-up regularly following renal surgery.

Urinary Bladder Injury

It should be noted that the narrow small pelvis of a child assumes the bladder located in an intra-abdominal position urinary bladder trauma may be associated with pelvic fractures. Bladder volume in children varies with age. In child below 2 years of age it is about 7 ml/kg, but above 2 years it is calculated as age in years × 30 ml.

Straddle Injuries

These are caused forcible compression of the perineal soft tissues against the bony pelvis. It is mostly due to falls, bicycle crashes or associated with sports equipment related trauma. Bleeding from the perineum is mostly evident. The cases should be examined very carefully. Missed injuries can lead to urethral and/or vaginal stricture afterwards.

ORTHOPEDIC INJURIES

Specific musculoskeletal injuries in children includes epiphyseal fractures, shaft fractures and dislocations. These injuries may cause various complications such as vascular and/or nerve involvement causing ischemia/vascular necrosis physeal (growth plate) involvement causing growth disturbances and joint instability.

Pediatric fracture can also be classified according to physeal (growth plate involvement):

Type I   : When the fracture is displaced or nondisplaced through growth plate.
Type II : Fracture involves small metaphyseal fragment.
Type III : Intra-articular fracture through epiphysis.
Type IV : Fracture through metaphysis and epiphysis
Type V   : Severe crush to growth plate.

These cases needs careful physical examination. Active and passive range of motion to be assessed to delete bone injury, ligamentous injury or muscle weakness. Peripheral pulse should be recorded. Sensory and motor function also needs proper evaluation. Radiographic studies and computed tomography (CT) are needed for exact diagnosis.

Treatment for fractures and dislocations include traction and splinting. Circulation must be reestablished before fracture stabilization. Immobilization of the limb can be done by splint, cast, traction, external fixation or internal fixation. Bone fractures complicated by vascular or nerve derangements require urgent surgical exploration. Distal humerus fracture in children may be associated with neurovascular injury and compartment syndrome. This may need urgent closed/open reduction.

Open fractures always threat for infection and even amputation. Thus these fractures should have extra caution in the early care. Extensive and appropriate early irrigation of gross contamination, proper debridment of necrotic and contaminated tissues and skeletal stabilization are most important. Antibiotics and prophylaxis against tetanus are essential. General supportive care including fluid resuscitation and even blood transfusion are indicated. Surgical intervention may be need in selected cases.

CHAPTER 23

Regional Anesthesia for Children

Regional anesthesia in pediatric patients is becoming increasingly popular in recent times. It provides the advantages of reduced drug requirements for other anesthetic agents and postoperative analgesia. Local blocks or regional anesthesia can well extend into the postoperative period. But it exposes the children to the risk of both a general and a regional anesthesia as the pediatric patients under regional block need to be kept quiet and still by light general anesthesia.

Various peripheral nerve blocks used for pediatric surgery include penile block, ilioinguinal and iliohypogastric block, brachial plexus block, and so on. Intravenous regional neural anesthesia can also be used for repair of injury or treatment of fracture of extremities. Caudal block is also a much popular technique for all operations upto and including umbilicus. Lumbar epidural anesthesia and spinal anesthesia can also be used in pediatric patients.

Regional anesthesia may be strongly recommended in the case of children with a family history of malignant hyperthermia. It may be useful in premature infants who require surgery below the umbilicus. Children with chronic airway diseases or hypotonic infants and children with neuromuscular diseases may tolerate regional anesthesia better.

The age of the child usually does not pose limitation to regional anesthesia. But lack of parental consent and infection at the site of injection are the absolute contraindications. However, relative contraindications may include lack of patient cooperation in older children, difficult airways, coagulopathy, anatomic anomalies at the injection site, hypovolemia, neurologic diseases, poorly controlled seizures, etc.

Local anesthetic agents should be used very carefully and cautiously in children. The dose should be accurate and because of small body mass of children, it is often necessary to use dilute solutions of local anesthetics to avoid overdose. As in the case of adults, the drugs in usual doses given on body weight basis are mostly sufficient and satisfactory. However, toxicity can occur in some cases for which sensible precautions have to be taken. It should be remembered that myelinization of the central nervous system is not complete until about 18 months of age, so effective neural block may be obtained with lower concentration of local anesthetic agent.

Some common techniques of regional anesthesia used in pediatric surgery are discussed in this chapter.

LOCAL OR SUBCUTANEOUS INFILTRATION ANESTHESIA

Local subcutaneous infiltration of the anesthetic agent is used to produce sensory anesthesia in the injected area without any attempt to block specific nerves. Lignocaine 0.5% is commonly used. A long-acting local anesthetic such as bupivacaine 0.25% can also be used. The suggested maximum dose of lignocaine is 5 mg/kg body weight and of bupivacaine is 2 mg/kg body weight.

ILIOINGUINAL AND ILIOHYPOGASTRIC NERVE BLOCKS (FIG. 23.1)

The ilioinguinal (L_1) and iliohypogastric (T_{12}, L_1) nerves are important branches of the lumbar plexus. These nerves pass in between transversus abdominis and internal oblique muscles. Ilioinguinal nerve becomes superficial as it approaches superficial inguinal ring and supplies cutaneous sensory innervation of scrotum and inner part of thigh. The iliohypogastric nerve supplies cutaneous innervation above inguinal ligament.

This nerve block causes skin analgesia over the inguinal region and it may be used for herniotomy, herniorrhapy, or orchidopexy in children. These nerves traverse beneath the internal oblique muscle, a little medial to anterior superior iliac spine. The nerves may be blocked by infiltration of the abdominal wall in the particular region.

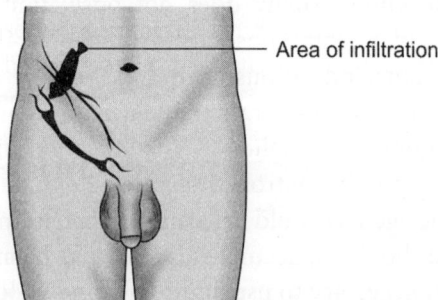

Fig. 23.1: Ilioinguinal and iliohypogastric nerve block

A point is taken at one child's finger breadth away from the anterior superior iliac spine along the line connecting the spine and umbilicus. A 22 gauge needle is inserted from that point perpendicular to the skin and then advanced until the external and internal oblique muscle is pierced. If the bone strikes, the needle should be withdrawn a little. Two-thirds of the solution is injected there and the rest as the needle is withdrawn leaving a skin wheal to block the perforating branches of T_{11} and T_{12}. Bupivacaine 0.25 or 0.5% (not more than 2 mg/kg) may be used satisfactorily. This block also provides postoperative analgesia after herniotomy.

PENILE BLOCK (FIGS 23.2 AND 23.3)

The dorsal nerves of the penis may be blocked to provide postoperative pain relief after circumcision. It may also provide analgesia to some extent after repair of distal hypospadius. The penis is innervated by pudendal nerves S_2–S_4 via two dorsal nerves. The dorsal nerves of penis pass inferior to the pubic bones (symphysis pubis) on either side of the midline alongside the dorsal arteries and veins deep to Buck's fascia. These supply

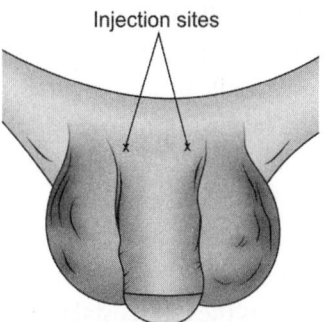

Fig. 23.2: Penile block

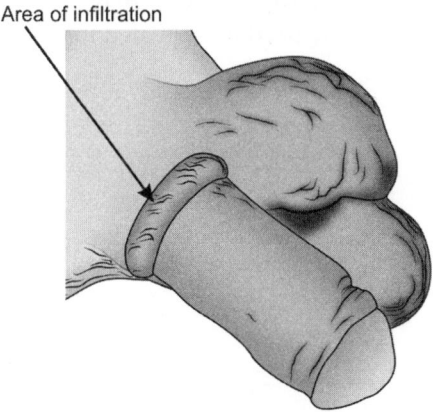

Fig. 23.3: Penile ring block

the dorsal surface of penis and foreskin. But the base of penis is innervated by branches from the genitofemoral and ilioinguinal nerves.

Usually, bupivacaine 0.5% solution without adrenaline is used. It should not exceed the maximum safe dose of 2 mg/kg. 1% plain lignocaine 0.8 ml may be used in case of neonates. Adrenaline should never be used as vasoconstriction may result in ischemia. With proper aseptic measures, bilateral injections are given caudal to symphysis pubis at the base of penis at 11 O' clock and 1 O' clock positions. The needle should be felt to pierce through Buck's fascia and the anesthetic solution should be deposited there. Penile block can also be performed by a ring block at the base of the penis. The ring block is mostly safe and easy. Care should be taken to keep the needle subcutaneous in the midline as urethra is very superficial at the base of penis.

INTERCOSTAL NERVE BLOCK (FIG. 23.4)

Intercostal nerve block may be indicated for postoperative pain relief after thoracotomy or some other abdominal operations. Bilateral T_{10} block may provide satisfactory analgesia following repair of umbilical hernia.

In children, the nerve in the intercostal space should better be approached by angling the needle posteromedially, as it lies almost parallel to the rib. Care should be taken not to exceed a total dose of 2 mg/kg of bupivacaine. The intercostal space is very vascular and there is risk of rapid absorption. Intravascular injection should be avoided. Pneumothorax is a major complication, particularly in children, as the nerve and pleura are very close to each other. Total spinal block may occur, if injection is performed near their origin as the intercostal nerves are sheathed in a dural layer posteriorly.

Indwelling intercostal space catheters may be helpful in long-term anesthesia, thus avoiding the need for repeated injections.

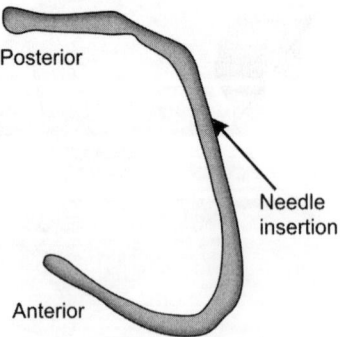

Fig. 23.4: Intercostal nerve block

BRACHIAL PLEXUS BLOCK (FIG. 23.5)

Axillary approach seems to be better as it is simple and easy to perform. It also lacks serious complications like pneumothorax. The arm is abducted and the head is turned to opposite side. It may be further simplified, if the hand is placed behind the head. With strict aseptic measures after skin analgesia or under general anesthesia a 25 gauge needle is introduced alongside and parallel to the axillary artery at a 45° angle to the skin. A slight give may be felt to enter the neurovascular sheath and the needle will move with the arterial pulsations. The guidance to paresthesia for proper placement is avoided. Response to electrical nerve stimulation may signal right placement. Arterial puncture should be avoided. After careful aspiration test, the local anesthetic solution should be injected carefully. Local anesthetics may include 0.5% lignocaine (7 mg/kg maximum) or 0.25% bupivacaine (2 mg/kg maximum) with 1 in 200,000 adrenaline.

The axillary block may be indicated for plastic surgery procedures of hand and forearm, manipulation of forearm fractures or for insertion of shunts for dialysis. It should be noted that the block does not include some areas of upper arm and part supplied by musculocutaneous nerves.

Interscalene approach to brachial plexus may also be used as it provides analgesia of the shoulder and upper arm. It is indicated for operations on the forearm and the outer upper arm including reduction of dislocated shoulders. But various complications, such as phrenic nerve or recurrent laryngeal nerve block, stellate ganglion block (Homer's syndrome), total spinal block and pneumothorax can occur.

The child should be supine, the head turned to the opposite side and a slight downward pressure is exerted on the arm. The interscelene groove is palpated at the level of cricoid C_6. Following aseptic measures and analgesia, a needle is advanced perpendicularly into the groove. Paresthesia may be obtained in the elbow and hand. A peripheral nerve stimulator may be

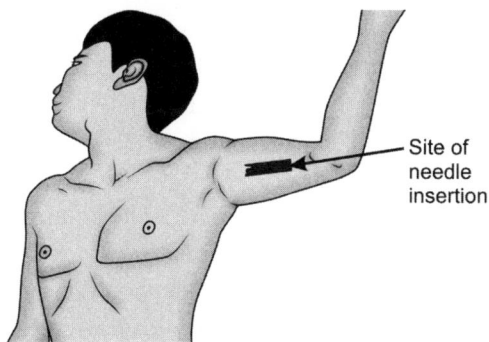

Fig. 23.5: Brachial plexus block (axillary method)

helpful to check proper placement of the needle. After careful aspiration test for blood or CSF, low injection of the local anesthetic solution (bupivacaine or lignocaine) should be made.

INTRAVENOUS REGIONAL ANESTHESIA (THE BIER BLOCK)

Intravenous regional anesthesia may be performed in older children. It is a simple method of producing anesthesia of the arm or leg. It is done by injecting a large volume of local anesthetic solution intravenously while the circulation to that extremity is occluded by applying tourniquet.

The common local anesthetic solution used for intravenous regional anesthesia is 0.25% lignocaine (but not exceeding 5 mg/kg). Bupivacaine should never be used in an intravenous block due to its systemic toxic effects, particularly on the heart, when it enters the circulation. Prilocaine can be used, but there is a risk of methemoglobinemia due to excessive dose.

A small venous catheter is placed in the distal part of the hand or foot. The arm or leg is exsanguinated by wrapping with an elastic bandage. A reliable double tourniquet should be used. The proximal cuff is then inflated and the local anesthetic solution is injected slowly. The block is usually established in about 5 minutes. The distal cuff is inflated and then the proximal is deflated. The remaining cuff should not be released before at least 30 minutes even if the surgery is finished earlier.

The Bier block may not be much useful for reduction of fractures as application of tight cast may be problematic in an ischemic limb.

FEMORAL NERVE BLOCK (FIG. 23.6)

This block may be useful in the case of fracture of the shaft of femur. It provides good analgesia, relieves muscle spasm (quadriceps) and allows painfree manipulation of femoral shaft fractures.

The femoral arterial pulse is palpated just below the inguinal ligament. After skin analgesia, a small needle is passed just lateral to the artery at 45° to the skin. Mild resistance may be felt while piercing fascia lata and the iliac fascia before entering the femoral canal. Following aspiration test, 1% lignocaine with 1 in 200,000 adrenaline or 0.5% bupivacaine should be injected slowly.

Continuous femoral nerve block may also be attempted for prolonged pain relief. Here a Tuohy needle is used through which a standard epidural needle is advanced for 5 to 10 cm within the femoral sheath. After placing the catheter in place the Tuohy needle is withdrawn gently and the local anesthetic solution injected through the catheter.

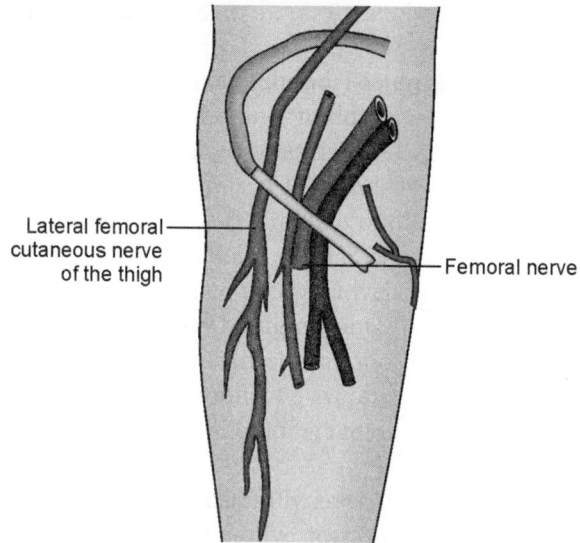

Fig. 23.6: Femoral nerve block

Lateral cutaneous nerve of the thigh may be blocked to provide analgesia over the lateral aspect of thigh. The needle should be introduced medial and inferior to the anterior superior iliac spine and passed in superior and lateral direction till it touches the iliac bone. The local analgesic solution (2 to 5 ml of 1% lignocaine with 1 in 200,000 adrenaline or 0.5% bupivacaine) is injected while the needle is being withdrawn.

SPINAL ANESTHESIA

Spinal anesthesia is also being used in pediatric surgical procedures. It is commonly used for surgery at or below the level of umbilicus. This is particularly beneficial to infants and children who are at risk of postoperative apnea or airway damage as it avoids the necessity of intubation and ventilation.

Some points special to pediatric cases should be considered. The spinal cord extends to L_3 in neonates and to L_1L_2 in older children. So lumbar puncture should be done at L_{4-5} or L_5S_1. The dural space extends to S_{3-4} in the neonate.

The volume of cerebrospinal fluid in infants is about 4 ml/kg while in adults it is about 2 ml/kg. Lumbar puncture may be done either in the sitting or lateral position. The sitting position makes the block technically easier. The assistant should help to keep the infant in right position gently. Neck flexion should always be avoided as it may compromise the airway. Head must be supported while the needle is being introduced. During insertion of the spinal needle, the bevel should face laterally until CSF appears.

Spinal anesthesia produces little change in hemodynamic status of infants. It provides satisfactory surgical anesthesia and lowers the incidence of postoperative cardiorespiratory problems in preterm and former preterm infants.

The needle should be 22 gauge with the length of 1 inch for neonates and infants. The dead space of the needle should always be measured using a tuberculin syringe. The volume may vary from 0.05 to 0.1 ml and it must be considered in the volume of local anesthetic solution the patient receives.

Bupivacaine 0.5% with 8% dextrose or lignocaine 5% with dextrose can be used. Addition of adrenaline may increase the duration of block to some extent. Tetracaine 1% with 10% dextrose is also being used.

Following injection of local anesthetic drugs the baby should lie supine in horizontal position. Patient's legs should not be allowed to be raised; otherwise, high block may result.

These cases should be prepared as for general anesthesia. No premedication is usually needed. The anesthesia machine, endotracheal tubes, laryngoscope, etc. should be kept ready. All aseptic measures should be taken carefully. A reliable intravenous line should always be established. It should be remembered that the time for return of the motor functions after spinal hyperbaric tetracaine is shorter in children. Thus, the technique requires a relatively quick surgery.

Spinal anesthesia is contraindicated in certain conditions like sepsis, or infected lumbar puncture site, coagulopathy, lack of parental consent, etc.

CAUDAL BLOCK (FIGS 23.7 AND 23.8)

This is the most popular and useful block in infants and children for all operations upto and including the umbilicus. It also provides postoperative analgesia, particularly following herniotomy, orchidopexy, circumcision, lower abdominal and perineal surgery, and orthopedic operations on lower limbs. This block is often much easier in children. Caudal analgesia may be used as an alternative to spinal analgesia for lower abdominal surgery in infants. Continuous caudal analgesia through suitable catheters may be used for prolonged surgery. Technical simplicity, reliability, safety and rapid performance make the caudal block widely accepted.

The absence of the fat over the sacrum of infants and children makes the technique rather easy. The dural membrane is usually very close to sacrococcygeal ligament. Thus, in pediatric caudal block, the needle is made to gently approach the caudal canal using loss of resistance test. The contents of the epidural space offer little resistance to the spread of local anesthetic solutions.

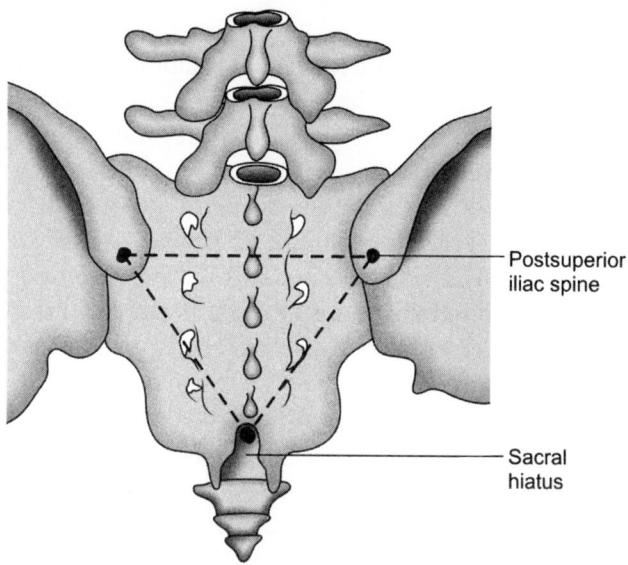

Fig. 23.7: Landmarks of caudal block over sacrum and coccyx

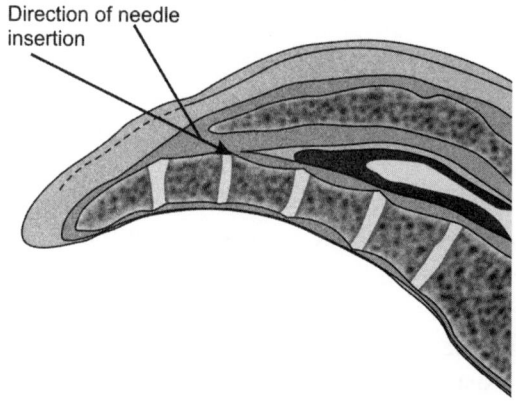

Fig. 23.8: Caudal block

A dose of 1 ml/kg of 0.25% bupivacaine with 1 in 200,000 adrenaline is mostly used for surgery below the level of umbilicus. The low concentration of 0.125% bupivacaine usually diminishes the motor block. This may be used for ambulatory surgery and the patients may be discharged provided no motor block is present; they can walk without assistance and hypotension is not evident.

Technical difficulties, unilateral and uneven spread of local anesthetic solution, and inadequate local analgesia can occur in some cases. Failures can occur and these are mostly due to the development of presacral fat pad.

Technique

The child should be placed in the left lateral position with the upper knee well flexed. The landmarks like the tip of coccyx, sacral cornua and sacral hiatus should be identified. Child is carefully prepared and draped in the usual manner. With full aseptic measures, the needle is inserted in the caudal space at 45° to the skin. It should not be advanced further after it pierces the sacrococcygeal membrane. The needle should be aspirated to check blood or CSF. Then, the predicted full dose of local anesthetic solution should be injected slowly. As the distal end of dura can be as low as S_3 level in neonates, adequate care should be taken to avoid dural puncture.

Addition of adrenaline 1 in 200,000 to bupivacaine 0.25% produces little increase in the mean duration of local analgesia. Clonidine can be used as an additive to caudal local anesthetics as it enhances and prolongs the anesthetic effect of local anesthetics.

Complications following caudal block may include urinary retention, intravascular injection and dural puncture. Caudal catheter increases the risk of infection because of proximity of anus. Motor block and paresthesia may sometimes be frightening for the child.

LUMBAR EPIDURAL BLOCK

This block is mostly used for postoperative pain relief in children. It can also be used for surgery in older children. The technique of epidural block is mostly similar to that performed in adults.

The spinal cord ends at L_3 in neonates. But at the age of 1 year the end of the cord is usually at adult position of L_1. The dural sac in neonates ends at S_3, but at the end of 1 year of age it ends at S_1. Thus, the lumbar epidural block should be safe at L_{4-5} or L_5S_1. The epidural space is best identified by the loss of resistance method. It is said that in children of over 10 kg body weight, the distance from skin to epidural space in millimeters, is numerically very similar to the child's weight in kg.

In children below the age of 5 years, use of a 19–9 gauge Tuohy needle and 21 gauge catheter is advised, while for children over 5 years of age, 18 gauge Tuohy needle and 20 gauge epidural catheter are recommended. A dose of 0.5to 0.75 ml/kg of 0.25% bupivacaine with 1 in 200,000 adrenaline can be used. For surgery, bupivacaine 0.5% may be needed for motor block. Preservative-free narcotics can also be given in this route for pain relief.

Epidural block causes little change in hemodynamic status of the children. Other advantages may include a reduction of total dose and volume of local anesthetic required to provide analgesia and a decrease in the endocrine stress response to surgery.

Placement of epidural catheter at the desired space is most important, particularly during epidural infusions. To ensure a high success rate for blind placement of the catheter tip, either fluoroscopic guidance or nerve stimulation guidance may prove useful. Wire wrapped styletted 20 gauge catheters are easily visible with fluoroscopy. Standard nonradiopaque catheter can be visualized by repeated injection of a little myelographic contrast agent. But it is expensive and disadvantages may include radiation exposure and lack of ready availability. Electrical nerve stimulation directly through the catheter may also be a useful guide to locate the catheter tip.

Special Note

While performing regional anesthesia in children some basic points should always be considered. Regional anesthesia alone may not be sufficient for the child due to overall nonacceptance and lack of cooperation of the child. Many times, light general anesthesia may have to be supplemented. Thus, all equipment and drugs are to be kept ready. Moreover, all resuscitative equipment and drugs should be available to tackle the emergency situations.

All patients should be prepared well as if general anesthesia is to be given. Patient should not be allowed any feed at least 4 hours before anesthesia.

The dose of local anesthetics should be properly calculated and the maximum safe dose of the drug should never be exceeded. A good block should be ensured before surgery is allowed. Intravascular injection should be avoided. Aspiration test should be carefully done frequently. The position of the patient should be carefully adjusted and the airway should always be secured. Initial needle insertion is always painful, so EMLA cream may be applied over the skin before injection. [Eutectic mixture of local anesthetics like lignocaine and prilocaine is the EMLA cream.]

Following regional anesthesia, the child should always be monitored to detect any toxic reactions. Signs of neurologic toxic reactions may be masked by general anesthesia. Halothane may augment the cardiac effects of local analgesic drugs.

The pharmacokinetics of local analgesic drugs are different to some extent in infants and smaller children. The absorption of drugs is usually rapid in children. The cardiac output and regional tissue blood flow are high. The epidural space contains less fat tissue to buffer uptake. The volume of distribution of the drug is larger in children and this may extend the elimination half-life.

The extent of protein binding is less in children. In neonates, serum albumin and alpha-1 acid glycoproteins are low. In jaundice, patient's bilirubin may further reduce the potential for protein binding. The rate of metabolism of local anesthetics is reduced in smaller children. Low plasma cholinesterase activity may prolong the metabolism of ester type local anesthetics. The hepatic pathways for the conjugation of the amide group of local anesthetics are also immature in neonates. However, older children may have rapid metabolism due to relatively large liver.

Adrenaline is being used to extend the action of local anesthetics. It may cause extensive tachycardia and may interact with halothane and precipitate arrhythmias. However, doses upto 10 µg/kg by infiltration may be recommended as safe in children.

CHAPTER 24

Miscellaneous

CROUP

It is a disease characterized by suffocative and difficult breathing. It is usually due to inflammation in the region of larynx. It may also be due to other causes like foreign body, laryngeal spasm and sometimes the formation of membrane.

The inflammation may be either supraglottic (epiglottitis) or subglottic (laryngotracheobronchitis).

Epiglottitis

Epiglottitis or supraglottitis is the infective condition of the epiglottis and supraglottic structures like arytenoid cartilage mucosa and aryepiglottic folds. It is mostly due to bacterial infection (*Haemophilus influenzae*, streptococci), but viral (parainfluenza virus) infection may also occur. It can occur at any age, but is common in children of 3 to 5 years of age. The child appears ill and toxic. Usual symptoms include dysphagia, dysphonia, dyspnea, high fever and severe sore throat. Inspiratory stridor may be present. The child sits upright, leaning foreword in a sniffing position to improve the airflow. Blood examination shows leukocytosis. Lateral X-ray of the neck shows "swollen thumb" sign at the level of epiglottis. These patients are usually toxic, drooling with dysphagia and stridor accompanied by a muffled cough.

Early recognition and appropriate airway management are vital to tackle such patients. Supplemental oxygen should be given as early as possible. An intravenous line should be established. It is not wise to try to visualize the pharynx, as it may cause acute obstruction. The child should be taken to operating room for better management of the airway. All anesthetics and surgical equipment should be checked and ready for use. Emergency bronchoscopy and even tracheostomy may be needed.

If the child becomes apneic, ventilation with oxygen can be done by bag and mask. If adequate oxygenation is not possible, laryngoscopy and intubation should be tried. If it fails, emergency tracheostomy is indicated.

General anesthesia should be induced with oxygen and halothane when the child is in the sitting position. When the patient loses consciousness, the position is changed to supine and then direct laryngoscopy and endotracheal intubation are to be tried. The endotracheal tube should be one size smaller than normal. Once the airway is secured, other supportive measures should be taken immediately.

The child should be taken to the intensive care unit. Antibiotic therapy should be started. Blood culture is also needed. The child may need to remain intubated for the next 48 hours. Adequate humidification of inspired gases should be ensured. Usually, the child is extubated when the pyrexia subsides and a leak has developed around the endotracheal tube.

Laryngotracheobronchitis

It is the acute inflammation of larynx, trachea and bronchi. It is mostly caused by virus and is common in children of 2 to 5 years of age. There is acute respiratory distress often with inspiratory stridor. Treatment should be immediate, but may vary according to the severity of the disease. In mild cases, simple measures like humidification of inspired gases, antibiotic therapy, etc. may prove useful. In some cases adrenaline inhalation delivered through intermittent positive pressure ventilation is needed. In severe cases, intubation or even tracheostomy may be a lifesaving procedure. Steroids are often useful to treat the inflammation despite the infective etiology. Tracheobronchial toilet is of utmost importance and suction clearance is often vital.

Postextubation Croup

It is a potentially dangerous complication in the postanesthetic recovery period in children. It is mostly due to laryngeal edema caused by the pressure, irritation and inflammation following endotracheal intubation. Management of such cases should be immediate and vigorous; otherwise, the condition may end fatally.

The treatment should include the following:
1. Adequate oxygenation. Administer oxygen as a cool mist.
2. Inspired gases should be humidified.
3. Adequate hydration by giving IV fluids.
4. Light sedation to calm the child.
5. Adrenaline through nebulizer and mask.
6. Steroids: Dexamethasone 4 to 8 mg/kg IV.

7. Reintubation may be indicated, if there is hypoxia.
8. Tracheostomy may be needed in extreme cases. Timely cricoid split procedure may avoid tracheostomy in large number of cases.
9. Antibiotics.
10. Other supportive measures. Granuloma, if present, may be removed with the help of bronchoscopy.

Complications of postextubation croup may include hypoxemia, hypercarbia, arrhythmias, aspiration of gastric contents and even cardiac arrest. Scarring may lead to subglottic stenosis.

LARYNGOSPASM

Laryngospasm causes obstruction of glottis and laryngeal inlet by action of the laryngeal muscles. Glottic closure may occur reflexly by intrinsic adductor muscles or by extrinsic muscles of larynx, particularly the thyrohyoid muscles. This may occur usually at the time of induction of anesthesia or emergence, during light anesthesia and, particularly, in presence of mechanical irritants in the airway. Foreign body, blood, secretions and airway in trumentation may initiate laryngospasm.

The condition is potentially hazardous and should always be prevented. Adequate depth of anesthesia should be maintained during airway instrumentation including endotracheal intubation, bronchoscopy, etc. Muscle relaxants should be used for intubation. Extubation should be done when the child is well awake or when the child is under deep anesthesia. Secretions should be well cleared prior to and after extubation.

Clinical manifestations may include stridor, hypoxia, tachycardia, tachypnea, intercostal suction, no phonation and no airflow even with respiratory efforts. The condition is usually critical and needs immediate vigorous management.

Ventilation should be instituted, particularly with continuous positive airway pressure (CPAP) with 100% oxygen using a bag and mask. Jaw thrust, head tilt and oral or nasal airway may sometimes be helpful to open the airway. The mouth and oropharynx should be cleared by adequate suction. If oxygenation is not adequate and laryngospasm is still present, suxamethonium is indicated IV in a dose of 0.3 mg/kg. Then the positive pressure ventilation should be established with PEEP by bag and mask and the patent airway should be maintained.

In extreme cases, reintubation following use of full dose of suxamethonium, cricothyrotomy with transtracheal jet ventilation or even tracheostomy may be indicated as a life saving measure.

Usual complications of laryngospasm include hypoxia, hypercarbia, arrhythmias, pulmonary edema and even cardiac arrest.

ANAPHYLAXIS

This is mostly due to penicillin, latex, radiological contrast media and so on. Early detection and adequate management are essential. In cases of airway obstruction, adrenaline IM may be indicated. It should be followed by nebulized salbutamol. Endotracheal intubation or even tracheostomy may be needed in advanced cases. Apnea also demands endotracheal intubation. In case of cardiac arrest, all resuscitative measures should be adopted according to appropriate protocol.

DOWN'S SYNDROME

Down's syndrome is a condition affecting the different systems of the baby. It often causes problems during anesthesia. The disease is often associated with hypotonia, mental retardation, duodenal atresia, airway problems (respiratory infection, congenital subglottic stenosis, etc.), high incidence of congenital heart disease, often with atrioventricular defects, patent ductus arteriosus and even tetralogy of Fallot. Sleep apnea is common. Thyroid hypofunction may also occur as the child grows older. Atlantoaxial joint is usually unstable and may lead to cervical spinal cord injury.

The child should be carefully assessed preoperatively. Pulmonary infection, if any, should be treated adequately. All the systems should be examined. Associated cardiac anomalies may be present. Mentally retarded children may be difficult to manage and need extra care. Airway problems like large tongue, small nasopharynx, subglottic stenosis, etc. should also be borne in mind. Routine investigations should be done. X-ray of neck may be needed in some cases. Polycythemia is common in neonates.

Anesthetic management should always be cautious. Heavy sedation in premedication is usually avoided. Excessive neck movements during laryngoscopy may be hazardous. Endotracheal intubation with correct size tube may be difficult due to subglottic stenosis. Hypoxia, hypercarbia and hypotension should be avoided. In the postoperative period narcotic analgesics, if needed, should be given in small doses. Respiratory problems may arise in early postoperative period and these should be detected early and tackled accordingly.

RETINOPATHY OF PREMATURITY

It is also known as retrolental fibroplasia. It is characterized by neovascularization and scarring of retinal vasculature, mostly found in premature infants. Other associated factors may include low birth weight, oxygen therapy, shock, sepsis, malnutrition, etc. Besides, abnormal vessel proliferation, retinal hemorrhage, scarring and even detachment of retina may occur. All these may lead to myopia, strabismus, glaucoma, amblyopia and lastly blindness.

Use of exogenous surfactants, continuous pulse oximetry, controlled oxygen therapy to maintain PaO_2 in the range 60 to 80 mm Hg, use of maternal antenatal steroids and improved neonatal nutrition—all these are helpful in reducing the incidence and severity of the disease.

As oxygen therapy is the most widely recognized contributing factor, it should be well controlled with continuous pulse oximetry. PaO_2 should always be maintained between 60 and 80 mmHg.

BRONCHOPULMONARY DYSPLASIA

It is a chronic lung disorder, mostly affecting the neonates. These patients are previously treated with increased concentration of oxygen and mechanical ventilation of the lungs at birth to manage respiratory distress syndrome. The etiology of the disease seems to include many factors like oxygen toxicity, volutrauma, barotrauma, endotracheal intubation, infection and so on. It is the result of a disturbed repair process following lung tissue injury. The characteristic findings may include hypoxemia, hypercarbia, increased airway activity and recurrent pulmonary infection.

Essential management should include the use of antenatal steroids by mothers, exogenous surfactants after delivery, controlled mechanical ventilation with lowest possible airway pressures to minimize barotrauma. Fluid management should be carefully judged. Fluid overload should be avoided. These patients may be treated with frusemide, inhaled bronchodilators and steroids. Chronic pulmonary hypertension and cor pulmonale are the common sequelae.

MALIGNANT HYPERTHERMIA

It is a hypermetabolic syndrome involving disorder of skeletal muscle with varied manifestations. The defect is mainly increased intracellular calcium. It is a rare inherited disease often triggered by volatile anesthetics and suxamethonium.

Onset is usually sudden but may be delayed in certain cases. Defective intracellular calcium control mechanism in muscle may cause sustained muscle contractions (Masseter muscle spasm). Manifestations of increased metabolism may include increased CO_2 production ($PaCO_2$ > 100 mm Hg, pH < 7.15), tachycardia, increased cardiac output, high rise of body temperature, cardiac dysrhythmias, arterial hypoxemia, anaerobic metabolism, metabolic acidosis, increase in plasma creatine kinase, cellular hypoxia, hyperkalemia, myoglobinemia, myoglobinurea and so on. Cardiac failure and renal failure follow eventually.

A careful examination of personal and family history is always helpful in detection of malignant hyperthermia prone subjects. A history of previous episode, a history of unexplained fever during or after anesthesia and any kind of muscular dystrophies should be carefully enquired. Myopathic syndrome may be associated with an increased risk. Routine estimation of plasma creatine kinase may be helpful in detecting the susceptible subjects. Skeletal muscle biopsy is the definitive test confirming the sensitivity to malignant hyperthermia.

Management of anesthesia in such cases needs extra caution and skill. Prophylaxis may be tried with administration of dantrolene preoperatively. Dantrolene can also be given IV prior to induction and every 6 hours thereafter. Induction and maintenance of anesthesia should be restricted to use of nontriggering agents. Triggering agents like volatile anesthetic agents, particularly halothane and depolarizing muscle relaxants like suxamethonium, should always be avoided. Regional anesthesia is mostly satisfactory, but stress-induced malignant hyperthermia can occur on rare occasions. Monitoring of vital signs, particularly body temperature, should be done during and after anesthesia. It will help in early detection and immediate treatment, if body temperature rises.

Treatment of malignant hyperthermia should be immediate. It is better to terminate inhaled anesthetics and conclude surgery as early as possible. Hyperventilation and adequate oxygenation should be started. Active cooling should be tried. Ice may be applied to groin, axilla and neck. Gastric lavage with iced saline is often helpful. Adequate hydration should be maintained. Metabolic acidosis should be corrected with sodium bicarbonate. Mannitol or furosemide is often needed to maintain urinary output. Cardiac dysrhythmias should be treated whenever indicated.

Dantrolene 2 to 3 mg/kg IV should be given. It should be followed by repeat dose every 5 to 10 minutes until symptoms are controlled. Total dose is usually less than 10 mg/kg.

In this context, some drugs are said to be safe and can be used in such cases. These are barbiturates, etomidate, droperidol, opioids, nondepolarizing muscle relaxants, except probably curare, anticholinesterases, local anesthetic agents, nitrous oxide, propranolol, catecholamines, etc. Known triggering agents are all inhalational anesthetics, except nitrous oxide, and depolarizing muscle relaxants like succinylcholine. The role of curare, phenothiazines and ketamine is mostly controversial and thus these should better be avoided.

CARDIOPULMONARY RESUSCITATION

Cardiac arrest is the sudden stoppage of the effective mechanical activity of the heart and in a spontaneously breathing child stoppage of effective ventilation. It may be due to ventricular fibrillation, or cardiac asystole (complete absence of cardiac activity), or electromechanical dissociation (lack of cardiac mechanical activity in response to cardiac electrical stimulation; Gaba, et al.1994).

Usually, there are three factors that determine successful outcome of cardiopulmonary resuscitation. The first is concerned with the rapid restoration and continuation of support of ventilation and circulation. This is often termed as basic life support. It aims to prevent clinical death from marching to biologic death before definitive treatment begins. The second includes rapid definitive remedial therapy such as defibrillation and the third involves detection and correction of predisposing factors.

Prevention of Cardiac Arrest

The primary cause may be uncertain and most commonly it may be extracardiac. But certain factors which may predispose cardiac arrest should be borne in mind. These may include overdose of analgesic or anesthetic drugs, bad anesthesia, hypoxia, hypocarbia, hypotension; fluid, electrolyte and acid-base imbalance, preexisting cardiac diseases, undue vagal reflex overactivity, instrumentations like cardiac catheterization, bronchoscopy, etc.

Prevention of cardiac arrest should be tried with proper preanesthetic assessment, determination of operative risk and skillful choice of safe anesthetic agents and techniques. Continuous monitoring of vital signs during and after operation is essential. Hypoxia, hypercarbia and hypotension should be avoided. Fluid, electrolyte and acid-base balance should be kept normal as far as practicable. Body temperature should be maintained at normal level. Awareness of the possibilities of cardiac arrest, constant vigilance and early recognition are most vital.

Manifestations

Common manifestations are as follows:

No peripheral pulse even in great vessels, absence of heart sounds, no respiration or gasping, unconsciousness, widely dilated pupils, cyanosis, darkening of blood in wound, sudden cessation of bleeding in operative area, pallor, abnormal rhythm on ECG, and asystole or ventricular fibrillation.

Management

It essentially includes initially the basic life support and then advanced life support. As soon as the diagnosis of cardiac arrest is made by palpating the pulse (carotid or femoral) and auscultating the heart, the basic life support should be started.

Basic life support

a. Airway should be cleared and a clear patent airway should be provided. Foreign bodies can be removed from the mouth by a careful single finger sweep. Chin lift is extremely helpful in opening the airway in the unconscious child.
b. Ventilation should be checked by looking for the respiratory movements of chest and listening to the breath sounds. If there is no effective breathing, artificial ventilation should be immediately started by expired air respiration. In children, the mouth and nose are covered by the mouth of the rescuer and he blows his expired air into the child. In infants, where the tidal volumes are small, only puffs are necessary. Respirations should be continued with 20 to 24 breaths/minute.
c. When the pulse is undetectable by precordial or carotid palpation, artificial circulation must be created by external cardiac massage. Chest compressions are carried out on the lower third of sternum. It is usually one fingers breadth below the internipple line. In children, the tips of two fingers or the heel of one hand may be used depending of the size of the child. In children, the rate of compression is 100/ minute, in infants it is 120/minute and in adolescents it is 80/minute.

The compression depth is usually 1 to 1.5 cm. Cardiac compressions can also be applied in neonates and small children by encircling the chest with both hands. This method is said to provide a larger cardiac output than anterior sternal compression.

After the initial minute and subsequent 5 minutes interval, the pulse should be checked and pupil size noted to assess the child. Resuscitation should be resumed within 10 seconds. Once the basic life support is started, it should be continued until the advanced life support becomes available.

Advanced life support

Advanced life support includes the use of equipment and advanced techniques in resuscitation and it must come next to basic life support. The sooner the advanced life support is available, the better is the outcome of resuscitative procedures.

Here the child needs ventilation with oxygen, preferably through endotracheal tube, definitive eletrocardiographic diagnosis of cardiac activity and defibrillation, if indicated. Supportive drugs including adrenaline, calcium, sodium bicarbonate, fluids, etc. are also needed as necessary.

Usually, there are three main changes in the cardiac rhythm in cardiac arrest, namely, ventricular fibrillation, asystole and electromechanical dissociation.

Ventricular fibrillation

It needs cardioversion by immediate defibrillation. For infants and children below 20 kg, pediatric defibrillator plates should be used. The electric shocks should also be appropriate to the child's size to get the optimum effect. Too much energy charge may induce myocardial damage. The initial defibrillation should always be set at low energy charge (2 watt-seconds/kg). The initial shock is followed by a second shock.

If it fails, adrenaline IV may be given in a dose of 0.1 ml/kg of 1 in 10,000 solution. The drug can also be given endotracheally. Adrenaline increases the peripheral vascular resistance and improves coronary circulation. After administering adrenaline, a further shock should be applied to produce reversal of normal rhythm.

Lignocaine 1 mg/kg can be tried. It acts as membrane stabilizer and thus prevents refibrillation following defibrillation.

Cardiac asystole

In children cardiac arrest is mostly associated with asystole in comparison to ventricular fibrillation. In this case adrenaline 1 in 10000 solution, 0.1 ml/kg should be given early as acidosis reduce the effectiveness of catecholamines.

In presence of acidosis, it should be corrected with IV sodium bicarbonate before giving adrenaline. The initial dose of sodium bicarbonate is 1 ml of 1 molar (8.4%) solution per kg body weight. It may have to be repeated after 5 minutes. Ultimately, the dose should be titrated with serial blood gas analysis.

Atropine sulfate 0.02 mg/kg IV and isoprenaline infusion may also prove beneficial in such cases. If all these fail and there is still p wave activity on ECG, then electrical pacing should be considered.

Electromechanical dissociation

This is not common in children. Primary electromechanical dissociation may occur when the excitation-contraction coupling mechanism fails. There is QRS complex in ECG, but there is no palpable pulse. It may be due to drugs (beta-adrenargic blockers, calcium antagonists), toxins, electrolyte imbalances (hypocalcemia, hyperkalemia, etc.). In such cases also adrenaline should be the drug of choice. Then specific therapy should be considered.

Calcium is indicated in cases of hyperkalemia, hypocalcemia and in patients with calcium antagonists. The dose is usually 10 mEq/kg. It may help to restore cardiac tone.

Secondary electromechanical dissociation may occur in cases with hypovolemia, cardiac temponade, etc. In such cases, specific measures and therapy are indicated.

Postresuscitation Care

The child should be taken to intensive care unit for better monitoring and care. Fluid therapy should be adequate. Artificial ventilation may have to be continued till the ventilation becomes spontaneous and adequate. Blood pressure should be kept at normal levels. Normothermia should also be maintained and hyperpyrexia must be prevented. Full neurologic assessment should be done early.

Complications of cardiac arrest

These include death, brain damage, pulmonary edema, renal failure and so on. Injury to liver, pneumothorax, hemothorax, rib fracture, etc. may be the complications of external cardiac massage.

Bibliography

1. Adams AP and Cashman JN. Anaesthesia, analgesia and intensive care. London: Edward Arnold, 1991.
2. Al-shaikh B, Stacey S. Essentials of anaesthetic equipment. New York: Churchill Livingstone,1995.
3. Atkinson RS, Adams AP. Recent advances in anaesthesia and analgesia. No. 15 Edinburgh: Churchill Livingstone, 1985.
4. Atkinson RS, Adams AP. Recent advances in anaesthesia and analgesia. No. 16 Edinburgh: Churchill Livingstone, 1989.
5. Atkinson RS, Hamblin JJ, Wright JEC. Handbook of intensive care. London: Chapman and Hall, 1981.
6. Atkinson RS, Langton Hewer C. Recent advances in anaesthesia and analgesia. No. 14 Edinburgh: Churchill Livingstone, 1982.
7. Basak BK. Pharmacology for the anaesthesiologist. Technornic Publishing Co. USA, 1987.
8. Beasley JM, Jones SEE. A guide to paediatric anaesthesia. London: Blackwell Publishing Co., 1990.
9. Campbell D, Spence AA. Anaesthetics, resuscitation and intensive care. Edinburgh: Churchill Livingstone.
10. Chambers WA, Patey R. Clinical scenarios in anaesthesia. Edinburgh: Churchill Livingstone, 1995.
11. Collins VJ. Principles of anaesthesiology. Bombay: Kothari Book Depot, 1972.
12. Condon RE, Deosse JJ. Surgical care. Philadelphia: Lea and Febiger, 1980.
13. Devenport HT. Paediatric anaesthesia. London: William Heinemann Medical Books Ltd., 1980.
14. Dorsch JA, Dorsh SE. Understanding anaesthesia equipment. Baltimore: William and Wilkins, 1985.
15. Gaba DM, Fish KJ, Howard SK. Crisis management in anaesthesiology. New York: Churchill Livingstone, 1994.
16. Gregory GA. Paediatric Anaesthesia. New York: Churchill Livingstone, 2002.
17. Hatch DJ, Summer E. Neonatal anaesthesia, London: Edward Arnold, 1981.
18. Hewer CL, Atkinson RS. Recent advances of anaesthesia and analgesia. Vol. 11, Churchill Livingstone, 1972.
19. Hewer CL, Atkinson RS. Recent advances of anaesthesia and analgesia. Vol. 12. London: Churchill Livingstone, 1979.
20. Hewer CL, Atkinson RS. Recent advances of anaesthesia and analgesia. No. 13. London: Churchill Livingstone, 1979.
21. Hewer CL Atkinson RS. Recent advances of anaesthesia and analgesia. No. 14. London: Churchill Livingstone, 1982.

22. Hutton P, Cooper G. Guidelines of clinical anaesthesia. Oxford: Blackwell Scientific Publication, 1985.
23. Kirby RK, Gravenstein N, Labato EB, Gravenstein JS. Clinical anaesthesia practice. Philadelphia: WB Saunders & Co., 2002.
24. Lebowitz PW. Anaesthesia for urological surgery. Boston: Little, Brown & Co., 1983.
25. Lee JA, Atkinson RS. A synopsis of anaesthesia. Bristol: John Wright & Sons, 1990.
26. Miller RD. Anaesthesia. Vols. 1,2 and 3. Edinburgh: Churchill Livingstone, 1986.
27. Micheal MZ, Goodman, NW, Aitkenhead AR. Essay plans for anaesthesia exam. Edinburgh: Churchill Livingstone, 1992.
28. Michelle BH. Anaesthesia Review. Philadelphia: Lippincot Williams & Wilkins, 1999.
29. Nunn JF, Utting JE, Brown BR. General anaesthesia. London: Butterworths, 1988.
30. Orland MJ, Saltman RJ. Manual of medical therapeutics. Boston: Little Brown & Co., 1986.
31. Paul AK. Drugs and equipment in anaesthetic practice. New Delhi: Elsevier, 2005.
32. Paul AK. Essentials of anaesthesiology. Calcutta: Academic Publishers, 2002.
33. Pearson GA. Handbook of paediatric intensive care. Philadelphia: WB Saunders & Co., 1999.
34. Pullerts J, Hotzman RS: Anaesthesia equipment for infants and children. Boston: Little Brown & Co., 1992.
35. Ravin MB. Problems in anaesthesia. Boston: Little Brown & Co., 1981.
36. Reed AP. Clinical cases in anaesthesia. 2nd ed. New York: Churchill Livingstone, 1975.
37. Rees GJ, Gray TC, Paediatrid anaesthesia. London: Butterworths, 1981.
38. Smith G, Aitkenhead AR. Text book of anaesthesia. London: Churchill Livingstone, 1985.
39. Steward DJ. Manual of paediatric anaesthesia. New York: Churchill Livingstone, 1985.
40. Stoelting RK, Dierdorf SF. Handbook for anaesthesia and co-existing disease. Edinburgh: Churchill Livingstone, 1993.
41. Stoelting RK, Miller RD. Basics of anaesthesia. New York: Churchill Livingstone, 1994.
42. Vickers MD. Medicine for anaesthetists. Oxford: Blackwell Scientific Publications, 1990.
43. Wylie Ed, Churchill-Davidson HC. A practice of anaesthesia. London: Lloyd Luke, 1988.
44. Yao FF, Artusio JE. Anaesthesiology. Philadelphia: JB Lippincott Co., 1982.

Index

Page numbers followed by *f* refers to figure.

A

Abdominal injuries
  intestinal 256
  liver 256
  pancreas 256
  spleen 256
Abdominal surgery 194
Abdominal wall defects 201
Acute abdomen 210
Adenoidectomy 156
Airencephalography 229
Airways
  laryngeal mask 70
  nasopharyngeal 70
  oropharyngeal 68
Alcuronium 111
Anaphylaxis 274
Anemia 117
Anesthesia
  equipment 47
  for pediatric trauma 248
  regional 259
Anesthetic agents
  intravenous
    diazepam 101
    ketamine 101
    methohexitone 100
    neuroleptanalgesics 102
    propofol 102
    thiopentone 100
  volatile
    enflurane 99
    ether 98
    halothane 98
    isoflurane 99
Anesthetic circuit 55
  closed system 53
  Mapleson A 48
  Mapleson D 49
  Mapleson E 49
  Mapleson F 52
  pediatric 55
Anesthetic gas, nitrous oxide 97
Anesthetic machine 47
Anesthetic technique
  Ayre's 50
  pediatric 127
Anorectal anomalies 209
Appendicitis, acute 210
Armored endotracheal tubes 61
Arnold-Chiari malformation 230
Atracurium 112
Atresia
  duodenal 208
  jejunal/ileal 208
Atropine 105
Axillary temperature 86
Ayre's T-piece 50

B

Bain circuit 54
Basic resuscitation
  airway 249
  breathing 250
  circulation 250
  management 249
Biliary atresia 2, 206
Bladder exstrophy 204
Bleeding tonsil 155
Block
  Bier 264
  brachial plexus 263
  caudal 266
  femoral nerve 264
  iliohypogastric 260
  ilioinguinal 260
  lumbar epidural 268
  penile 261

Blood
    gas analysis 92
    loss assessment 92
    pressure monitoring 82
    replacement 35
    transfusion 251
    volume in children 14, 35
Body fluids 34
Bowel obstruction 207
Brachial plexus block 263
Bronchography 164
Bronchopulmonary dysplasia 275
Bronchoscope 73
Bronochoscopy 73, 163
Brown adipose tissue 24
Bullard laryngoscope 68
Bupivacaine 115
Burns
    dressing 184

C

Capnography 85
Cardiac
    arrest 277
    catheterization 18, 240
    surgery 241
Cardiopulmonary resuscitation 276
Cardiothoracic surgery 236
Cardiovascular system 11
Catheter
    epidural 77, 268
    mount 65
    suction 72
Caudal block 266
Cerebral
    blood flow 224
    tumor 233
Cerebrospinal fluid pressure 224
Chest injuries 254
Choanal atresia 157
Cholinesterase plasma 96
Circumcision 214
Cisatracurium 113
Cleft lip and palate 180

Coarctation of aorta 244
Cole tube 62
Condylectomy 187
Congenital heart defects 246
Connections
    Cobb 65
    Magill 64
    Rowbatham 64
Craniectomy 186
Craniofacial dysostosis 184
Croup 146, 271
CVP monitoring 89
Cystic hygroma 185
Cystoscopy 215

D

Day case surgery 188
Defibrillation 279
Dehydration 37
Dental surgery 175
Diaphragmatic hernia 9, 194
Diazepam 101
Difficult intubation 138
Disorders of heartbeat 18
Down's syndrome 274
Droperidol 103
Ductus arteriosus 12

E

Ear surgery 157
Electrocardiogram 81
Electrolyte balance 34
Encephalocele 231
Endoscopy 162
Endotracheal tubes
    armored 61
    Cole 62
    laser 63
    microlaryngeal 63
    Oxford 62
    PVC 63
    RAE 61
Endtidal CO_2 estimation 85
Enflurane 99
ENT surgery 153

Epidural
  block 268
  catheter 77
  needle 77
Epiglottitis 271
Epistaxis 161
Equipment, pediatric 47
Esophageal
  atresia 197
  stethoscope 81
  temperature
    monitoring 87
Esophagoscopy 165
Ether 98
Etomidate 102
Exomphalos 203
Expiratory valve 57
Extubation 134
Eye injury, penetrating 174

F

Face mask
  Rendell-Baker Soucek 58
Fazadinium 112
Femoral nerve block 264
Fentanyl 103
Fetal circulation 11
Fibreoptic laryngoscope 139
Filling and reconstruction of teeth 177
Fluid
  balance 33
  management 36
  resuscitation 250
  therapy 37

G

Gallamine 111
Gastroschisis 202
General surgery 194
Genitourinary tract injury
  renal 257
  straddle 257
  urinary bladder 257
Glaucoma 173
Glycopyrrolate 106
Guedel airway 69

H

Halothane 98
Head injury 235, 253
Hemoglobin 16
Herniotomy 213
Hirschsprung's disease 209
Hyaline membrane disease 9
Hydrocephalus 230
Hygroma, cystic 185
Hyoscine 105
Hyperpyrexia 28
Hypoglycemia 122
Hypospadius 216
Hypotension
  induced 228
  postoperative 149
Hypothermia 30

I

Ilioinguinal and iliohypogastric
  nerve block 260
Incisional hernia 205
Infusion
  pump 76
  set 75
Inhalational anesthetics 97
Intercostal nerve block 262
Interdental wiring 187
Intestinal obstruction 207
Intracranial surgery 227, 234
Intraocular surgery 173
Intravenous
  access 250
  catheters 75
  regional anesthesia 264
  therapy 40
Intubation
  blind 139
  difficult 138
Intussusception 207
Invasive monitoring 88
Isoflurane 99

K

Ketamine 101
Kidney disease 218

L

Laryngeal mask airway 70
Laryngomalacia 163
Laryngoscope
  Bullard 68
  Macintosh 66
  Magill 66
Laryngoscopy 131, 162
Laryngospasm 146, 273
Laryngotracheobronchitis 272
Laser
  endotracheal tube 63
  microsurgery 165
Lighted stylet 72
Lignocaine 114
Lobar emphysema, congenital 238
Lung
  surgery 236
  ventilators 73

M

Macintosh laryngoscope 66
Magill
  breathing system 66
  connections 64
Malignant hyperthermia 275
Mapleson system
  A 48
  D 49
  E 49
  F 52
Mask
  for anesthesia 130
  for pediatric 58
  Rendell-Baker-Soucek 58
Maxillofacial surgery 186
Meatotomy 214
Meckel's diverticulum 208
Meconium ileus 209
Mediastinal tumors 239
Methohexitone 100
Metoclopramide 106
Midazolam 102
Middle ear surgery 160
Monitoring 79

Morphine 103
Muscle relaxants
  atracurium 112
  gallamine 111
  pancuronium 112
  suxamethonium 109
  tubocurarine 111
  vecuronium 112
Myelography 230
Myelomeningocele 231
Myringotomy 159

N

Naloxone 105
Nasal surgery 160
Nasolacrimal duct probing 173
Nasopharyngeal airway 70
Neck
  contracture 184
  injury
    cervical spine damage 254
Needles
  intravenous 75
  spinal 76
Neonatal cold injury 30
Neostigmine 114
Neuroleptanalgesia 102
Neuromuscular
  blocking agents 113
  function
    monitoring 91
Neuroradiology 228
Nitrous oxide 97
Nonrebreathing valve 48

O

Oculocardiac reflex 170
Omphalocele 203
Ophthalmic surgery 169
Oral airway 69
Orchidopexy 213
Oropharyngeal airway 68
Orthopedic injuries 257
Oscillotonometry 83
Outpatient surgery 188
Oximetry, pulse 84

P

Palatoplasty 180
Pancuronium 112
Patent ductus arteriosus 243
Penile block 261
Pentazocine 104
Pethidine 104
Phenoperidine 103
Pheochromocytoma 212
Pierre Robin syndrome 7
Plastic surgery 179
Porphyria 100, 117, 124
Postanesthetic
  care
    recovery score 141
  complications
    convulsion 148
    hypotension 149
    nausea and vomiting 148
    pain 147
    pyrexia 150
    restlessness 147
    shivering 148
Postoperative
  analgesia 143
  sedation 143
  shivering 148
Preanesthetic assessment 116, 189
Precordial stethoscope 81
Premedication 121
Preoperative preparation 198
Preoxygenation 131
Prochlorperazine 106
Promethazine 106
Propofol 102
Prune belly syndrome 203
Psychological problems 42
Pulmonary artery pressure
  monitoring 90
Pulse rate 20
PVC endotracheal tubes 63
Pyeloplasty 217
Pyloric stenosis 199
Pyrexia 27

R

RAE tube 61
Recovery
  score 141
Rectal polyp 214
Rees modification of Ayre's T-piece 52
Regional anesthesia 259
Renal
  disease 218
  function 33
Reservoir bag 56
Respiratory
  distress 6
  physiology 1
Retinopathy 274
Rocuronium 112
Rowbatham connection 64

S

Secondary survey 252
Sevoflurane 99
Shunt
  ventriculoatrial 230
  ventriculoperitoneal 230
Spinal needle 76
Splenctomy 211
Stethoscopy
  esophageal 81
  precordial 80
Strabismus 172
Stylet 71
Subglottic stenosis 180
Suxamethonium 109

T

Temperature
  monitoring 86
  regulation 25
Thalassemia 211
Thermometry 86
Thermoregulation 21
Thiopentone 100
Thoracic anesthesia 236
Tongue-tie 215
Tonsillar abscess 156

Tonsillectomy 153
T-piece system 50
Tracheoesophageal fistula 9, 197
Tracheostomy 166
Treacher Collins syndrome 8
Trimeprazine 106
Tubocurarine 111
Tympanic temperature 87

U

Umbilical polyp 201
Urinary output 84
Urological surgery 216

V

Vecuronium 112
Venepuncture 128
Ventilators 73
Ventriculography 229
Voiding cystourethrogram 216
Volvulus 208

W

Water balance 35
Wilms tumor 217
Worcestor connection 65f